Impotence

A CULTURAL HISTORY

Angus McLaren

The University of Chicago Press   Chicago and London

ANGUS MCLAREN is professor of history at the University of Victoria, British Columbia. He is the author of eleven books, including *A History of Contraception: From Antiquity
to Present Day* and *Prescription for Murder: Victorian Serial Killings of Dr. Thomas Cream*, the
latter also published by the University of Chicago Press.

The University of Chicago Press, Chicago 60637
The University of Chicago Press, Ltd., London
© 2007 by The University of Chicago
All rights reserved. Published 2007
Printed in the United States of America

16 15 14 13 12 11 10 09 08 07   1 2 3 4 5

ISBN-13: 978-0-226-50076-8 (cloth)
ISBN-10: 0-226-50076-4 (cloth)

LIBRARY OF CONGRESS CATALOGING-IN-PUBLICATION DATA
McLaren, Angus.
    Impotence : a cultural history / Angus McLaren.
      p. ; cm.
    Includes bibliographical references and index.
    ISBN-13: 978-0-226-50076-8 (cloth : alk. paper)
    ISBN-10: 0-226-50076-4 (cloth : alk. paper)
    1. Impotence—History.   2. Impotence—Social aspects.   I. Title.
    [DNLM: 1. Impotence—history.   2. Men—psychology.   WJ 11.1 M478i   2007]
    RC889.M345   2007
    616.6′922—dc22

                                                        2006021188

♾ The paper used in this publication meets the minimum requirements
of the American National Standard for Information Sciences—
Permanence of Paper for Printed Library Materials, ANSI Z39.48-1992.

CONTENTS

ILLUSTRATIONS

ACKNOWLEDGMENTS

Why impotence? My first books were devoted to studying how men and women in past generations attempted to control their fertility. This study is in some ways a new departure. It is true that in looking at early modern discussions of reproduction I frequently came across instructions on how individuals—concerned by some sexual infirmity—could seek to enflame their lusts and assure their fecundity. I was surprised by the number of references to aphrodisiacs made in medical books and herbal texts, but tended to skip over many of the reports, preoccupied as I was by my search for evidence of contraceptive practices. Some of these readings nevertheless lodged themselves in the far reaches of my brain and eventually I began to wonder if they did not warrant more systematic examination. We risk being left with a distorted view of the past if we have only accounts of how partners tried to limit their fertility and none of how they sought to increase it, and only histories of women's bodies but none of men's. Such musings led me to go back more carefully over a number of the sources I originally perused decades ago. In this roundabout way the research was launched that resulted in this study.

I owe an enormous debt of gratitude to the many friends and colleagues who assisted me in this undertaking. I first have to thank Brian Dippie for subjecting the manuscript—like so many earlier ones—to a careful and insightful reading. I only wish I had the space to respond to his many challenging ripostes. Special thanks goes to Michael Finn for putting me up in Toronto and generously sharing with me his research notes on the French decadents. Countless students and colleagues provided me with encouragement and assistance, but I particularly value the intellectual support offered by Robert Nye, Lesley Hall, Chandak Sengoopta, Barbara Marshall, Hera Cook, Ralph Dose, and Christian Graugaard. Over the years Roger Davidson, Jennifer Evans, Simon Szreter, Bruno Wanrooij, and Pat Thane kindly passed on references. Stephanie Olsen and Heather Stanley were cheerful and industrious research assistants. I received useful feedback from friendly audiences when portions of the study were delivered as part of the Horning Lecture Series at Oregon State University and at the European Social Science History Conference held at Humboldt University, Berlin.

I am very appreciative of the generous support of the Social Science and Humanities Research Council of Canada, which enabled me to make the numerous overseas trips that this project required. My repeated stays in London were brightened by the hospitality and kindness of Susannah and Richard Taffler and Aimée and Michael Birnbaum. Thanks to Bill Benzie, I have for many years been perfectly situated in London in Upper Woburn Place, halfway between the British Library and the Wellcome Institute. Christine Delphy saw to it that in Paris I was even more centrally located on the rue Jean-Jacques Rousseau.

For their unflagging service I owe a debt of gratitude to the staffs of the University of Victoria Library, the Woodward Medical Library at the University of British Columbia, the Cambridge University Library, the British Library, the Wellcome Institute for the History of Medicine, the Bibliothèque Nationale, and the Kinsey Institute. At the University of Victoria Andrew Rippen has been a supportive dean, Eric Sager and Tom Saunders understanding history department chairs, and Karen McIvor an ever helpful departmental secretary. No one writes more engaging letters than Doug Mitchell; he and Tim McGovern made the production process a pleasure.

I am as ever indebted to Brian and Donna Dippie, whose boundless generosity makes my continual shuttling between Victoria and Vancouver possible. Although now in residency in Montreal, Jesse still keeps me from taking myself or my projects too seriously. Arlene remains my main critic and supporter.

INTRODUCTION

Who today hasn't heard of Viagra? The little blue pill has garnered billions for the Pfizer corporation and made male impotence—now reconfigured as erectile dysfunction—a topic of public discussion. What most participants in the current debate ignore is that impotence has a history. Have men always suffered from impotence or the fear of it? Strictly speaking they have not, given that the *Oxford English Dictionary* states that the word "impotence" to denote an absence of sexual power only came into common usage in the seventeenth century. Nevertheless in preceding centuries men lamented their loss of "courage," lack of desire, and debilitated loins. And more important than the changes in vocabulary were the changes over time in the ways in which male sexual incapacity was culturally conceptualized and the social meanings it was given. The purported causes of impotence (the term we will resort to for simplicity's sake) varied and so did its impact. In Mesopotamian texts from the seventh century BCE, historians have found references to men consuming roots and plants to restore their potency. They also recited protective spells to counter sorcerers' attacks on their virility.

> Get excited! Get excited! Get an erection!
> Get excited like a stag! Get an erection lik[e a wild bull]!
> Let a lio[n] get an erection along with you![1]

Centuries later the inquisitors of sixteenth-century Venice reported that by tying three knots in a rope while repeating a spell, a jilted lover could sexually incapacitate the man who had abandoned her. In nineteenth-century England quacks claimed that the main cause of impotence was masturbation. "As in man, so in woman, this pernicious habit takes away the *inclination* for those pleasures with which the multiplication of the species is connected, sometimes it destroys the actual *power* of effectual communion."[2] Today urologists and pharmaceutical corporations blame erectile dysfunctions on poor blood circulation.

In some senses the history of male incapacity appears to have come full circle. Historians tell us that until the twentieth century the public commonly assumed that sex, marriage, and procreation were inextricably linked and so impotence was long discussed in the context of a man's ability to marry and have children—not in the context of merely being able to have sex. In early modern Europe when patriarchal power depended upon a man producing heirs, the public openly discussed the problems posed by impotence. Doctors, wise women, and priests prescribed a variety of herbal and magical remedies. Family fortunes and dynastic stability demanded successful coition. Charles II's lack of success in siring an heir led to the Hapsburgs' loss of Spain. On the one hand rumors about Louis XVI's initial failure to consummate his marriage fed the public unrest that ultimately resulted in the French Revolution; on the other hand the fledgling American republic was strengthened by George Washington's inability to found a dynasty. Impotence could be both a metaphor for, and an actual cause of, failures of the body politic. In the nineteenth century the concern for family privacy and male sensitivities led the respectable to avoid such topics. These decades of discretion were anomalous. In the early twentieth century psychoanalysts attributed rising rates of impotence to Oedipal desires, endocrinologists blamed an insufficiency of "male" hormones, and novelists targeted henpecked males' fear of cocksure feminists. By the 1990s guaranteed medical cures were heralded and impotence was once again front-page news. But the sellers of Viagra, Levitra, and Cialis did not suggest that their purpose was to overcome problems of infertility. In a small-family culture male potency was no longer proven by siring children, but by being an accomplished sexual partner.

A disease, according to Michael Solomon, "is a social construct and, as such, is dependent on a complex codification of patterns, images, and forms that are produced within the conventions of an interpretive community. To become diseased is less a process of being ill than one of putting our ills—or having our ills put for us—into categories, fables, fictions, and myths that offer explanations for suffering, strategies for coping, and hopes for cure."[3] Although in this study impotence is regarded as a problem rather than as a disease, a similar perspective has been adopted. The goal is to locate impotence in the context of changing social expectations and cultural givens. In providing a constructionist history of impotence, we trace Western discourses and theories to understand the cultural forces that structured representations of masculine sexual inadequacy. The result is something akin to what Foucault would term a genealogy of a specific modern issue. Beginning with the premise that language always mediates the material world, we have paid special attention to the sexual vocabulary of each age. The ways in which the body was described obviously affected the ways in which the body was actually experienced. In other words impotence in an age that believed in witchcraft was quite different from impotence in an age that believed in science. Such comparisons help reveal why different cultures took their particular approaches in conceptualizing and dealing with such a problem. What at first glance might seem a bizarre view of the body's workings can—when placed in its cultural context—reveal itself as a rational and understandable reflection of the society's values. The notion of impotence can accordingly serve as a heuristic device in rethinking the history of Western sexuality, particularly in posing the question of how this category related to the masculine ideal.

To write a history of impotence entails a survey of changing models of masculinity.[4] Though every era has employed discourses to represent and control sexuality, certain ages clearly manifested a heightened anxiety about the issue of male sexual dysfunction. But what did one mean by the term "impotence"? When reproduction was highly prized it was often confused or equated with sterility or barrenness. Even in modern times it has had a variety of meanings—failure to achieve an erection, failure to penetrate, and either failure to ejaculate or ejaculating prematurely. Such failures might be chronic or intermittent; they could have physical or psychological causes. They could arrive with old age.

Why such a concern for the erection? It was obviously essential when the purpose of sex was propagation, but modern sex surveys revealed that much if not most of the male's sexual pleasure came from means other than penetration. Nevertheless it was taken as a given in Western culture that sex was synonymous with intercourse, a man penetrating his partner. The implication of such a belief is that a man feared impotence, not so much because it might deprive him of pleasure, but because it would prevent him from providing proof that he could perform as a male should. Potency was long linked to maturity. The close association of sexual virility with youth is a relatively recent phenomenon.

Whom were men's erections for? Where does the issue of women's pleasure figure in the discussion? It is important not to conflate cultural representations with practices. If one is to believe today's pharmaceutical advertisements, men's desire to overcome sexual dysfunctions is driven by their concern for their partners. Asking whether or not this is true today or ever was in the past highlights the fact that sexual practices can have a range of meanings. For many men intercourse became reified and was made synonymous with "sex" because it represented social dominance.

We have been talking about men, but this study focuses on notions of manhood in Western cultures. Yet even within these narrow confines it is impossible to ignore the ways in which discussions of sexual dysfunctions by whites played a role in their construction of ideas about race and ethnicity. Such discussions created the racial "other" partly by attributing to nonwhite men either an animal-like, primitive potency or an exhausted lack of virility. Historians have begun to track the role played by such beliefs in the process of racialization.[5]

What societies make of male sexual problems is naturally of great interest to the historian of gender. The way in which impotence was treated and discussed always affected both men and women. No better example could be given than the writers of *Playboy* and *Penthouse* heralding the arrival of Viagra as somehow freeing men from feminist oppression. Despite such assertions, the history of impotence is perhaps even more about power relations among men. Who traditionally decided what was normal and healthy masculinity? Men. Who set the standards? Men. Who communicated them? Men. Though there has never been a universal, biologically determined standard of male potency, when discussing impotence men in every culture made clear what they felt most threatened male potency, what they recognized as the signs of the loss of masculinity, and how "remasculinization" could be attempted. Gender identity, in short, was something that they believed could be both threatened and protected.

Here, the traditional medical historian might protest that a history of impotence shows that no matter what earlier quacks might claim, men unable to attain an erection had no hope of cure until the emergence of modern biochemistry. Yet the story is obviously more complicated than that. The cultural historian—while not denying the improvements in treatment—would argue that the history of impotence demonstrates how every age has culturally framed the discussion of male incapacity.[6] Fiascoes in the bedroom have been attributed at one time or another to witchcraft, masturbation, homosexual desires, shell shock, sexual excesses, feminism, and the unconscious. The arrival of new explanations did not necessarily displace older ones. Even in a scientific age some would still attribute failures to irrational forces. As made clear in songs, plays, novels, and movies, Western culture has simultaneously regarded impotence as life's greatest tragedy and life's greatest joke.

The debates over Viagra have brought home to the public that the pursuit of normative sexuality has both its benefits and its costs. A history of impotence not only allows us to locate these discussions in their cultural context; it provides a compelling way in which to understand male power and the configurations of male desire. What precipitated ideas of masculine vulnerability? How was male anxiety assuaged? What sorts of women were regarded as posing a threat to virility? In seeking to answer these questions we are led to see how cultures constructed their particular notions of sexuality's pleasures and dangers, its private and public functions. Every age turned male sexual dysfunctions to its own purposes; every culture created, combated, and in some fashion cured the forms of impotence it found most alarming.

What do we learn in investigating the history of impotence? Most importantly we discover that male sexuality does have a history. Countless studies have tracked the ways in which women's sexuality was "constructed" or repressed or policed. We have, for example, histories of hysteria, pregnancy, orgasms, and breasts. In contrast, next to nothing has been said about how normative standards of male performance were established. "It is noteworthy," a legal scholar recently observed, "that an expanding and exciting feminist literature which discusses images of the female body as leaky, volatile, and permeable has provoked far less comment on the implicitly or explicitly contrasted construction of the male body as bounded, stable, and non-permeable."[7] But was the male body assumed to be stable? Most histories of sexuality seem to take that position. In his pathbreaking study *Making Sex: The Body and Gender from the Greeks to Freud* (1990) Thomas Laqueur all but ignored men. "It is probably not possible to write a history of man's body and its pleasures," he asserts, "because the historical record was created in a cultural tradition where no such history was necessary."[8] Yet the study of impotence reveals that a vast and changing cast of characters were interested in men's sexual capacities. Their private problems were implicated in the discussion of a range of important public issues including marriage, divorce, reproduction, illness, and aging. Such discussions naturally reflected societies' changing views of men's bodies and appropriate masculine behavior, but they were also entangled in preoccupations with sex, race, gender, age, and class. Though some recent studies give the impression that until the twentieth century impotence was almost unknown, an investigation of what earlier cultures regarded as the causes and cures of male dysfunctions reveals that male potency was rarely taken as a given; each culture sought in its own fashion to nurture and protect it. Only by understanding the responses made to impotence in the past can we fully appreciate (and perhaps anticipate) the ways in which it will be dealt with in the future.

   We begin in chapter 1 by surveying Greek and Roman discussions of sexuality. This was a world in which penetration proved manhood; it mattered little whether the penetrated was a woman or a boy. Given the importance of potency to reputation, doctors provided recipes for restoratives yet at the same time ribald writers produced comic accounts of men who failed the crucial test. Unlike the Romans, Christians could neither laud potency nor regard impotency as a joke. Yet, if the gloomy Augustinian view of the purposes of marriage placed a new stress on celibacy and "inner masculinity," Christians could not ignore the problem posed "when desire refused service." Chapter 2 follows the long line of celibate church doctors who made themselves experts on erection, penetration, and emission. When the power of the church declined, as in Restoration England, wits once again made impotence a laughing matter. Chapter 3 demonstrates how jokes about sexual humiliations played a vital part in a common male culture of the seventeenth century. Male sexual dysfunctions appeared distinctly different when viewed through an eighteenth-century prism. Chapter 4 shows how quacks and philosophes—in attempting to cure, counter, and explain away male sexual problems—embraced the new notion of men and women inhabiting separate sexual spheres. The nineteenth-century culture that craved privacy found discussions of such disasters distasteful, but given the middle-class fixation on the notion of the active male and the passive female, I argue in chapter 5, the issue of impotence could not be ignored. The writers of middle-class marriage manuals popularized the notion of a "spermatic economy" in which excesses led to a loss of manly vigor and bankruptcy resulted ultimately in impotence. Physicians, chapter 6 demonstrates, showed a new concern for youthful indiscretions, highlighting the dangers of masturbation, spermatorrhoea, prostitution, and venereal disease. Quacks employed the new cheap press both to create anxieties and to sell their nostrums to cure "lost manhood." As the Victorian model of masculinity that valorized restraint was displaced by a more relaxed ideal, the early twentieth century witnessed a shift from moral to psychological explanations of impotence. Chapter 7 contrasts the writers of marriage manuals who increased pressures on males to perform with Freudians who attributed impotence to Oedipal guilt, and the resulting incapacitating male view of women as either Madonnas or whores. Chapter 8 argues that the rise of endocrinology in the 1920s finally legitimized the scientific study of the male reproductive system and dramatically revealed a twentieth-century hostility to aging. New operations and patent medicines indicated how far a culture would go in egging men on in the desperate pursuit of a particular sign of manliness. Following World War II, marriage counselors and sex therapists declared impotence to be a problem from which not one but two people suffered, and both would have to be treated. Chapter 9 shows that it was hardly a coincidence that in the 1970s reports of a "new impotence" followed the emergence of second-wave feminism and the discovery of the multiorgasmic female. We conclude in chapter 10 by analyzing the furor created by Viagra. Its backers claimed that pharmaceuticals had trumped surgery, psychoanalysis, sex therapy, and feminism. The corporations did make billions, but did the new impotence pills "revolutionize" sexuality?

The medicalization of sexuality has displaced, but not entirely banished older beliefs in the noxious influence of sin, guilt, bad habits, and even evil spells. A layer of biomedical reasoning has in effect been added to the earlier stock of arguments used to explain sexual dissatisfactions. The gist of this study is that every age has turned impotence to its own purposes, each advancing a model of masculinity that informed men if they were sexual successes, and if not, why not. Nothing is more revealing of a culture's social and ideological preoccupations than the enormous pains it takes in goading men on in the often painful pursuit of the "normal" and the "natural."

THE IMPENETRABLE PENETRATOR
Manhood in Greece and Rome

Ovid's *Amores* and Petronius's *Satyrica* provide the two most famous literary accounts of the ancients' view of impotence. In *Amores* 3.7 the Latin poet amusingly describes his inexplicable inability to perform with a woman he has long lusted after.

> Yes, she was beautiful and well turned out,
> The girl that I'd so often dreamed about,
> Yet I lay with her limp as if I loved not,
> A shameful burden on the bed that moved not.
> Though both of us were sure of our intent,
> Yet could I not cast anchor where I meant.

Following this disastrous encounter the narrator is enraged to find his refractory member suddenly full of vigor.

> But notwithstanding, like one dead it lay,
> Drooping more than a rose picked yesterday.
> Now, when he should not be, he's bolt upright,
> And craves his task and seeks to have his fight.
> Lie down in shame and see you stir no more!
> You've caught me with your promises before.
> You've tricked me, got me captured weaponless,
> And I've endured great shame and sore distress.[1]

Coming across such a familiar scenario it is tempting to assume that men in ancient Greece and Rome regarded impotence in exactly the same way as do men in the twenty-first century. Indeed it would be easy to produce a history of impotence by simply totting up every reference to what today we might interpret as concerns for erection. The obvious danger of such an approach is that one begins with the assumption that there actually exists such a thing as "impotence" that can be tracked over time. Even in our scientific world different people mean different things in employing the term. Accordingly there is all the more reason to be sensitive to the fact that earlier cultures constructed, explained, and gave special significance in quite different ways from ours to what could in general terms be described as male sexual failures. To make the story even more complicated, it also has to be admitted that we cannot know if such failures actually existed; relying on written sources produced by the literate elite, all we really we know is how such events (or nonevents) were culturally represented.

Some sense of the importance of cultural framing is given by a reading of Petronius's *Satyrica*. His hero Encolpius tries to bed Circe, but at the crucial moment he too goes limp.

> Three times I whip the dreadful weapon out,
> And three times softer than a Brussels sprout
> I quail, in those dire straits my manhood blunted,
> No longer up to what just now I wanted.[2]

Again, this sounds very familiar to the modern ear. The cultural resonance of impotence is only made clear when Petronius goes on to deal with the possible causes, cures, and import of the problem. Encolpius is humiliated not simply because he is unready for sex, but because he appears less able than a *cinaedus*, a passive homosexual whose status is lower than his. Encolpius's lack of erection is thus shameful inasmuch as it signals a loss of both masculine and social status. And why does he suffer such a fate? Is it because of his boyfriend whom Circe says he should drop? Is it due to an unhealthy regimen that he seeks to ameliorate by continence, diet, and a restriction on wine? Might he be bewitched? An elderly crone helps him counter the evil eye. In chapter 138 when he is finally cured, it is by a sadistic old priestess who buggers him with a leather dildo smeared with oil, pepper, and nettle seeds.[3]

In providing a comic account of impotence, Petronius is not attempting to document all the ways in which his contemporaries viewed the problem. Nevertheless a reading of his masterpiece reminds us that to appreciate earlier societies' understandings of the workings of the body we have to make a conscious effort to avoid assuming that they shared our views and values. Certain acts employed by the Greeks and Romans no doubt either curbed or encouraged potency, but what mattered was not so much the act as the social construction of meanings given to it and the individual responses to such meanings. How are we to understand the ancients' discussion of impotence? The construction of both the problem and the cure directly related to their notions of sex and gender. To place the issue of impotence in its social setting we begin this chapter with an analysis of the roles assigned to men and women in the ancient world, then turn to Greek and Roman attitudes toward intercourse and procreation; we will examine the many ways in which they sought to control desire, and review how their notions of manhood accommodated biology and behavior.

To be a man in the ancient world a vigorous character was essential. The Romans were positively fixated with an ideal of the self-controlled, aggressive, virile male. They had an extravagant concern for winning recognition through public achievement. According to what has been called the Mediterranean notion of manliness, men had to appear strong and active. A man manifested proper male behavior by expressions of his righteous anger, powerful desires, and personal autonomy. Even humor was seasoned with a strong element of sexual aggression, as opponents in law and politics were commonly abused as soft or effeminate. Hence the poet Catullus threatened to rape or bugger his critics.[4]

Of course, given that almost all the sources available to us were written by men, the portrayal of the aggressive, virile, emotionally cool male was obviously an ideal or cliché rather than a reality. The ancients admitted as much in stressing the importance of performance. One might be born male, but to prove one's manhood one needed to walk and talk in a certain way. Rhetorical skills, for example, played a key role in establishing gender identity. Gender was in effect learnt. "Masculinity in the ancient world was an achieved state," one scholar has noted, "radically underdetermined by anatomical sex."[5] There were few hard rules.[6] Though gender norms existed, deviations were accepted. Male reputation and honor were not predetermined; men learned how to manipulate community expectations and the norms of masculinity to their own advantage.

Notions of assertive male behavior were projected onto the genitals. Thus Plato personified the penis as "disobedient and self-willed, like a creature that is deaf to reason, and it attempts to dominate all because of its frenzied lusts." Indeed the assertion that masculinity was for the ancients not simply determined by anatomy sounds counterintuitive, given their acceptance of public male nudity, the attention paid to male genitalia, and the displays of the phallus. Greek nurses molded the baby's body, even using swaddling to shape the scrotum and stretching to elongate the foreskin. To judge by illustrations and statuary, the ideal penis was small, thin, and had a pointed foreskin. The Greeks believed a dainty penis was not only more attractive but more serviceable in reproduction, since its semen, not having to travel as far, would suffer less heat loss. They represented Satyrs with huge penises as sign of their ugliness. The Romans, however, preferred big penises, or at least that was the case of the emperors when choosing their favorites.[7]

In the ancient world the erect penis was a symbol of maturity and power. The Romans celebrated a boy's first ejaculation. Representations of the penis were found everywhere. Artificial penises were used on the comic stage of Athens until the fourth century BC. A phallic stele of Hermes stood at the doorway of every Greek house and during ritual processions the men carried an enormous phallus through the community. In Roman gardens, instead of a scarecrow, a representation of the god Priapus, complete with erect penis, threatened intruders with rape.[8]

The ancients moreover employed an elaborate vocabulary to describe the male genitals. "People will laugh aloud at you," warned an early Greek epigram, "if you venture to sail unequipped, a rower who has lost his oar." In common parlance the erect penis was described as one's equipment, tool, spear, ram, goad, or drill. In its flaccid state it might be called a snake or rope. A woman accordingly cursed her younger rival "may you find a snake in your bed." The Romans believed the sparrow to be lecherous, so in Latin "sparrow" was a synonym for penis. In Catullus 2 and 3 the narrator talks about his girlfriend's sparrow being dead, that is, himself as impotent. In literature the phallus was frequently personified, especially the impotent prick as in Ovid's *Amores* 3.7.[9]

The flaccid penis represented failure since for the virile in the ancient world sex could only mean penetration. A man had either to penetrate or be penetrated. Martial (*Epigram* 3.73) for example accused Gallus of not being able to stand and thereby implied that he was a fellator. The real man was an "impenetrable penetrator." The special resonance this concept held can only be fully appreciated when it is recalled that this was a resolutely inegalitarian society in which elite men always had at their disposal submissive and sexually available male and female slaves. Sexual relationships were embedded in social relationships. Respectable men necessarily took the accusation of being sexually passive as the gravest insult, implying as it did that one was no better than a slave. Male character assassination fed on such innuendos that one was "soft." In the musings of philosophers such as Seneca as well as in popular lampoons, graffiti, and satires appeared the same expressions of distaste for effeminacy.[10]

The genitals represented the man. Potency represented power, hence the number of literary references to the penis as a weapon. Loss of potency meant loss of manhood and defeat. Catullus in one poem refers to a groom whose "short sword hung like a strip of limp beet / between his legs, never / cocked navelwards." In Petronius's *Satyrica* the narrator lamented, "I was a ready soldier, but I had no weapons." The poet Martial wielded the inability to have an erection as amongst the most wounding of charges to hurl at his opponents. He derided one victim (*Epigram* 11.46): "You no longer rise, Mevius, except in your sleep, and your penis begins to piss onto the middle of your feet; your shriveled cock is stirred by your weary fingers and, thus solicited, does not lift its useless head." In stating that cunts and asses could no longer serve Mevius, Martial implied that mouths were his last resort. And indeed Martial made just such a charge (*Epigram* 11.25) against Linus. "That over-active cock, well known to girls not a few, has ceased to stand for Linus. Tongue, look out!" Finally Martial asserted (*Epigram* 11.61) that Nanneius was so weak that even his tongue was impotent.[11]

Penetration was central to the ancient world's notion of healthy male sexuality, but whom might the man penetrate? Historians are largely now in agreement that the concept of sexuality is a discourse—a way of organizing and controlling desires—that only came into being in modern times. Consequently we have to be wary of ahistorically reading back into the ancient world our notion of "sexuality," in particular the idea that every individual would have a sense of self as being either heterosexual or homosexual. To guard against such presentist thinking, historians of ancient Greece have recently spoken of an age of presexuality, an era in which there was no such thing as "sexual identity." It has been similarly suggested that Greek homosexuality should be more precisely called pseudohomosexuality or male-to-male intercourse, since few in the ancient world had the concept of a desire for only one sex.[12]

In the Mediterranean world a man who penetrated and dominated either men or women proved his manhood. The man who sought to please or was the passive partner of either man or woman was considered effeminate. Failure to be aroused by either girls or boys concerned the ancients. Martial scoffed (*Epigram* 12.86) at the man who despite having thirty boys and thirty girls could not get his cock to rise. Strato had a laugh at himself in ending a poem with a pun on the name of Hector's son and the word for failing to make erect (12.11): "Yesterday I had Philostratus for the night, but was incapable, though he (how shall I say it?) made every possible offer. No longer, my friends, count me friend, but throw me off a tower as I have become too much of an Astyanax." And later (12.216) he complained: "*Now* you're upright, damn you, and stiff, when nothing is here. But when there *was* something yesterday, you heaved no breath at all."[13]

The Greeks sustained a somewhat ambiguous pederastic model of chaste courtship in which the honor of both male partners could be retained. This culture accepted what we might describe as homosexuality though such relations were at times a source of anxiety. In Rome who penetrated whom was crucial. Anal rape was feared. There were no discussions of the boy's pleasure, indeed the assumption was made that the passive male could not be pleasured. Those who brandished accusations of effeminacy tended to liken passive men to slaves and women. Yet the worst thing a man could be accused of—even worse than servicing another man by fellatio—was, as noted in Martial (*Epigram* 2.28), that of servicing a woman by cunnilingus.[14]

The ancients' concerns for potency can only be fully understood when viewed in the context of a culture that lauded male dominance and feared the mythical, sexually voracious female. This culture supported a specific sort of sexuality that assumed inequitable, often violent, relationships in which women and slaves were necessarily subordinate. Men in the ancient world were supposed to be sexually aggressive. They were believed to swell with both anger and desire, doctors viewing the two passions in men as related. Women were objectified, and their use by men—like the taking of food—was often presented by writers as little more than a hygienic necessity.[15]

The position women enjoyed in the Greek family is still very much a subject of debate. Those who opt for the darker view of the Attic character stress the themes of male dominance and violence that permeated the ancient myths. The countless references to patriarchy and misogyny in much of Greek literature are difficult to ignore. Zeus had, according to Hesiod punished man for Prometheus's theft of fire by creating woman and endowing her with crafty speech, thievish habits, and a licentious mind. Semonides, in what has been considered the earliest work in European literature devoted to women (c. 640 BC), portrayed the female as rivaling in vice the sow, vixen, bitch, ass, ferret, mare, and monkey. Male mortals were, for their part, candidly outspoken defenders of a sexual double-standard. "We have," asserted an Athenian orator, "courtisans for pleasure, concubines to look after the day-to-day needs of the body, wives that we may breed legitimate children and have a trusty warden of what we have in the house." The public tolerance and, in the Greek case, the lauding of male homosexuality undercut the importance of heterosexual intercourse. Poets praised the buttocks of both beautiful boys and women, but the vagina was not lauded like the boy's anus.[16]

Depending on whether one looks at the portrayal of women in the law, theater, or medicine one comes away with distinctly different views of their status.[17] Perhaps the best that can be said is that for a variety of reasons men and women often lived quite separate lives. Males dominated the public world of the political forum, the gymnasium, and the symposium. Women oversaw the domestic sphere. The difference in the age of spouses presupposed different outlooks on life. In the Greek cities men married at close to thirty (when their own fathers, if still alive, were preparing to make way for the next generation) whereas brides were often in their early teens. The Romans assumed that family order was best assured if an age gap of about ten years separated the bride and groom.

Aristotle regarded late marriage as healthy because, "to abstain from early marriage conduces to self-control; for women who have sexual intercourse too soon are apt to be wanton, and a man's body also is stunted if he exercises the reproductive faculty before the semen is full grown." He believed semen and the menses started and stopped at the same ages, but men only became fertile at twenty-one. He contradicted himself later, acknowledging men could be still be potent in old age. An older husband presumably could more easily control a young wife, but Aristotle voiced the fear that she might prove sexually demanding. To dissuade men from entering into marriages in which there would be too great an age disparity, Plutarch claimed the Athenian law allowed the wife a legal right to demand her husband be physically capable of fulfilling his conjugal duties at least three times a month.[18]

Given the sexual double standard, the ancients regarded heterosexual intercourse somewhat ambiguously. Discussions of the use of pleasure inevitably raised the specter of dangerous over indulgence. There was no particular sexual practice or activity—not masturbation nor sodomy nor same-sex intercourse—that especially aroused their concerns; rather it was the idea of excess that preoccupied them. At first glance they seemed to view the problems posed by sex like those of thirst and hunger. That does not mean, as has often been claimed, that unlike Christians, the pagans accepted the "naturalness" of sexuality. What counted for them was gender, not sexuality. That is to say, almost anything an elite male did was, by definition, acceptable. Elite behavior was regarded as being confirmed by rather than being a result of biology. The early medical texts accordingly said much about diet, regime, and self-control. In these accounts orgasm was analyzed not because of the pleasure it gave but out of concerns for control, utility, and hygiene. As long as a man was dominant, the ancients were not so much interested in whom he had sex with or how, but with the dynamics of desire. Those who believe that the ancients had no notion of forbidden acts are mistaken. They might not have sought the complete renunciation of desire as would the Christians, but they felt the need to demonstrate mastery of their desires.[19]

Women were told that to be healthy they needed sex—even if they did not find it pleasurable. In men lust was taken as a given. For Plato desire emerged in the seed itself. In Greek medical thinking heat was necessary for life; cold brought death. Only men were hot enough to produce semen. For Diogenes the Cynic air was the life principle and male semen the "foam" of the blood; the mother simply reared in the womb the offspring produced by the father. Similarly the Hippocratic text "On Generation" held that semen was transported from brain to loins, thus a cut above the ear could render one sterile. Since it looked like spinal fluid the seed was thought to come from the head and the essence of life from the knee. Given the Hippocratic idea that sperm came from the marrow of the spine, hunchbacks with their exaggerated backbones were thought especially lecherous.[20]

For Aristotle semen was a residue concocted from the blood; further concoction occurred in coition, which explained the child's resemblance to the parent. He argued that the presence of *pneuma* (air) in the semen turned it white and also expanded the penis. Holding one's breath supposedly helped to release sperm. Though Aristotle located semen in the scrotum, he saw no need for the testicles except as weights to keep the vesicles extended. While Herophilus investigated the vas deferens, the seminal vesicles, and prostate gland, he too retained the notion that blood turned into semen. Rufus of Ephesus was the first to assert that semen was formed in the testicles.[21]

The Hippocratic authors argued that women, like men, produced seed or semen though of a weaker nature. Aristotle argued in a circular fashion that because women lacked heat they could not produce semen and their failure to produce semen proved they lacked heat. Moreover since they could not emit semen it followed that, unlike men who had to reach orgasm if conception were to take place, women's pleasure was not required. "A sign that the female does not emit the kind of seed that the male emits, and that generation is not due to the mixing of both as some hold, is that often the female conceives without experiencing the pleasure that occurs in inter-course." Indeed Aristotle held that a woman's colder physiology was most influenced by the moon: "the menstrual discharge in the natural course tends to take place when the moon is waning . . . that time of the month is cooler and more fluid." Women—being weak, cold, and passive—could be likened to eunuchs or young boys. The female was incomplete at the bio-logical level and accordingly could not resist the male who would make her complete.[22]

Discussions of reproduction were colored by this general assumption of female inferiority. In Aeschylus's *Eumenides* woman was presented as little more than a nest for the growing conceptus: "She who is called the mother is not her offspring's Parent, but nurse to the newly sown embryo. The male—who mounts—begets. The female, a stranger, guards a stranger's child if no god bring it harm." Anaxagoras claimed that males provided the seed and females only the "ground" in which embryos were reared. Aristotle noted, "Anaxagoras and some other philosophers hold that sex is already determined in the sperm. They say that while the father provides the seed, the mother only provides a place for the fetus to develop; that male offspring come from the right testis and female from the left; and that furthermore, male offspring develop in the right side of the womb, females in the left." Similarly Plato argued, "for the woman in her conception and generation is but the imitation of the earth and not the earth of the woman." Aristotle likened the male element operating on inactive female matter to a carpenter working on wood or to rennet changing milk into cheese.[23] If the seed succeeded in impressing form on matter a male was produced; if it failed a female resulted.

The Romans relied heavily on Greek medicine for their understanding of reproduction—indeed the leading physicians of the empire were Greek—but the Romans tended to take a more pessimistic view of health. They were clearly preoccupied with corporal fragility and exhibited an intense interest in diet and regimen. For Galen sexual intercourse was necessary for health. "It is evident," he concluded, "that a chaste person does not indulge in sexual intercourse for pleasure, but with the intention to relieve this urge, as if this were not associated with pleasure." Galen, like the Hippocratic writers, believed women produced seed and their hysteria resulted from a surplus. Men suffered even more from retaining semen. Masturbation might have been recommended as a therapy. The ancients said little about the topic, but the act certainly posed no ethical problem. Galen repeated the famous story of Diogenes the Cynic bringing himself off, not for pleasure but to avoid bodily disturbances.[24]

The medical sources contained many references to cures for barrenness, which could be taken as evidence of a widespread fear of sterility. The barren wife certainly risked being divorced. But what if the man failed to complete the sexual act? As Plutarch made clear, sterility and impotence were often confused. "Diocles holds that sterility in men ariseth from some of these causes,—either that they cannot at all ejaculate any sperm, or if they do, it is less than nature doth require, or else there is no generative faculty in the sperm, or the genital members are flagging; or from the obliquity of the yard."[25] The fact that the ancient texts contain extended discussions of how such situations might have arisen and how they could be remedied is the most striking indication of the anxieties provoked by fears of impotence.

The ancients recognize a wide range of causes of male failures. The Greeks believed that a male child would be made impotent if placed on tomb. Firmicus Maternus cited the influence of the planets as a cause. Others attributed men's failures to the work of the gods. In the *Odyssey* (10.299–301) Hermes warns Odysseus of Circe's magical power to render him impotent. The *Odyssey* also made reference to Melampus, the first mortal to understand the language of animals. Phylacus offered to free him and to give him his cattle if Melampus would cure his son, Iphiclus, of impotence. Melampus discovered the antidote to Iphiclus's impotence from two vultures. Dionysus purportedly punished the Athenians with impotence for dishonoring his cult. But the vengeful might also appeal to the gods. An enemy could make a man impotent by inscribing on obsidian the figure of a castrated man and have the victim touch it. For a similar purpose some resorted to casting spells on wax effigies.[26]

A man could always attribute his failure to such witchcraft. More commonly the woman would be blamed for the sort of inexplicable inability to perform that in modern times would be called his psychic impotence. Martial (*Epigram* 1.146) castigated a partner for simply shattering the aura of romance.

> Hedyle, when you say, "I'm rushed. Do it if you're going to,"
> My weakened equipment droops right away and stops.
> So tell me to hold on; I'll go faster if I'm held back.
> Hedyle, if you are in a hurry, tell me not to hurry.[27]

Horace portrayed the man who defensively attributed his failures to the woman who was too ugly or too fat but had the temerity of accusing her exhausted victim of being a "sluggardly bull." The historian Herodotus more sympathetically described the plight of Amasis, king of Egypt, who was only impotent with Ladice. Ovid and Strato in poems noted above commented on the frustrations of the man who mysteriously found himself unable to perform with his beloved. Martial (*Epigram* 3.70) presented a man who now desired the same woman whom he had spurned when she was his wife. "Is it that when secure you lack appetite?" The Stoics attributed sterility to temperament, noting that one could be barren with one partner but fruitful with another.[28]

Commentators also listed a number of organic causes of sexual dysfunctions. Hippocrates (*On Airs*) referred to the Scythians' impotence being due to their horse riding. Aristotle wrote that men who put on flesh "emit less seed and have less desire for sexual indulgence." "Fat people too, both men and women, appear to be less fertile than those that are not fat, because the residue when concocted in well-nourished bodies becomes fat; for fat too is a healthy residue caused by good feeding."[29]

To be potent a man had to be healthy. It was commonly believed that wine was an aphrodisiac, though in excess it led to sleep. According to Aristotle, "the man must not be drunk, nor should he drink white wine, but strong unmixed wine, eat very strong food, not take a hot bath, be strong, in good health, abstain from unhealthful foods." Commentators warned that cooling foods could abate lust. Plutarch asserted that wine was cool and countered the need for heat. The ancients claimed that a variety of cooling vegetables could serve both as contraceptives and as anaphrodisiacs. Pliny the Elder noted that Homer called the willow "fruit losing" because it lost its seeds quickly; for that reason, continued Pliny, "it is well known that willow seed taken as a drug produces barrenness in a woman." Bryony mixed with ox urine caused impotence. Soranus described the cooling effects of wine, rue, wallflower seed, myrtle, myrrh, and white pepper. Dioscorides listed nine plants endowed with contraceptive properties and the water lily that caused impotence. Aelian claimed that usually lustful male animals could be rendered coy by the use of a certain herb.[30] Ovid (*Amores* 3.7) referred to chilling anaphrodisiacs such as hemlock that prevented erections.

> She round my neck her ivory arms did throw,
> Her arms far whiter than the Scythian snow,
> And eagerly she kissed me with her tongue,
> And under mine her wanton thigh she flung.
> Yes, and she soothed me up, and called me sire.
> And used all speech that might provoke and stir.
> Yet like as if cold hemlock I had drunk,
> It humbled me, hung down the head, and sunk.[31]

In literature there were many references to men's fears of women tampering with their food. Doctors believed the man had to be inflamed in order to be potent. It followed that narcotics that calmed and soothed his spirits could in effect unman him. Wives who sought to keep the affection of their husbands, women attempting to bind a lover to them, and enemies seeking to lull an opponent into complacency would, it was reported, use spells and narcotics to lessen a man's anger and thus his potency. Plutarch warned women against using love potions and magic on their spouses. He claimed Antony failed as general since he was always thinking of Cleopatra, as if bewitched by a spell or certain drugs.[32]

Commentators attributed most common forms of impotence to the bodily failures associated with either old age or youth. The elderly, and those on dry and cool diets were thought to bear sex least well. The ancients took it as a given that old men would become impotent. According to Aristotle emitting seed helped the young but hurt the old. He asserted that the age of procreation for men ended at seventy and for women at fifty. The semen of the elderly was less concocted. The Greek poet Antiphanes drew the moral that one had to enjoy life when young. "Thenceforward is the heavy winter of old age; you shall not make love, not even for a thousand drachmas, such is the impotence that awaits you."[33]

The Greeks and Romans cruelly joked about the incapacities of the elderly. Juvenal (*Satire* 10.204–209) coolly captured the sexual frustrations that often accompanied aging.

> For intercourse is already long distant in memory;
> Or should you try, your tool lies small and vessel-swollen.
> And although it be stroked all through the night,
> It will lie unresponsive.
> So can this old age of debilitated loins hope for anything?
> And isn't desire without ability,
> Which actually impairs passion, truly suspect?[34]

Satiric writers' references to the limp members of old duped, ugly, impotent men are, according to one historian, "of course in the grand tradition of comic scurrility and appear often." Aristophanes' lost play *Amphiareus* concerned an old man with a young wife seeking vigor either through lentils or erotic incantations. Lucilius ridiculed weak old men. Martial (*Epigram* 11.81) compared the geriatric to the eunuch: "Lack of strength makes the one, length of years the other useless for the job; so each labours in fruitless desire."[35] The sixth-century writer Maximianus Etruscus (Maximian) in *Elegies of Old Age* produced the most extended tragic/comic account of old age in which the hero finds himself unable to perform with a Greek beauty.

> I wish't, I ask't, and gain'd the Beautious She;
> But, oh! What Witchcraft did Enervate me!
> Lifeless I on that mass of Beauty lay,
> Nor the due debts of Sacred Love could pay.
> All vigorous warmth my languid Limbs forsook,
> And left me cold, like an old sapless Oak.
> My chief, yet basest Nerve, did then prove lank,
> And, like a Coward, from the Battle shrank;

Shrivell'd, and dry, like a dead wither'd flow'r.
Depriv'd, and void of all vivisick pow'r.
No fertile Moisture, no prolifick Juice,
Could the enfeebled Instrument produce;
No unctious Substance, no kind Balm emit;
Balm, nourishing as Milk, as Honey sweet.
At last cry'd out the Disappointed Fair,
Thy dull unactive weight I cannot bear;
Thy heavy Limbs press me with joyless pain,
And all thy faint Endeavours are in vain.

. . . such was my first sad Night,
That I could neither give nor take Delight.
But a base conscious shame possest each sence,
Nor left me pow'r to make the least defence,
Dash'd with the Guilt of my own Impotence.

. . . .

For what, alas, can those Defects supply,
Which weaken'd Nature do's to Age deny?
But then I blush't, and stupify'd became,
Much more debilitated by my Shame.[36]

Such wistful portrayals countered the philosophers' argument that man was not to fear old age, but welcome it for freeing him from fleshly preoccupations.[37]

Doctors in turn warned young men that they could become old before their time if they over indulged. As lassitude followed emission of semen, sexual excesses were believed to result in impotence. The general concern of medical writers was that a balance be retained and excesses avoided. For example, the Hippocratic writings asserted that the wasting disease of tabes was due to unrestrained lust: "This consumption originates in the spinal marrow. It chiefly attacks newlywed husbands and lechers. . . . If you ask such a patient, he will tell you that he has a sensation like ants crawling from the head down his spine, and copious seminal discharge with urination and defecation. There is also infertility; and in his dreams, whether sleeping with his mate or without her, he is plagued by love's mockery." According to Galen semen was the finest blood, which in being injected with the breath or *pneuma* essential to life, became white and frothy. Excesses led to loss of vital spirit. Epicurus said all coitus was dangerous. Rufus came close to agreeing and pointed out that the accompanying loss of heat suffered by men—but not women—resulted in indigestion, memory loss, spitting of blood, and fading of sight and hearing. Soranus agreed that excessive coition was dangerous. Caelius Aurelianus, who translated and abridged Soranus, claimed that venery contributed to pleurisy, apoplexy, madness, paralysis, nephritis, and hemorrhaging. He went on to assert, in attacking Asclepiades' argument that coitus could cure epilepsy, that coition was itself "minor epilepsy." "For it causes a motion of the parts like that in epilepsy; various parts are subjected to spasms, and at the same time there occur panting, sweating, rolling of the eyes and flushing of the face. And the completion of coitus brings with it a feeling of malaise along with pallor, weakness, or dejection." Coition, he concluded, exacerbated mania, "for it not only deprives the body of strength but also agitates the soul."[38]

There are no references to same-sex acts endangering Greek males, yet a long line of thinkers portrayed sex with women as dangerous. According to the Hippocratic corpus women were dried out by too little sex; men were dried out by too much. Women relied on intercourse with men for their health. Men could thus be exhausted, but women were inexhaustible, having no self-control. Some seasons posed special dangers. "In general the sexual appetites of animals are keenest in spring-time"; asserted Aristotle, "the time of pairing, however, is not the same for all, but is adapted so as to ensure the rearing of the young at a convenient season." In the heat of summer men were soon exhausted; women's appetites remained unsatiated. According to Hesiod women were then "at their most wanton, while men are completely enfeebled." The woman could render a man impotent and he would soon find himself in "raw old age." She "withers him up and brings old age on youth too soon."[39] Even the god Priapus complained:

> The sexed-up neighborhood womenfolk,
> Hornier than sparrows in Spring,
> Endlessly wear me out.[40]

Men had to protect themselves from demanding women whom Aristotle likened to mares in heat. "Coition," warned Democritus, "is a slight attack of apoplexy. For man gushes forth from man and is separated by being torn apart with a kind of blow." Semen, according to the pessimistic Pythagorians, was a "clot of brain containing hot vapor within it" and consequently every sexual pleasure was harmful. Plato, Aristotle, and the Hippocratic corpus similarly stressed the need for sexual moderation. In *On the Nature of Things* Lucretius portrayed sex as a trap for men: "Add that they waste their strength, they strain, they die; add that the will of a woman rules their life."[41] In such texts, men were endangered by intercourse; women, however, were prescribed it. Hippocratic medicine thus validated male domination in its assertion that women's health depended on the sexual services of their partners.

Ancient men's fear of women—capped by the nightmarish belief that in losing bodily heat and vigor one could for all intents and purposes become a woman—explains the seriousness with which they regarded displays of virility. There was accordingly no shortage of advice for the man concerned about his flagging sexual abilities. The sheer volume of material devoted to the discussions of how impotence could be cured dramatically demonstrates how preoccupying the Greeks and Romans found the issue. The ancients produced sex manuals providing suggestions of positions and techniques. These texts, resolutely phallic and heterosexual, though no doubt penned by men, were usually attributed to prostitutes, thus sustaining the myth that aside from the odd impotent emperor, real men did not need instructions. In fact from the scraps that survive (and Ovid's parodies) these cookbook-like manuals appear to have listed positions and stressed the active male, passive female scenario.[42]

The extensive literature on sex—produced by men for men—explained what to do in case of declining sexual abilities. Some suggested the use of arousing books and pictures. Theodorus Priscianus (2.11) advised "reading tales of love" This fourth-century medical man went on to suggest: "Let the patient be surrounded by beautiful girls or boys; also give him books to read, which stimulate lust and in which love-stories are insinuatingly treated." References to stimulating or erotic images were mentioned by Ovid. The pornographic wall paintings of Pompeii appear to have decorated both brothels and private homes.[43]

Martial (*Epigram* 3.75) noted a range of possible cures, including purchasing the services of youths. Dancing girls were hired to arouse old men. In his biography of Tiberius, Suetonius described the court's turning to voyeurism and pedophilia to stumulate desire. Fellatio offered impotent old men a last resort. Yet putting such advice into practice did not always work. Ovid scoffed: "and my girl didn't even disdain to incite you / softly with the motion of her hand. / But . . . she saw no skill could make you rise."[44]

To judge by the literature, men's most common response to fears of impotency was to consume an inciting herb or beverage. We know that aphrodisiacs were commonly used. There are records of court cases in which women, accused of poisoning their lovers, claimed to have only given them love potions. According to Suetonius, Caligula's wife gave him such a concoction. Plutarch called on men to avoid the use of aphrodisiacs. In his writings on the life of Lucullus he reported, "but Cornelius Nepos says that Lucullus lost his mind not from old age, nor yet from disease, but that he was disabled by drugs administered to him by one of his freedmen, Callisthenes, in order to win more of his love, in the belief that they had such a power, but they drove him from his senses and overwhelmed his reason."[45] The many recipes for inflaming lust were usually meant for men. Pliny, for example, did not see arousal of the female as posing a problem, though assuring that she conceived might be.

Anything that looked like a penis or that warmed the body as did arousal was thought to work. According to the Hippocratic texts legumes, cereals, and nuts, contained air and heat, and so raised the passions. Oils, liquids, and foods were similarly ingested. In particular, as male anger and sexuality were linked, so it was thought that irritants raised a man's ardor. Accordingly the Greeks used nettles, peppers, and erection-producing drugs like cantharides (crushed blister beetles). Theophrastus listed many such cures in his *Historia plantarum*. Dioscorides, in the *De materia medica* added to the earlier herbal information of Theophrastus, discussed love-making, and listed a number of aphrodisiacs, prescribing them according to theories of similarity or contrariety. Paulus Aegineta recommended mollusks, pot herbs, rocket, turnip, pulses, peas and beans, and for the impotent narcissus root, seed of nettle, anise, pepper, satyricon and saffron, chick peas, pine nuts, honey, and wine.[46]

The most extensive catalog of stimulants was provided by Pliny the Elder in his *Natural History*. The leek, he asserts, "is an aphrodisiac" (20.47). The turpentine tree or terebinth "is a gentle aperient and an aphrodisiac (24.28)" Garlic "is believed to act as an aphrodisiac, when pounded with fresh coriander and taken in neat wine" (20.57). The water of boiled wild asparagus serves the same purpose (20.110). "The Cyprian reed, called donax . . . taken in wine is an aphrodisiac" (24.87). The leaves of clematis "eaten with vinegar . . . act as an aphrodisiac" (24.140). "Sexual desire is excited by the upper part of the xiphium root given in wine as a draught; also by the plant called cremnos agrios and by ormenos agrios crushed with pearl barley" (26.94). "Democritus thinks that as a food radishes are aphrodisiac; for this reason, perhaps, some have maintained that they are injurious to the voice" (20.28). "Orpheus said that there is in staphylinus a love-philtre, perhaps because it is a proved fact that when eaten it is an aphrodisiac; for which reason some have declared that by it conception is aided" (20.32). Pliny cites Hesiod and Alcaeus on the use of golden thistle (22.87). "They have written that when it is in blossom the song of the cricket is shrillest, women are the most amorous and men most backward in sexual unions, as though it were through Nature's providence that this stimulant is at its best when badly needed." That is, in the heat of summer. He says of chervil, "Its special merit is that it gives strength to a body exhausted by sexual indulgence, and revives sexual virility when flagging through old age" (22.80). Dioscorides had asserted that rocket "eaten raw in great quantitie doth provoke Venery" (2:170),[47] Pliny recommends it as well: "It is believed that desire for mating is also stimulated by articles of diet, for instance rocket in the case of a man and onions in the case of cattle" (10.182). Elsewhere he writes of rocket, "Its properties are quite different from those of lettuce, and it acts as an aphrodisiac" (19.154).

Many such herbal cures were attributed to their visual and magical associations, following the so-called doctrine of the signatures. Vegetables and plants that were penis-shaped were esteemed. Orchid-like plants with two testicle-like tubers were similarly thought useful for genital problems and as aphrodisiacs.[48] In addition bulbs like onions and garlic produced gas that was thought to be needed for erection. Accordingly Martial advised: "If envious age relax the nuptial knot / Thy food be scallions, and thy feast shallot." Dioscorides recommends a number of bulbs. Orchis, in goat's milk "to provoke venery" (19.154); Saturion, a type of orchid, "use it, if he will lie with a woman. For they say that this also doth stirr up courage in ye conjunction" (3.143); Saturion Eruthronion " is storied that the root being taken into ye hand doth provoke to Venerie, but much more, being drank with wine" (3.144); Orminon Emeron (Salvia Horminum) is also "thought being drank with wine to provoke conjunction" (3.145); and Gladiolus communis: "They say also that the upper root being drank with wine doth provoke venery, but that ye undermost doth make them lustless" (4.20).

Pliny agrees. "But very high on the list of wonders is the plant orchis. . . . The root has two tubers, like testicles, so that the larger, or, as some put it, the thinner, taken in water, excites desire" (26.94). "Megarian bulbs [a type of onion?] are a strong aphrodisiac" (20.105). Asphodel, another bulbous plant, was used against poisons. "It is also been held that it is an aphrodisiac if, with wine and honey, it is used as an ointment or taken as a medicine" (22.71). Cynosorchis has, notes Pliny, two roots. "If men eat the larger of these roots, male children are said to be conceived, but female if the smaller is eaten by women. In Thessaly men take in goat's milk the softer roots as an aphrodisiac, but the harder as an antaphrodisiac. The one part neutralizes the other" (27.65). Pliny claims that Sea-holly does more than counteract poisons. "Marvellous is the characteristic reported of it, that its root grows into the likeness of the organs of one sex or the other; it is rarely so found, but should the male form come into the possession of men, they become lovable in the eyes of women" (22.20). "Satyrion is a sexual stimulant." One has "a double root shaped like human testicles, which swells and subsides in alternate years . . . [which] taken in the milk of a farm-yard sheep, causes erections; taken in water, however, it makes them subside" (26.96).

The ancients assumed that what worked for animals might work for humans. According to Aristotle humans first learned how to use herbs by watching animals; the herbals in turn advised the same treatments for men and beasts. Pliny asserts "yet another kind of satyrion they call erythrai-con. . . . They tell us that sexual desire is aroused if the root is merely held in the hand, a stronger passion, however, if it is taken in a dry wine, that rams also and he-goats are given it in drink when they are too sluggish, and that it is given to stallions from Sarmatia when they are too fatigued in copulation because of prolonged labour; this condition is called prosedamum" (26.97–98). Buprestis was poisonous, at least for oxen, but Pliny suggests that those driven by lust might seek it out since taken in drink it "is the most potent aphrodisiac known" (22.78).

Some proceeded to seek cures through the use of animal parts associated with potency. Snakes (since they were popularly believed to rejuvenate themselves), and the genitalia of roosters and goats were consumed. On the forehead of a newborn foal was found a growth called the *hippo-manes*, which, reported Aristotle, was a powerful aphrodisiac.[49] The penis was often likened to the lizard, which leads Pliny to note the powers of a large one known as the skink (28.120): "Its muzzle and feet, taken in white wine, are aphrodisiac, especially with the addition of satyrion and rocket seed. . . . One-drachma lozenge of the compound should be taken in drink." Pliny then proceeds to provide a survey of other popular beliefs in how one might tap into the potency of the animal world.

> Aphrodisiacs are: an application of wildboar's gall, pig's marrow swallowed, or an application of ass's suet mixed with a gander's grease; also the fluid that Virgil too describes as coming from a mare after copulation, the testicles of a horse, dried so that they may be powdered into drink, the right testis of an ass taken in wine, or a portion of it worn as an amulet on a bracelet; or the foam of an ass after copulation, collected in a red cloth and enclosed, as Osthanes tells us, in silver. Salpe prescribes an ass's genital organ to be plunged seven times into hot oil, and the relevant parts to be rubbed therewith, Dalion the ash from it to be taken in drink, or the urine of a bull after copulation to be drunk, or the mud itself made by it applied to the pubic parts. (*Natual History* 28.261–62)

As Pliny noted not all cures were taken orally. The Greeks attempted to increase potency with various salves, plasters, and creams. A number of magical recipes listed lotions to rub on the penis "for an erection," "to play with a woman," and in order "to have fun with a woman." The Egyptian magical papyri also listed incantations, potions, and salves including one of carrot juice for premature ejaculation. In his *Medical Collection*, Oribasius drew on Rufus in recommending suppositories to treat paralysis of the virile member (8:39). One recipe for those whose humors had thickened and member had cooled was made of mustard, which led to Oribasius warning the patient of the danger of burning the anus.[50]

Many of the various herbal or animal concoctions were presumed to work by a sort of sympathetic magic. Impotence was, of course, often believed to be caused by witchcraft. Ovid spoke of the nefarious effects of black magic carried out by effigies, poisoned drinks, and incantations.

> What, am I poisoned by some witch's charms?
> Do spells and drugs do me, poor soul, such harms?
> Did she my image in red wax procure,
> And with her needles' points my liver skewer?
> Charms transform wheat to weeds, and make it die,
> Charms make the running streams and fountains dry.
> Through charms oaks acorns shed, from vines grapes fall,
> And fruits from trees when there's no wind at all.
> Why might not then my sinews be enchanted,
> And I grow faint as with some spirit haunted?[51]

In response, urine could be used medicinally (28.64), suggested Pliny, especially "that of eunuchs to counteract the sorcery that prevents fertility." He also recommends Southernwood a powerful, warming plant, useful to fight off chills. "They say that a spray of it, laid under the pillow, acts an aphrodisiac, and that the plant is a most effective countercheck of all magic potions given to produce sexual impotence" (20.162). To protect himself against impotence a man might wear a stone talisman or amulet. It was claimed that the "right molar of a small crocodile worn as amulet guarantees erection in men." In Rome males wore as protection against the evil eye a replica of the penis, called the *fascinum* from the word to "bewitch." And finally one could make an appeal to the gods. "While you're alive I'm hopeful rustic guard / Come. Bless me, stiff Priapus: make me hard."[52]

Did the aphrodisiacs, lotions, and talismans work? This is an ahistorical question inasmuch as when we moderns talk of medicines "working" we

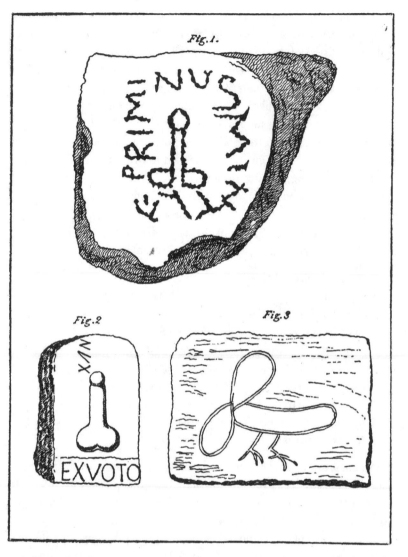

1. Phallic carvings from Roman Britain, depicted in Thomas Wright, *On the Worship of the Generative Powers during the Middle Ages of Western Europe* (London: Chiswick Press, 1865), 23. Inscriptions 1 and 2 served as votive offerings for those appealing to Priapus to overcome a sexual infirmity. Carvings such as figure 3, found at entrances or gateways, were employed to protect dwellings from evil influences.

mean in a scientifically provable way, whereas the Greeks and Romans regarded many herbal potions having magical qualities. Having said that, it has to be acknowledged that the ancients knew quite well that restoratives did not always have the desired effect. Martial (*Epigram* 3.75) laughed at one man's futile expenditures in medicines.

> Scallions, lustful rockets nought prevail,
> And heightening meats in operation fail;
> Thy wealth begins the pure cheeks to defile,
> So venery provoked lives but a while;
> Who can admire enough, the wonder's such
> That thy not standing stands thee in so much?

When commenting on cures of which he was dubious Pliny often signaled his skepticism by the phrase "they say" or by attributing his account to another chronicler.[53] For example, he reported, "Again, those carrying on their persons the pith of tithymallus branches are said to become thereby more excited sexually. The remarks on this subject made by Theophrastus, generally a weighty authority, are fabulous. He says that the lust to have intercourse seventy times in succession has been given by the touch of a certain plant whose name and kind he has not mentioned" (26.99). Obviously many of the methods could not "work" in the sense of having a direct, desired physiological effect, but many no doubt played a positive psychological role. Men refused to see themselves as passive beings and sought to have some control over their fates. Whatever the effectiveness of the various therapies, their use demonstrates the serious intent with which the ancients sought to control biology.

In the ancient world the attention paid to potency stemmed from the enormous importance of every free man marrying and having children. For the Greeks and Romans a male heir was essential. In Greece only a man could be the owner or *kyrios* of his lands, children and spouse. In the Roman Empire bachelors were penalized and large families rewarded. Martial asserted that if one was a real man one would have heirs, and joked about Almo who was impotent yet complained his wife produced no children (*Epigram* 9.66, 10.91). What if a man could not sire children? One might presume that the impotent man would been disbarred from both marriage and fatherhood, but in the ancient world, social status trumped biology. What counted in being a man was, as one scholar has noted, "the male's gender role—his legal capacity both to marry a wife and to adopt. Anyone who had a penis, even if not in full working order, or who used to have one, was classified as a man, and therefore, once recognized as legally adult, had the legal capacity of a man."[54] In Rome a male was someone with a penis; only they had heirs. Girls were automatically of age at twelve; boys only when inspected and shown capable of procreation, but if impotent, at fourteen.

Marriage confirmed status and status was dictated by elite males. Women over fifty could not marry. Slaves, forbidden to marry, were permitted unions but no inheritance rights and their owner could break up their families. For free Romans premarital sex was unimportant and not an impediment to marriage, though consanguinity and class barriers were. But for the purposes of this study what is essential to understand is that in Rome, a marriage did not have to be consummated—it was a simple contract. In the first and second centuries sexual potency was "not a legal prerequisite for lawful marriage" as it would be for Christians. Ulpian stated that the castratus could not leave a will, that is, he could not marry and name heirs. There was no problem if a man only suffered from temporary impotence. Even the physical deficiencies of the *spado* (a natural eunuch who could not reproduce) were not a bar to marriage, though insanity was. Consent was always the key issue. The ancients' concern was not with the sex act per se, which usually posed no ethical issue, but with whatever might possibly jeopardize the social hierarchy and family property.[55] The same deference shown the concerns of elite males explained the workings of divorce. A Roman man could repudiate his spouse with no cause given. Only with Constantine were causes needed; only with Justinian was male impotence noted.

Since the purpose of marriage was to have children—indeed under the Julian Laws childlessness was penalized in inheritances—what point was there in the impotent marrying? Some men would, of course, insist that the barren marriage was the wife's responsibility. Seneca the Elder noted such arguments. The married man lacking children could become the butt of humor because they, as Juvenal notes (9.85), are "proofs of your manhood." But such failures could be overcome by partner swapping. Plutarch noted that in Greece impotence led to wife lending or husband doubling (*Lycurgus.* 15.4–7). Spouses were shared to beget children, for example, an "elderly man with a young wife" might choose a noble young man for her. On an informal level complacent husbands allowed others to do their work for them. Juvenal has a character protest: "had I not been a loyal and devoted client, your wife would still be a virgin?" (9.71–72).[56]

Adoption provided another solution. Even if one were a *spado*, one could adopt. So too could the unmarried. Indeed the Augustan legislation that required one to be a "father" to fill certain posts sometimes necessitated such a strategy. The Augustan marriage laws gave some flexibility, a man could be paterfamilias even without natural children. In Rome since males alone could be effective heirs, a man with only daughters might adopt a young man for this purpose. The new heir in turn would be obliged to marry one of the daughters. Adoption was common in the ancient world, but those adopted were usually adults; the purpose was not to provide for the poor, but rather to obtain a suitable claimant to protect the family's property. As one's own children were often a disappointment, adoption was, asserted the overrational Democritus, the most reasonable way in which to assure oneself of worthy inheritors. Seneca expressed the view that conceiving a child was the least part of fatherhood: "The generation of me was the least part of the benefit: for, to live is common with the brutes; but, to live well is the main business." In the Greek comedies it was suggested that barren, wealthy wives passed off foundlings as their own. On children depended the conservation of the household, the maintenance of the estate, the carrying on of the family name, the forging of family alliances, the provision for the elderly in old age, and the performing of funeral rites after their passing.[57] By not relying solely on biological fatherhood to sustain the family, the Greeks and Romans skirted what could have been the most disruptive effects of male sexual dysfunctions.

How are we to understand the ancients' discussion of impotence? It obviously reveals contradictions in their notions of masculinity. On the one hand it asserted that to be considered a real man one had to be potent; on the other hand it acknowledged that sexual failures were not an uncommon occurrence. To have sex demonstrated one's vigor; to have it too often threatened exhaustion. Elite males whose powers flagged turned to a range of therapies in attempts both to restore their virility and to shore up their position in society.[58] The construction of both the problem and the cure directly related to Greek and Roman notions of sex and gender. As we have seen they did not identify themselves according to their "sexuality," a concept that did not yet exist. The desires of ancient men, though they often sound similar to ours, are not what we usually associate with manliness. A man could be alarmed that neither women nor boys stirred his passions. If a lack of an erection shamed him, the feeling would not be sparked by his sense of having failed to pleasure a female partner. To have such a sense of guilt was to be effeminate. Normative male desire, the ancients believed, was fueled by aggression and anger; female desire by passivity. Penetration was likened to a beating, representing the domination of one partner and the submission of the other. Men were explicitly taught to use sex not for intimacy but control. They used herbs, potions, and magic to inflame their passions. And even if these failed, they could, because of the powers they enjoyed as free males, marry and become, through adoption, fathers. In the Greco-Roman world masculinity

WHEN "DESIRE REFUSES SERVICE"
Impotence in the Christian West

When deciding whether a marriage should be annulled on the grounds of the husband's impotence, fifteenth-century English church courts sometimes employed "honest women" to examine the man. One woman was reported as giving the following account to the courts of York and Canterbury.

> The same witness exposed her naked breasts, and with her hands warmed at the said fire, she held and rubbed the penis and testicles of the said John. And she embraced and frequently kissed the same John, and stirred him up in so far as she could to show his virility and potency, admonishing him that for shame he should then and there prove himself a man. And she says, examined and diligently questioned, that the whole time aforesaid, the said penis was scarcely three inches long, . . . remaining without any increase or decrease.[1]

That men who were otherwise virile might fail such a test is hardly surprising. "Under the stressful circumstances of such an inspection, men who were being examined might well have failed to show arousal—particularly after being cursed for failure by the examiners—regardless of their sexual capacities in less frightening situations."[2] What is surprising is that churchmen should have been involved in such confrontations. Christians had to know whether or not a marriage had been sexually consummated. But, pondered celibate church doctors, what was consummation? Was it simple penetration? Or did it require emission? Might it even necessitate the wife's orgasm? Michel Foucault tartly observed that the pagans were too reserved to leave such a full and intrusive discussion of conjugal rights, methods, and duties.[3] Why then did the church ultimately so immerse itself in the messy discussion of impotence? Why did churchmen, at first embarrassed by the issue of male potency, eventually come police it?

Some historians have suggested that a cultural shift occurred in the late Roman world, when sexuality became a topic of discussion in poetry and advice literature, as well as a privileged source of pleasure. Whereas once the intimate lives of the members of the social elite were dictated almost solely by the demands of clan, property, and honor, they were increasingly displaced by concerns for privacy and sexual preferences.[4] The rise of Christianity represented another aspect of this turning inward, shifting attention from the public to the private. The difference was that the early Christians mirrored the Stoics' distrust of fleshly appetites; indeed many regarded sex as inherently sinful. Unlike the Romans they could neither laud potency nor regard impotency as a joke.

In the first instance the early Christians were understandably hostile to the discussion of impotence, focused solely as it was on bodily desires. Yet in seeking to set themselves off from pagans, they were part of an evolution rather than a revolution in mores. Christians did not so much create a new morality as act as its conduit. Already the Stoics had put in place a "puritanical" creed and the metaphysics of the Neoplatonists and mystery cults had popularized an otherworldliness. The passions were suspect; sexuality was regarded as necessarily pitted against reason. Many of the attacks on the old style of life launched by the Stoics were simply continued by Christians converts. John Chrysostom was preceded in his opposition to public baths and nudity by pagan moralists. Seneca had condemned adultery because of the trouble and disorder it caused; Jerome attacked it as immoral and dangerous. Musonius Rufus's critique of pursuit of sexual pleasure was followed by those of Jerome, Origen, and Clement.[5] Clement of Alexandria, Tertullian, and Lactantius vividly portrayed the dangers of lust. Oribasius noted the dangers caused by sexual excesses. Most condemned the spells and aphrodisiacs employed to stimulate the passions and lauded the "feminine" virtues of restraint.

Though most Christian virtues had been anticipated by the ancients, Christians were not simply philosophers. They also formed a social movement: they practiced and preached. Especially striking was the vigor with which they listed and attacked a vast range of vices. They carried over the Jewish abhorrence of sexual perversions and prided themselves on "avoiding porneia," which, as cataloged in the first-century Syrian Christian teachings called *Didache* or *Teachings of the Twelve Apostles*, included abortion, infanticide, magic, and same-sex acts. *The Book of Barnabas*, in drawing on Hellenic natural history, likened the adulterer to the hyena, which changed sex each year; the fellator to the weasel, which conceived through the mouth; and the corrupter of children to the hare, which "increases unduly its discharge each year, and thus has as many holes as it is years old."⁶ Adultery was particularly associated with the *philtres* or love potions that the ancients employed to increase lust.

For the Greeks and Romans desire was not often discussed as a problem, though performance was. In Christian Europe desire increasingly was viewed as a danger—something to be restrained. Church fathers declared themselves shocked by the attempts made by some to actually inflame male arousal. They opposed wine for causing sexual excitement. John Chrysostom condemned couples' recourse to libations, incantations, and love-potions. Clement of Alexandria attacked pictorial pagan lewdness intended to raise desires. Christians particularly abhorred the means employed by the Greeks and Romans to spur on procreation. Clement of Alexandria denigrated women's use of charms. Caesarius attacked the Gallo-Romans for their employing an "impious drug" to cure barrenness. "Therefore," he wrote, "those to whom God is unwilling to grant children should not try to have them by means of herbs or magic signs or evil charms."⁷

The more extreme Christian thinkers ultimately objected to almost every manifestation of sexuality from abortion, contraception, divorce, and adultery to the wearing of wigs and the use of make-up. The purported intent of condemning such acts was to end debauchery. Similar concerns had been voiced by some pagans, but a new shift in emphasis was evident. What had been primarily proprietary concerns were made ethical issues. The ancients sought to police sexuality for the conservative purpose of subjecting every individual to a family patriarch; the Church sought to police sexuality for the radical purpose of freeing Christians from the entangling world of secular ambitions and family squabbles. The asceticism of many of the early Christians was due to their apocalyptic expectations. Their contempt for intercourse was not so much due to a hostility to sex per se, as it has been argued, but to the perceived need to prepare for the next world.⁸

Key to the Christians' morality was a reappraisal of masculinity. Sexual difference had been crucial to the Romans. To be a man was to be dominant; lesser men were regarded as feminized. If notions of masculinity remained central to the intellectual life of the Christian era, certain anxieties resulted as they were incorporated into the new belief system. Some behaviors previously regarded as unmanly were now regarded benignly. Demonstrations of sexual prowess had been central to the Roman concept of masculinity. For Christians it was not unmanly to be celibate. With a shift in power from political to clerical office, new notions of sexual and marital renunciation cohered with the Christian ideals. Christianity was better equipped to defend a fresh form of masculinity focused on the image of the "Soldier of Christ." The virginity of women was exalted by zealots like Jerome who praised those who had not "soiled" their garments. And by the fifth century it was not just female virginity that Christians treasured. Church fathers argued that renunciation of sex was a sign of superior manliness. Such preachers, though they attacked the sexual exploitation of women, were intent on shoring up male authority and excluding women from the public realm. A man had to demonstrate self-control if he was to control others. Reminding their flocks that Roman athletes wore clamps to prevent erection and ejaculation, priests called on men to likewise become athletes for Christ.[9]

A concern for a victory over the powers of the flesh preceded Christianity and should not be confused with it; the pagans' goal was hygiene, not holiness. The Greeks were not interested in the who or how of sex but with the ability to demonstrate a mastery of one's own desire. Christians made sexuality the symbol of the difference between themselves and pagans; it was the key indicator of individual morality. The married and the celibate, the rich and the poor all were subject to a new moral common denominator: the importance of controlling sexual urges. An enormous ethical burden was now borne by acts heretofore considered hardly more significant than eating or drinking. Though pagans had not been unthinking hedonists, the idea of viewing mundane sexual practices as the privileged indicators of one's spiritual condition had previously been unthinkable. The Christians made a nuance the basis for a fundamental cultural cleavage.[10] They advanced the modern view of sex as the essence of one's being.

The eunuch was the most striking symbol of the campaign to subdue the male body. Pre-Christian groups throughout Asia Minor and Egypt had performed cultic castration. Pythagorus's assertion that sex was injurious to men due to the accompanying loss of energy was a common belief among Greeks. Stoics similarly expressed a desire for sexual self-control. Christians—like Jews—opposed mutilation but they lauded celibacy. Jesus noted that some eunuchs were born, others made by men, and finally "there be eunuchs which have made themselves eunuchs for the kingdom of heaven's sake" (Matt. 19:12). Eastern Christians were sharply ambivalent in their views on eunuchs. In the Byzantine Empire castration was condemned but eunuchs were imported. The sort of abstinence eunuchs owed to their mutilation, Christians sought to obtain through faith. Origen envied men who by nature were cool and could easily control their passions.[11] Though he argued that eunuchs simply provided a metaphor for such self-control he was suspected of having castrated himself. Other early Christians certainly did. One could go no further in repudiating concerns for potency.

In this distaste for sex Christians distanced themselves from their Jewish roots. Judaism was, of course, not without its defenders of sexual renunciation. Maimonides, for example, reflected a platonist-like pessimism as regards sex. Some rabbis stressed the production of spiritual rather than corporeal children. In main, however, Judaism plumped for the importance of sex and reproduction. Sex was not regarded as due to the fall.[12] Jews regarded impotence as a curse. In the book of Genesis, God was portrayed as imposing it on Abimelech for taking Abraham's wife Sarah. He informed Abimelech that "therefore suffered I thee not to touch her" (20:6). After Abimelech released Sarah, "God healed Abimelech, and his wife, and his maidservants; and they bare" (20:17).

Jews viewed virginity negatively and took the notion of the marital debt as a given. Most rabbis called for the separation of the barren. The purpose of marriage was procreation and therefore a man had the right to divorce his wife if she proved infertile. Divorce and polygamy (allowed until medieval times) were used to assist in the duty to "be fruitful and multiply." Some scholars stated that at minimum two sons were needed. Procreation was monotonously reported in the long genealogical passages of the Old Testament. Celibacy was frowned on and masturbation condemned. Some rabbis thought that self-abuse—like wet dreams—was a result of men not marrying. The Talmud even has a passage in which rabbis' members are compared.[13]

Unlike the Jews, Christians lauded continence, celibacy, and life-long virginity. Unlike the ancients who were proud of the body, the Christians found themselves embarrassed by it. Tertullian asserted that part of one's soul was lost in orgasm. Desire was a sin in itself. The devil tried to ensnare the celibate; erections or nocturnal emissions were signs of evil thoughts. Clement of Alexandria likened semen to epileptic froth, though he did not think intercourse was inherently sinful if the intent was to have children. He used Hippocratic and Aristotlian notions to explain conception while also asserting that angels assisted in the process. Lactantius similarly drew on Aristotle in his natural theology when attacking those who sought to turn sex into an "empty and sterile pleasure." According to Lactantius procreation was the only reasons the genitals existed.[14]

For St. Augustine the "disease of lust" was a result of the fall. Did Adam have erections? Augustine argued that in Eden the body must have obeyed the rational will. Sex, like urination, would have taken place rationally. After man disobeyed God, his body disobeyed him and he found himself in bondage to sexual desires. For Augustine the genitals were the "shameful parts" that had to be covered "because they excite themselves just as they like, in opposition to the mind which is their master, as if they were their own masters."[15] The first erection was the result of eating the forbidden fruit. The penis was often in a rebellious state, hence Adam was ashamed. Sex was not in itself bad but, according to Augustine, the "autonomy of the penis" was. The libido was uncontrolled. "At times the urge intrudes uninvited; at other times, it deserts the panting lover, and, although desire blazes in the mind, the body is frigid. In this strange way, desire refuses service, not only to the will to procreate, but also to the desire for wantonness; and though for the most part, it solidly opposes the mind's command, at other times it is divided against itself, and, having aroused the mind, it fails to arouse the body." Augustine guiltily described himself as "seduced" by his own sexual feelings. In Greco-Roman culture the erect phallus had been a sign of power. For Augustine the erection was both the sign of man's fallen state and the means of transmitting original sin.[16]

Christian apologists undercut the Jewish stress on the innate value of procreation, presenting it instead as a result of humanity's sinful condition. Adam and Eve should have been able to have children without sin but they did not. St. Augustine's importance lay in his crystallizing the doctrine of the "marriage debt"—that sex in marriage could only be justified if it produced offspring, fidelity, and continence. He did not mention mutual love. Love was viewed by Christians, as it had been by pagans, as a subversive and destructive passion and therefore dangerous in marriage. The church was more interested in assuring *charitas conjugalis*—amity, charity, and fidelity. Augustine contrasted a respectable marriage "contracted for the sake of issue, and the compact of a lustful love."[17] Sex continued to symbolize the fall from grace and the coming of disorder. Impotency, frigidity, and erections were, asserted Augustine, all uncontrolled; all demonstrated man's enslavement to lust. Marriage was good, but celibacy was better.

Thus, far from being worried about impotence, early churchmen feared excessive marital intercourse; it was considered beyond the need to reproduce, overly passionate, or took place in an unnatural fashion. The Decretists argued that sex for procreation was blameless and that the married had a right to intercourse. Others asserted intercourse always involved sin and certainly was not a positive act. The Christian suspicion of sex cast a long shadow over marriage. It was regarded by some as a sort of slavery, entailing as it did a loss of liberty. All St. Paul could say was that it was better to marry than to burn. Many early Christians like Jerome expressed clear antifamilial sentiments. St. Joseph's position as the patron saint of marriage was an eloquent testimony to Christians' ambivalent view of male sexuality. He was always portrayed as an old man and a virgin, his marriage with Mary never consummated. Nevertheless priests instructed couples having trouble conceiving to pray to him.[18]

If the gloomy Augustinian view of the purposes of marriage placed a new stress on celibacy and "inner masculinity," Christians could not altogether ignore the subject of impotence, the problem posed "when desire refused service." Their German converts regarded sexual consummation as making a marriage, a view that ultimately overrode the traditional Roman stress on consent. And once it was accepted that a marriage was created by the act of sexual consummation, the argument could be made that if the man were impotent the marriage was either invalid or should be annulled. A long line of celibate church doctors soon found themselves debating the finer points of such subjects as erection, penetration, and emission in their efforts to spell out how to determine if consummation had occurred.

Whereas Greco-Roman and Arab cultures did not prioritize impediments to marriage, Catholic Europe was forced to take up this onerous task. Under the Christian emperors the first attempts were made to restrict divorce. Wife beating was no longer accepted as a cause and divorce by mutual consent was ended except in cases where a man wished to enter a monastery. Adultery was the main justification of a husband seeking to divorce. A wife could also be cast aside for aborting, wantonness, or attempted bigamy. The Romans ignored the issue of impotence until Justinian in AD 528 allowed a divorce if a marriage was not consummated after two years. He thereafter restricted divorce. In 556 divorce by mutual consent was ended.[19]

In the Middle Ages positive discussions of sexuality were crowded out by references to sin, lust, and lechery. Marriage was described in the *Hali Meidenhad* as "that beastly copulation, that shameless coition, that foulness of stinking ordure and uncomely deed." The Penitentials assumed that all sex was polluting. Given that churchmen viewed almost all sexual desires as unnatural, they regarded heterosexuality almost as bad as same-sex acts. The married were instructed that they sinned in seeking inordinate pleasure, but that an unconsummated marriage was not a true marriage. Did impotence invalidate a marriage? Anglo Saxons scholars said it did. Vinnian and Cummuan counseled continence in such cases. A letter of Archbishop Rabanus Maurus attributed to Pope Gregory the Great, allowed couples who could not have sex to separate. The Canons of Theodore permitted a woman to take another husband, a notion revived by the abbot of Fulda. The Teutons only allowed a man to repudiate a wife. The Carolingians in the eighth century allowed a woman's remarriage if her spouse's impotence was proven. Hincmar, the ninth-century archbishop of Rheims, had to judge the marital squabbles of King Lothair II and Queen Teutberga, and those of Count Stephen of Aquitaine and the daughter of Count Raymond of Toulouse. In doing so Hincmar contrasted natural and acquired impotence. In the first case the remarriage of the healthy partner would be allowed. In the latter case in which the impotence (perhaps due to a spell) might be reversible, remarriage was not permitted.[20] Such discussions of impotence usually focused on marriages that had not been consummated. If impotence occurred later it obviously posed more complicated questions.

Impotence loomed large in the medieval church's attempt to establish some logic in its treatment of sex. After the fall sexual relations were necessarily imperfect, but as Peter Lombard argued in his *Four Books of Sentences*, the goods of marriage—the production of children and avoidance of concupiscence—excused marital sex. Sexual excesses were, of course, to be avoided for both physical and spiritual reasons, but partners owed each other the "marriage debt." In practice, though, priests clearly assumed that the conjugal debt was owed the man, rather than the woman. In divorces involving impotence, asserted Burchard of Worms, the husband's statement should be accepted; the wife's needed corroboration.[21]

Impotence especially preoccupied canon lawyers. In the mid-twelfth century Gratian completed his textbook of canon law, providing a coherent view of marriage. Marriage required consent and coitus. It was a sacrament that by the act of consummation was made indissoluble. Afraid of licensing promiscuity, Gratian's *Decretum* (1140) held that impotence could justify a marriage annulment, but the man could not subsequently remarry. Most clerics advised caution. Rolandus asserted that if one spouse was unable to have sex, the other did not have the right to seek it elsewhere. Yet if sorcery was recognized as the cause of impotence remarriage was allowed.[22]

Thomas Aquinas continued the line that procreation was the primary end and avoidance of fornication the secondary end of marriage. He argued that an inability to consummate a marriage rendered it void. "In marriage there is a contract whereby one is bound to pay the other the marital debt: wherefore just as in other contracts, the bond is unfitting if a person bind himself to what he cannot give or do, so the marriage contract is unfitting, if it be made by one who cannot pay the marital debt. This impediment is called by the general name of impotence as regards coition, and can arise either from an intrinsic and natural cause, or from an extrinsic and accidental cause, for instance spells, of which we shall speak later."[23] Both partners could be too young; the woman could be too narrow; the man could suffer from *frigiditas*, *maleficium*, or *sectio* (lack of testicles or penis). Aquinas also recognized that a woman might simply say her husband could not give her children because modesty forbade her to say he was impotent. Aquinas regarded the issue of consent as vital. If a woman knew of her spouse's impotence before the marriage she could not later seek an annulment on the basis of having been defrauded. Moreover, Aquinas held that sterility was not a sufficient cause of nullity. Marriage only required a *satiative copula*. That is, the male simply had to be able to penetrate the vagina, neither emission nor ejaculation had to occur.[24] Female impotence was assumed to be less a problem; in some cases a surgeon might remove the hymen.

The impotent should not marry because they could not pay the conjugal debt, yet Aquinas saw no reason to oppose the marriages of the elderly who were past child-bearing age. Was this a contradiction? For Aquinas the act of penetration rather than the possibility of conception was vital. Amazingly enough, Huguccio asserted that the church recognized that the elderly could have sex "by nature, by artifice or with the help of medication," stratagems he denied young couples.[25]

Here it should be noted that Thomas Aquinas, like Huguccio, argued that impotence might not prevent a true marriage—as long as the couple decided in advance not to consummate it. The church long defended the concept of such "spiritual marriages." Virgin wives were lauded in the thirteenth century, and their mates portrayed as being compensated with mystical rapture. In hagiographies, female saints were often described as torn between God and husband. In the early 1400s Margery Kempe appealed to Christ to stop her husband from having sex with her during Holy Week and as a result he was made impotent. "Then on Wednesday in Easter week, after her husband would have knowledge of her as he was wont before, and when he came near her, she said, 'Jesus, help me,' and he had no power to touch her at that time in that way, nor never after with fleshly knowing." John Nider reported a similar case of a wife's efficacious prayers.[26]

In ordinary cases church writers like Gratian accepted that impotence ended a marriage, but the issue became more complicated if the problem was not permanent. The lay model of marriage allowed break ups; the church advanced an indissoluble model. In cases of impotence Peter Lombard preferred probation to annulment. John of Salisbury was suspicious of wives' claims and annoyed at the scandals produced by court revelations. If divorce was granted, could the couple remarry? French canon lawyers said yes; the Romans said only the healthy spouse could wed. Popes had various opinions, on some occasions allowing divorce and remarriage. Pope Innocent III in 1207 concluded that Philip Augustus could divorce Ingeborg of Denmark if prayer and alms giving did not overcome witchcraft. Gregory IX

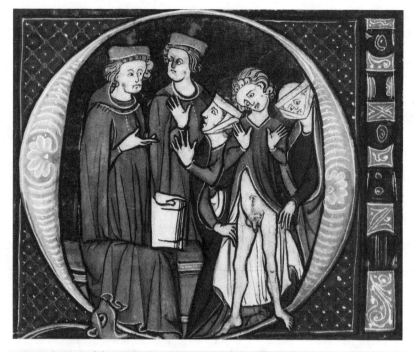

2. "Examination of the parties." A thirteenth-century Flemish illumination of Gratian's *Decretum* depicting a canonical court's determination of a husband's impotence. By permission of the Walters Art Gallery, Baltimore, MS W.133, fol. 277.

in *De Frigidus et Maleficiatis* spread the notion to the whole church that "the capacity to have sexual relations was deemed so central that where it was absent an otherwise valid marriage could be dissolved."[27] Yet churchmen, in seeking to impose on lay persons Christian marital regulations, were always suspicious that nobles, in search of easy annulments and lucrative remarriages, might turn the argument of nonconsummation to their own purposes.

In preparing for divorce cases, canon lawyers totted up all the possible causes of impotence including age, youth, filth, disease, cold, and inhibiting passions. Courts implicitly adhered to a sexual double standard. If the man denied he was impotent, his word was generally taken over that of his wife, as he was lord. Concerned that a wife might be moved by self-interest to claim her spouse was deficient, the authorities proceeded to insist that she alone be subject to physical examination. The woman would be inspected by a jury of matrons and witnesses were heard. The reasoning was that the state of the wife's hymen would best reveal whether or not the marriage had been consummated. Moreover it was held that the burden of proof lay with her as the conjugal debt was really owed by the wife. A virgin bride might herself insist on an examination to prove nonconsummation and so obtain a divorce. In an interesting 1443 English case, a woman brazenly defended her breaking of a marriage contract on the grounds that she discovered her intended's impotence before they were to marry. "And afterwards within a fortnight, she tried him, and because he could not she dismissed him and contracted with [another suitor] Thomas Ricard."[28]

Guy de Chauliac, while noting that impotency could have either natural or magical causes, reported that sometimes it was faked by men seeking to free themselves of a mate. Churchmen always suspected collusion in divorce cases and, coming to recognize that some shameless men might pretend to be impotent in order to end a marriage, demanded their examination as well. A copy of Gratian's *Decretum* contained an illuminated illustration of just such an impotent spouse being judged. The examination of husbands began in England in the thirteenth century. Even prostitutes were allowed to testify to the man's abilities, the one rare occasion when they played an official role in a church court. In practice, whether or not a husband or non-virgin were examined depended on the whim of the court. Quarrels were not ended with the granting of an annulment. An additional question was soon raised. If separated partners found themselves cured of their impotence or frigidity, would they have to take back their old spouses? Innocent III in 1206 argued that a woman who failed to consummate her marriage with her first spouse, but was successful with a second, should try again with the first. Similarly John Poynant of Ely in 1378–80 was forced to give up his second wife and child and return to his original partner.[29]

On June 27, 1587, Sixtus V declared that even spados who had erections were impotent. Sanchez the theologian explains that it was because such men could not produce *verum semen*. Sanchez went on to argue that it was not sufficient for the man to simply deposit his semen at mouth of the vagina even though that could result in generation. Penetration was required. Only a copula apt for generation counted. The marriages of the elderly were nevertheless defended on the grounds that their semen was only "accidentally" improlific. According to the church every man now had to produce *verum semen* (semination) to be declared potent. From the sixteenth century onward the Catholic Church was to maintain that consummation of marriage required both penetration and emission. In theory at least, men were under greater pressure to perform. As far as the church doctors were concerned, a woman only needed organs to receive the sperm, not necessarily a womb or ovaries. A man without testicles was deemed impotent but a woman lacking ovaries was not.[30] She only needed a vagina.

These contentious and embarrassing questions resulted from the church attempting to reconcile its distaste for marriage and childbearing with the Europeans' fervor for fruitful families. On the outcome of a marriage rested more than the happiness of two individuals. Property, power, and family pride were also involved. Large dowries might have to be returned. A case in point surfaced when the count of Urgel claimed his marriage of 1253 had not been consummated. He had only been fourteen at the time. His lawyers asserted that he was impotent, but witnesses testified that he consorted with prostitutes. The count, who ultimately had children by two wives, clearly launched his suit as part of a squabble over property.[31]

The process by which a marriage could be broken in cases of impotence was slowly institutionalized. In 1317 a woman in Normandy was granted a divorce because of her husband's impotence, and "whereas she is a virgin and wants to be a mother." By the fourteenth century court records were noting doctors acting as special witnesses. Thomas of Strasbourg wrote that a judge could cut the customary three years of failure needed before a court could grant an annulment, "if there is certainty about this frigidity, based on the observation of doctors." We know of two annulments granted in 1385 in which physicians acted as witnesses. A matron would observe the marital congress and in turn report to a doctor. Demands for annulments based on impotence were fairly frequent, ten being made in Augsburg in 1350.[32]

When Pope Alexander VI sought in 1497 to break the marriage of his daughter Lucrezia Borgia, he had her assert that she had been married for three years "and was still without any sexual relation and without nuptial intercourse and carnal knowledge, and that she was prepared to swear and submit herself to the examination of midwives."[33] Her husband Giovanni Sforza refused to prove his capacity before a papal legate and other witnesses in Milan. A commission under two cardinals accordingly declared that the marriage had never been consummated and Lucrezia was still a virgin. All Italy laughed. Though Sforza's first wife had died in childbirth he was ultimately forced to say his second marriage had not been consummated, and return Lucrezia's dowry.

Such disputes over impotence also took place at the other end of the social scale. A graphic account of a man's attempt to disprove his partner's assertions was recounted to the patriarchal court of Venice in the 1470s. Nicolo's wife claimed to be still a virgin and therefore unfulfilled in her desire to be a good Christian and mother. In rebuttal the priest of San Stefano gave a detailed history in defense of Nicolo's normality. He reported that after Nicolo kissed a prostitute named Magdalena, the accused said to the priest, "'Look here, I am a man, even though some say I cannot get it up.' And he made this witness feel his member, which was erect just like the member of any other man." The priest testified that he also witnessed Nicolo having sex with Magdalena and another prostitute named Maria. The witness had felt Nicolo's sperm on his hand.[34]

Sixteenth-century Protestants had to wrestle with the same issues. They lauded marriage as the basis of society yet stripped it of sacramental quality. Martin Luther went so far as to suggest a woman with an impotent husband could have children by a surrogate and so save the marriage. Protestants denied that marriage was a sacrament, but otherwise shared the Catholic view of impotence. Luther recognized three basic grounds for divorce, after which the innocent party might remarry: impotence, adultery, and failure to cohabit or to fulfill one's conjugal duties. Remarriage was allowed to provide an outlet for lust. Nonsexual discord provided grounds for a judicial separation only.[35]

Protestant reformers Ulrich Zwingli and Martin Bucer stressed the need for the married to have an active sex life. In Basel, impotence was a cause for legal action when one party was rendered unable to have intercourse. Divorce was not allowed if the healthy spouse had previous knowledge of the affliction or if impotence were the result of advanced age. The *Ehegerichtsordnung* of 1533 specified a careful procedure for the legal detection of impotence. First, the parties had to wait a year in the hope that the affliction would be corrected. After a medical examination by two court-appointed physicians, the court could grant a divorce. Both Catholic annulments and Protestant divorces followed the same procedures of marital jurisprudence.[36]

Protestants extended the grounds for divorce while maintaining Catholic provisions on impotence. Between 1550 and 1592, the *Ehegericht* or marriage court of Basel heard a total of 244 petitions for divorce or judicial separation. In seven cases, impotence was a factor. Ninety-five cases of impotence appeared in the *Officialatus* of Constance between 1551 and 1600. Such courts, like their Catholic counterparts, would not be moved by a woman's argument that she was sexually unfulfilled. To succeed she had to assert that her desire to be a mother had been frustrated. Proof of her husband's inability to perform could result from his failure to impregnate his wife during a court-ordered three-year trial period, a seven-handed compurgation of the oath by the parties that the man could not engage in sexual intercourse, or medical inspections of the husband and/or the wife.[37]

How did notions of masculinity emerge from the church's redrawing of the rules of marriage? In theory the aggressive masculinity of the ancient world fell into disrepute in the Middle Ages. Carolyn Bynum has argued that Christianity helped blur gender boundaries. The church praised holy women for their masculine qualities. Contrariwise some male saints were lauded for demonstrating feminine virtues. Christ himself was represented at times as a lactating female. Yet Christ was also represented as having a penis. Indeed some painters showed it erect. Feminist scholars have asserted such representations should be interpreted as signifying Christ's humanity rather than his sexuality. For Christians, bodily sensations were not the problem. The question was whether their source was demonic or godly. Yet the number of medieval castration stories suggests that the church regarded the genitals as an impediment. Abelard was, of course, castrated by a man seeking revenge. A heavenly saint castrated Hugh of Lincoln to give him peace. The church drew the moral that such men, once freed of the temptations of the flesh, demonstrated by their subsequent actions a superior "inner masculinity." [38]

Moving from the realm of the spiritual to the everyday, the evidence suggests few men were tempted by the thought of relinquishing their genitals. In the Middle Ages virility was prized and only fully proven by siring offspring. Relatives and friends put newlyweds to bed, brought them warming drinks, and celebrated the consummation of their marriage. Egged on by the community to prove their manhood, new grooms were in a sort of limbo until their first child was born. A man's duty was to be erect and ejaculate; the woman's duty was to gestate. Males were thought to play the more important role in conception; the woman was generally held responsible for a barren marriage. Masculine potency was sometimes regarded as a vice, yet the ancient notion of masculine ardor (and the danger of effeminate cooling) persisted. In effect a third gender might emerge. Young men were challenged to prove themselves, as reflected in the bawdy story of Jean de Condé in which a woman informs a poorly bearded knight, "it is easy to judge from the state of the hay whether the pitchfork is any good." [39] The elderly were not spared teasing. Italians joked that sodomy could cure old men's impotence. Wild male sexual behavior might be reprimanded yet was seen as integral to masculinity. We know of a case of 1515 in which a man bedded a woman "simply to prove that he could, because otherwise Katherine might tell women in the parish that he was impotent and scuttle his courtship of a wealthy widow." Charivaris, common on the continent from the fourteenth century, were aimed at those in defective marriages and must have added to the shame of impotent males. [40]

The penis remained a perennial source of crude humor. Medieval badges worn to ward off the evil eye depicted copulating couples, erect penises (sometimes dressed as pilgrims), penis animals, winged penises, and vulvae carried by penises. In Anglo-Saxon riddles attempts were made to embarrass others into naming the shameful member by asking what was "stiff, strong" (a key), a "boneless wonder" (bread dough), and "rooted I stand on a high bed" (an onion). Shakespeare exploited similar double entendres. In the *Merry Wives of Windsor*, Ford declares himself afraid of being cuckolded and bewitched. He refers to having "lost my edifice by mistaking the place where I erected it" (2.2.194–217). Falstaff—whose very name suggested either the *fallusstaf* or flaccid member—asserts if it is heard he dressed as a woman he will be "crestfall'n as a dried pear" (4.5.93–99).[41]

Churchmen told those worried by the specter of impotence that it could have "natural" or "accidental" causes. In the Middle Ages classical treatises on reproduction that provided information on the former subject began to resurface in Europe. In *The Merchant's Tale* Chaucer presented "oold Januarie" who wedded "freshe May" taking aphrodisiacs. "He drynketh ypocras, clarree, and vernage / Of spices hoote, t'encressen his corage" (563–64). Chaucer drew his information on such drugs from the work of Constantinus Africanus, a writer he condemned as lewd. In the eleventh century Constantinus Africanus's *De Coitu* introduced Europe to the Arab translations of Greek medicine. Though his Latin translations were fairly discrete he conveyed the Greco-Roman argument that sexual activity was both a symptom of health and cure for illnesses. Because anatomy had not progressed in the past thousand years, he repeated the Greek notion that erection was due to warm air or spirits. Drawing on Hippocrates, Galen, and Dioscorides, he listed the aphrodisiacs of the ancient world and a number of cures for impotence. He described the windy, warm, and wet foods like pepper, pine nuts, egg yolks, and ginger that provoked desire and gave recipes for oils and ointments that would prolong it. One prescribed the brains of male sparrows mixed with filberts and billy goat grease.[42]

William of Auvergne wrote in *De matrimonio*: "Fat men are sometimes frigid . . . we have learnt this same thing from women, not from men's rumours or [general] opinion, [but] from experience itself and with certainty, in statements given in confession." This moralist's observation that obesity impeded intercourse was given medical backing in Trotula's *On Treatments for Women*. Purportedly the work of an eleventh- or twelfth-century woman physician of Salerno, the text stated that to aid conception one should employ the ancients' recipes of warming herbs, strengthening medicines for "cold men," and fumigations for frigid women.[43]

The Christian world thus rediscovered the classical humoral theories of medicine in which impotence was attributed to an imbalance, the man being too cool or too dry, and regurgitated such remedies. Information on promoting conception was popularized in such tracts as *De secretis mulierum*, attributed to Albertus Magnus. This text followed an Aristotlian line that matter sought form; therefore women sought men. Intercourse had a therapeutic purpose. Indeed Albertus Magnus defended masturbation as a way of getting rid of excess seed. In *De Animalibus* he provided exotic remedies for impotence: "If a wolf's penis is roasted in an oven, cut into small pieces, and a small portion of this is chewed, the consumer will experience an immediate yen for sexual intercourse" (22.117). Since sparrows were given to frenetic copulation it followed that: "sparrow meat being hot and dry enkindles sexual desire and also induces constipation" (23.136). He described the starfish as a violent aphrodisiac that could lead to the ejaculating of blood but could be cured by cooling plants such as lettuce (24.55).[44]

In John XXI's *The Treasury of Healthe* (1276) of one hundred and sixteen prescriptions, thirty-four were for aphrodisiacs, twenty-seven were for anaphrodisiacs, fifty-six ensured fertility, and twenty-six were for contraception. Instructions were also given on dealing with "pustules in the yard," "inflamation of the yarde," and "swelling of the coddes." In such works the bean, resembling as it did the testicle and causing flatulence, was often prescribed to provoke lust. Wine and bathing were also said to increase heat. The fifteenth-century Spanish treatise *Mirror of Coitus* (*Speculum al Foderi*) advised the impotent to "eat chick peas, turnips, and carrots." A 1525 English herbal promised that skirret "stirreth a man to lechery"; a 1565 treatise asserted that "rocket stirreth up lust," while a 1567 text recommended coriander, which "provoketh a man to much venery."[45]

Aldobrandino of Sienna's *Régime du corps* (1265), written in French, was the first hygienic treatise in the vernacular. His chapter on "How to Cohabit with a Woman" drew on Galen and Aristotle to argue that sex in moderation was good for the health. A man who was too young or too old or too fat or too drunk might fail. He had to know the right time and the right position. Bernard de Gordon, a fourteenth-century Montpellier doctor, was the purported author of works that also provided advice on how herbs, potions, and ointments, as well as "enlarging massages and plasters," could overcome impotence due to either malefice or the smallness of a man's member.[46]

There was thus an active interest in the subjects of sterility and impotence in the later Middle Ages; almost all medical works dealt with them. A 1326 court case in Provence revealed that a market existed in which doctors offered cures to men and women. Practitioners attributed impotence and frigidity to heat or cold, to the waning of the moon, to an imbalance in one's constitution, or marital incompatibility. Doctors accepted that some sterility—such as that caused by the cutting of the veins behind the ears that took sperm from the brain to the kidneys and genitals—could not be cured.[47] But impotence and sterility were not strictly defined in the medical literature, which devoted far more attention to ways in which to respond to the problem.

Sex was also said to be good for women's health. Antonius Guainerius's *Treatise on the Womb* (1481) described how—if the husband were incompetent—the doctor's female assistant could arouse the woman in order to expel the womb's humors. In cases of sterility due to the man's penis being too short, suggestions could be given on the most advantageous positions to assume. Guainerius recommended warming plasters of opium and pepper for the testicles and pessaries for the vagina to ensure conception. Such texts generally agreed that loss of heat caused by "much venery, labour, traveyl" was itself the cause of aging.[48]

Handbooks also recognized the role imagination could play in stimulating desire. John of Freiberg cited Albertus Magnus's advice that if a man had problems in consummating his marriage, his wife should provocatively attire herself. A Spanish writer suggested a sort of "conditioning" for shy men by advising them to "imagine the act of coitus until the organs of sexual appetite begin to obey." John of Gaddesden and Michael Savonarola in the fifteenth century likewise recognized how erotic stories could help prepare a man for coitus. Once the body responded, the blood in the liver evaporated, and the resulting hot air spread to the heart and lower organs, so stiffening the penis.[49]

Such classic accounts of the workings of the male anatomy continued to be published right through the sixteenth century. In his 1577 anatomy text Thomas Vicary followed the body from head downwards to the feet, paying particular attention to the haunches and "the secret members." The man's bladder was connected to the yard. His testicles were on the outside of the body. The "coddes" provided the purse for their "custodie & comfort." The woman had testicles as well but they were on the inside of the body. Her matrix was cold and dry. Both sexes produced seed. A man's sperm was hot, white, and thick while the woman's was "thinner, colder, and feebler." The man's yard had two passages, one for urine and one for seed. The penis became erect due to wind. Thomas Cogan's *The Haven of Health* (1584) carried on Galen's account of the blood being concocted into semen and a man's health depending on its "moderate evacuation." A woman would not conceive if a man's seed were cold and thin, so oils and ointments could be used to heat the "privie member." Though doctors described the health benefits of intercourse, they also warned that excess enjoyment, in depleting bodily moisture, was dangerous. Many texts accordingly provided cooling recipes to control lust. "Also if a mans flesh arise to much, let him drink often vervain and his flesh shall not rise, nor hee shall have no likinge unto a woman." Rabelais had Rondibilis joke that the various ways to abate the passions included the excessive drinking of wine, the consumption of cooling drugs and herbs, exhausting work, hard study, and finally, sexual intercourse.[50]

In the Middle Ages there was no clear line between medicine and magic. For churchmen, sin and sickness were related. They regarded disease as normal or natural to fallen man: perhaps a punishment for sin, a test given by God, or even the result of demonic forces. While Constantinus Africanus helped reintroduce ancient medical ideas into Europe, he also noted witchcraft as a cause of impotence. Even earlier the Anglo-Saxons used magic to cure impotence. One Leechbook advised, "If a man is (sexually) constrained by means of herbs, give him springwort to eat and let him drink holy water." In the late Middle Ages, Lyndal Roper informs us, "impotence was the bodily ill for which men most often appear to have sought magical assistance, and which they feared women had brought about. Unlike womanhood, manhood was experienced as a fragile achievement, and masculine superiority was perceived as constantly subject to threat. Women who threatened 'that he should neither go up or down with any love' were fearsome creatures."[51] Men were believed to be the usual victims of sexual magic, and jealous or vengeful women the manipulators of harmful incantations.

Priests condemned the desperate mistress who used magic to incite love. Successes were claimed to have been accomplished by the woman who served a man bread she had kneaded with her buttocks or a fish she had previously inserted in her vagina. Burchard referred to women's magic employed to "change from hate to love or vice versa the passions of the man." Women were also accused of causing impotence. "Has thou," he asked, "done what some adulteresses are wont to do? When first they learn that their lovers wish to take legitimate wives, they thereupon by some trick of magic extinguish the male desire, so that they are impotent and cannot consummate their union with their legitimate wives." Hincmar of Rheims referred to the exorcisms, prayers, tears, and penances employed by the anxious to counter impotency caused by witchcraft, such as the tying of magical knots. Sterilizing spells were purportedly turned to malicious purposes. Guibert of Nogent in his early twelfth-century *Memoirs* stated that magic was commonly employed by the laity and certainly believed to be the cause of unconsummated marriages. His own father's impotency, which lasted for seven years, was only ended by the "aid of a certain old woman."[52]

Therapeutic "white magic" was not condemned by the church. The first church involvements in marriage—the blessing of bed, and so on—were in fact forms of exorcism. Pilgrimages and prayers, made to seek cures for barrenness, were common. The church even turned a blind eye to attempts made by magic to determine sex and promote fecundity. Indeed Guibert referred approvingly to a case in which magic was employed to end impotency. A man asserted that his misfortune was obviously caused by black magic because, "to sleep with a former concubine for pleasure was possible, and with his legally chosen wife impossible." Eventually "churchly medicine" restored his potency. Philip II of France suffered a similar complaint.[53]

Georges Duby suggests that the medieval tradition of hypergamy—aristocratic men marrying women of a superior status—underlay fears of impotence and led to projection of defilement. But men's concern for, as well as fear of, women's reproductive power fueled much of the pronounced misogyny of the Middle Ages. Ordinary intercourse was said to have ruined men's health and driven some to retire exhausted to monasteries. Guibert referred to one such noble "advanced in years and worn out in body, having—what is deadly for such men—a wife with more vigor for married life."[54]

The most important "accidental" cause of impotence was witchcraft and it was believed to primarily strike men. The church promulgated the belief that God allowed Satan and his followers to prevent consummation. The medieval clergy thus took up Augustine's fear of the undisciplined body, which the devil sought to attack at night with filthy thoughts and pollutions. The notion that the devil would employ witches as his intermediaries fully crystallized in High Middle Ages. Those who claimed that women and demons posed a real danger bore the responsibility for the witch hunts, which ultimately led to the execution of perhaps 100,000 victims, most of them women.[55] A central role in this crusade was played by experts who instructed men that, if they suffered from impotence, it was likely due to the vengeful spells cast by women they had betrayed.

The idea of devils causing impotence first appeared in letter of 860 sent to confessors by Archbishop Hincmar of Rheims and Burchard of Worms. They referred to wanton women who, when a lover married sought to "mortify his desire so that he can have no intercourse with his wife." These claims were expanded by Ivo of Chartes, Gratian, and Peter Lombard.[56] The devil could cause impotence, argued Thomas Aquinas, because God allowed him to inhibit intercourse, an act corrupted by original sin. A number of synods between 1217 and 1434 proceeded to condemn impotence-causing sorceresses. The church conceded that a man's impotence was obviously due to natural causes if his penis had never been erect. If he only failed on certain specific occasions, it might be a sign of witchcraft.

The work of the Dominican inquisitor Heinrich Kramer, the *Malleus Maleficarum*, or *Hammer of Witches* (1487), was the most important rational for the rise of witch hunting in the early 1400s. For Christians a marriage was a sacrament and proof of God's blessing would be the birth of children. Witchcraft explained why some marriages failed. Kramer chronicled the many ways in which witches attacked marriage: making it impossible for men and women to copulate, rendering them sterile, and inducing miscarriages and still births. He was most preoccupied by impotence. The argument (1.8) proceeded as follows. Witchcraft existed. It was not just a question of the imagination. Witches were recruited by the devil who, with the permission of God, were allowed to obstruct one natural act, the venereal act. It was susceptible because of its inherently corrupt and sinful nature. God permitted the devil to afflict in particular the lustful, but all were at risk. Kramer cited Peter of Pallude on the five ways in which the devil could do his work. By interposing himself as a phantom lover, by freezing a man's desire, by making the woman appear loathsome to him, by directly preventing the erection, and finally by closing the seminary ducts so ejaculation could not take place. Though women could also be rendered frigid, men were more commonly the victims of such attacks since most witches "being women, they lust more for men than for women."[57] Employing his arguments both Catholics and Protestants attributed male failures to women's maliciousness.

The *Malleus* (1.9) went on to discuss the means by which witches could make a man believe that his penis had been spirited away. They could "through some prestige or glamour" give the illusion that the male organ had been removed. A man would "see and feel nothing but a smooth body with its surface interrupted by no genital organ."[58]

> Peter's member has been taken off, and he does not know whether it is by witchcraft or in some other way by the devil's power, with the permission of God. Are there any ways of determining or distinguishing between these? It can be answered as follows. First, that those to whom such things most commonly happen are adulterers and fornicators. For when they fail to respond to the demand of their mistress, or if they wish to desert them and attach themselves to other women, then their mistress, out of vengeance, causes such a thing to happen, or through some other power causes their members to be taken off. Secondly, it can be distinguished by the fact that it is not permanent. For if it is not due to witchcraft, then the loss is not permanent, but it will be restored some time.[59]

The *Malleus* was a dramatic demonstration of powerful men's fear of poor women. The usual scenario would be for a man to find himself incapable of performing with his wife but able with his mistress. Why would this be?

An obvious explanation was that the jealous mistress was seeking her revenge. Kramer drew on St. Bonaventura's argument that the devil did not actually harm the man's organ but only artificially rendered it useless for one woman.[60]

The tying of knots was believed an especially effective way in which sympathetic magic could cause the impotency of one's enemies. Joannes Andrea and Nicholas de'Tudeschi expressed the common fear that discarded concubines and prostitutes could thus revenge themselves. Such knot tying—lace tying or "nouer l'aiguillette"—was noted by Bacon and Montaigne. The French jurist Jean Bodin in 1580 argued that causing impotence by black magic was a "detestable" crime that merited a "painful death." He wrote that "of all this filth there is none more frequently found everywhere, nor hardly more pernicious, than the impediment given to those who marry, which is called 'tying the codpiece string,' including even children who make a practice of it, with such impunity and license that it is not even concealed and many boast about it." He referred also to a spell to prevent procreation, but not copulation. There are some people with whom it is impossible to tie, "while there are others who can be tied before marriage, and also after it is consummated, but with more difficulty."[61]

Italian folk tales dating from the Middle Ages describe a woman's rival using witchcraft to bind her man making him wretched and impotent. While muttering a spell she would employ a padlock.

> Now here I close the lock,
> Yet 'tis not a lock which I close;
> I shut the body and soul of this ungrateful lord,
> Who would not meet my love.[62]

To lift an evil spell the church suggested a variety of means, from employing the sacraments to finding the witch and either killing her or forcing her to end her enchantment. The famous Martin Guerre (b. 1525) married at fourteen, but for eight to nine years due to "malefice" could not carnally cohabit with his wife. The common belief in southern France was that impotence due to magic could end with time, with the use of a countercharm or, especially in Gascony, by a recantation by the person who cast the charm. In Martin's case the spell was lifted after he followed the advice of saying four masses and eating some hosts and cakes (*fouaffes*). Johann Weyer, one of the most important critics of witchcraft, reported that upon finding her husband impotent, a woman in Germany hung a wax representation of his penis upon the church altar, much to the anger of the parish priest.[63] Like cases of natural impotence, if not cured within three years, impotence by curse was assumed permanent and would also prevent or annul a marriage contract. The induction of impotence and sterility was in the eyes of the inquisitors both a violation of the sacrament of marriage and a form of homicide. It accordingly warranted the death penalty.

Innocent VIII's bull of 1484 *Summis Desiderantes* reported that in Upper Germany wretches used incantations, charms, and conjurings to cause all sorts of evils, in particular "that they hinder men from begetting and women from conceiving, and prevent all consummation of marriage." Such beliefs swept across Europe in the sixteenth century. In *On the Demon-Mania of Witches* (1580) Jean Bodin claimed that the Devil and witches had no power to bind the other senses, nor to remove any member from men "except the virile organs, which they do in Germany, causing the shameful parts to be hidden and withdrawn into the abdomen." James I of England also entered the fray. He began his *Daemonologie* (1597) by asserting, "I say and proue by diuerse arguments, that Witches can, by the power of their Master, cure or cast on diseases: Now by these same reasons, that proues their power by the Deuil of diseases in generall, is as well proued their power in speciall: as of weakening the nature of some men, to make them unable for women: and making it to abound in others, more then the ordinary course of nature would permit."[64] The cure had to entail the death of the witch.

The argument that impotence was caused by witchcraft did not go unanswered. In his autobiography, Girolamo Cardano, the renowned sixteenth-century mathematician, encyclopedist, astrologer, and doctor, described the impotence from which he suffered.

This incredible evil happened to me in my twenty-first year. Then . . . I first began habitually to lie with a girl, and was already as it seemed to me sufficiently strong and ready for sex. But the thing ended otherwise. For being obliged to return [*in patriam*], from that time until my thirty-first year was completed, that is, for a whole decade, it was never permitted to me to lie with a woman. For even though I took many to bed with me, especially in the year in which I was rector [of the student] University [of Arts and Medicine] of Padua, when I was carefree, at the most flourishing age, and had strong forces for everything else—in the case of foods, I used abstinence and enjoyment with equal industry—yet I left them all dry. So that as since I often did the same thing with tedium, shame, and despair I decided totally to desist from this experience. For indeed sometimes I had little women with me for three whole nights and I could not do anything. Frankly, I think this one thing was to me the worst of ills. Not servitude to my father, not poverty, not illnesses, not enmities, quarrels, injuries from citizens, rejection by the medical profession, false calumnies, and that infinite heap of troubles could drive me to despair, hatred of life, contempt of pleasure and perpetual sadness; this one certainly could.[65]

His biographer pertinently notes: "Given the almost universal belief in Renaissance society in the power of spells to cause impotence, a problem from which he himself suffered for years at a time, Cardano's apparent reluctance to attribute impotence to preternatural causes is especially striking. He noted that men were sometimes impotent because they believed themselves to be enchanted; in such cases, supposedly magical remedies worked simply because they substituted hope for the patient's despair."[66] He attributed such complaints to the patient's imagination, which in effect could cool the passions. Cardano believed in witches but did not believe they caused impotence.

In *De praestigiis daemonum* (1579) Johann Weyer stated that there were melancholy men who simply thought their testicles had been magically removed. In Italy many believed knots caused impotence. He also reported the belief that if an ill-wisher knocked on the bedroom door and called out the groom's name while breaking off the point of the knife on the door, the groom—if he answered—would be made impotent. Weyer concluded, "But this is all nonsense." Men could only be made impotent by natural causes. Weyer observed useless charms would no doubt cure the impressionable. "It is plausible and frequently observed in practice, that a man who is harmed by false credulity is also thus relieved by the same credulity." Though Weyer's book was put on the Vatican's Index of Prohibited Books and he was attacked by Bodin, he found an eloquent supporter in Reginald Scot. In his *Discoverie of Witchcraft* (1584) Scot reported that some claimed that "the vertue of generation is impeached by witches both inwardlie, and outwardlie: for intrinsecallie they represse the courage, and they stop the passage of the mans seed, so as it may not descend to the vessels of generation: also they hurt extrinsecallie, with images, herb, etc." Such claims, like the stories of the loss of genitals or monks gelded by angels, Scot declared to be all "bawderie and lies."[67]

In his *Essays* (1580) Michel de Montaigne produced the most famous sixteenth-century discussion of the power of the imagination to both cause and cure impotence. He thought it likely that many miracles, visions, and remarkable events were similarly produced. "I am moreover of the opinion that those ridiculous attacks of magic impotence by which our society believes itself to be so beset that we talk of nothing else can readily be thought of as resulting from the impress of fear or apprehension." He proceeded to describe how one friend who was so impressed by a story of magical spells that he was soon convinced that he too was bewitched. To cure such delusions Montaigne suggested one have recourse to what could be called a placebo. When a count on his wedding night found himself incapable of an erection, Montaigne came to the rescue by providing him with a talisman. Believing that the flat medal inscribed with symbols would ensure his potency, the groom proved successful in the marriage bed. What he did not know was that the talisman was actually meant to protect against sunstroke. This little drama, Montaigne pointed out, was proof that "our thoughts cannot free themselves from the convictions that such strange actions must derive from some secret lore."[68]

The workings of the penis, Montaigne conceded, much preoccupied men. "We are right to note the licence and disobedience of this member which thrusts itself forward so inopportunely when we do not want it to, and which so inopportunely lets us down when we most need it; it imperiously contests for authority with our will: it stubbornly and proudly refuses all our incitements, both mental and manual."[69] Here he sounds very much like St. Augustine, but Montaigne went on to ask why only this one organ was accused of rebelliousness. When trying to hide our anxiety did not our face, heart, lungs, and pulse, our hands and voices similarly betray us? So why unfairly single out for condemnation our privy member? In this playful defense of the penis, Montaigne surreptitiously attacked 1500 years of Christian teachings. To suggest as he did that the penis was an organ much like any other was to undercut both the church's assertion that intercourse was inherently sinful and that impotence resulted from diabolical spells. Accordingly in 1676 Montaigne's book, like Weyer's, was placed on the Index.

We began this chapter by asking why the church was so interested in the mechanics of intercourse. We found that unlike the pagans, Christians believed that except for the special case of a "spiritual marriage," it was expected that one wed to produce children and avoid concupiscence. Adoptions were no longer recognized. A marriage that was not or could not be sexually consummated was not a marriage. Impotence, in threatening such partnerships, posed a real threat to social and economic stability, inheritances, family alliances, and even dynastic powers. The ancients had discussed the situation of the man unable to perform with either women or boys. Churchmen, having condemned sodomy, could not investigate such issues. Greek and Roman writers often joked about impotence because they were usually describing a man's embarrassment when involved in an extramarital or adulterous relationship. Christians primarily discussed impotence in the context of marriage and consequently it was no laughing matter. They attributed it to a range of anatomical, physiological, behavioral, and demonic causes, their medical and moral injunctions supporting each other. Having first declared the subject of sexuality disgusting, churchmen were ironically led on to delve ever more deeply into its complications. In theory, their discussions resulted in the establishment of more explicit and verifiable standards of manhood. By 1600 a man in Catholic Europe seeking to prove his potency might have to demonstrate in public his powers of erection, penetration, and emission. In practice, however, women were most threatened by the inquisitors' interest in impotence. Fear of female desire primarily motivated the church's discussion of sexuality. Churchmen provided men with a way of working through their anxieties by attributing their sexual failures to vengeful ex-lovers. Of course, in the ancient world some fellows had also attributed their sexual shortcomings to spells and magic. With the witchcraft craze, Christian Europe fanned such misogynist sparks of suspicion into a blaze. Yet the discussions of male sexual failings were not always framed by such worrying preoccupations. In the popular culture of early modern Europe men and women also employed comic accounts of impotence to police gender boundaries.

THE "INFIRMITY OF OTHERS"
Laughing at Fumblers in Early Modern Europe

In a letter which she wrote to her daughter in April 1671, Madame de Sévi-gné, the famous chronicler of French court life, shared what she regarded as the hilarious account of her son finding himself impotent in the arms of his mistress:

> A favorable occasion had presented itself, and yet . . . dare I say it? "He could not get his dada up at Lerida." It was a very strange situation: the demoiselle had never before found herself in such a predicament. The cavalier made his exit, in disarray, convinced that he had been bewitched. But what you will find amusing is that he could not wait to tell me about his mortification. We laughed uproariously. I told him that I was delighted that he had been punished for his sins at the precise point of origin![1]

A century later well-bred Europeans would be outraged to hear that a mother would pass on to a daughter such a scandalous portrayal of her brother's humiliation. Nevertheless, a cursory review of high and low literary references to "unperforming husbands" and "eunuchs or impotent fellows" makes it clear that many people in early modern Europe found the subject of impotence inherently funny. To understand why requires an understanding of both popular notions of the workings of the sexual organs and the functions served by jokes of bedroom fiascoes.

Before turning to the reasons why some would treat the issue of impotence lightly, it has to be stressed that right through the seventeenth century, there were those who still regarded it as caused by witchcraft. In the Middle Ages there always had been some who attributed sexual dysfunctions to problems of diet, regimen, and excesses, but only in the eighteenth century did such views supplant the Christian notion that sexual problems were sign of man's fallen state. Even the innocent might be bewitched. Though his archbishop might object, James I insisted that "if the Devil hath any power, it is over the flesh, rather over the filthiest and most sinful part thereof, whereunto original sin is soldered." Through the 1600s references continued to be made to magical knots or the *esquillette nouée* as noted by Ramble Cotgrave in *A Dictionarie of the French and English Tongues* (1611). Thomas Middleton in *The Witch* (1615–16) portrayed a wife's lover as having had a spell cast on the unfortunate husband. In the play a witch proclaims

> So sure into what house these are conveyed,
> Knit with these charmed and retentive knots,
> Neither the man begets nor woman breeds;
> No, nor performs the least desires of wedlock,
> Being then a mutual duty.
>
> (1.2.155–59)[2]

In his 1620s classic *Anatomy of Melancholy*, Robert Burton noted "diabolical means" employed to cause or cure impotency and sterility including "Spells, cabalistic words, Charmes, Characters, Images, Amulets, Ligatures, Philatures, Incantations, etc." Inquisitors in seventeenth-century Venice described in detail women's use of incantations and rituals. Three knots were tied in a rope along with a recitation. In one case, the goal was to bring Alvise Foscari back to his ex-mistress Barbara and that until then he was to be deprived of sleep and bodily powers. It ended with the line "Alvise Foscari's sleep and his member shall be bound for Barbara." The historian who reports this case also discovered that in Venice one saint was appealed to for similar purposes. "For some reason, the prayer of Sant' Orsola was a favourite where the impotence of the victim was the main aim, though unfortunately there is no surviving example of a complete version of this prayer from this period. . . . A man's 'faithfulness' was secured by rendering him impotent with all others rather than by actually eliminating the competitors for his attentions."[3]

The most famous victim of seventeenth-century sexual witchcraft was supposedly Charles II of Spain. Unable to produce an heir with two wives—probably because of premature ejaculation—the church declared that he was bewitched and carried out elaborate investigations to track down the culprit. The inquisitor general and king's confessor concluded that he had been given a charm that had corrupted his semen. Recourse made to holy oil, fastings, exorcism, and medicine all failed, and with his death in 1700 the Spanish Hapsburg line came to an end.[4]

And though the rational increasingly condemned such notions as vulgar errors, belief in a variety of types of sympathetic magic to cure impotence were commonly met within France and England right through the seventeenth century. In *The Compleat Midwife's Practice Enlarged* (1698), John Pechey suggested that an enchanted husband should drink water from the mouth of a "young Stone horse." Astrologer-herbalist Nicholas Culpeper and midwife Jane Sharp recommended that a man, who due to magic could not give his wife "due benevolence," should piss through her wedding ring. In France the man was enjoined to piss or pour white wine either through the wedding ring or through the keyhole of the church in which he had been married. A large painting titled *Venus and Cupid* by Lorenzo Lotto (c. 1480–1556) portrayed one version of this belief in sympathetic magic.[5]

The enlightened in Britain and France turned against such beliefs. In 1677 John Webster could in *The Displaying of Supposed Witchcraft* declare that he found it bizarre that the belief in knots still held on. Even some churchmen such as Paolo Zacchia downplayed the likelihood of maleficium causing impotence. Zacchia argued that men who claimed to be cursed needed to prove they had been potent before. Their weakness could be caused by eating cooling herbs such as lettuce, mint, rue, and thyme or they might have been blocked by some psychological barrier, perhaps by a preoccupation with some defect or lack of hygiene of their partners. At the very least men had to try to overcome their failing. Nevertheless, on the continent the Catholic Church continued to denounce those who used spells to cause impotence. The church also condemned the superstitious means employed to counter such incantations such as having the priest whip the newly weds and put them to bed fortified with wine. The faithful were enjoined to show patience and follow the church's teachings by relying on the sacraments, exorcisms, pilgrimages, fasts, and good works. Of course, the use of holy water, the sign of cross, and imploring the favor of Mary and the saints were themselves obvious forms of white magic. Some churches had their own peculiar rituals. In the late eighteenth century Sir William Hamilton was astounded to discover that in Isneria near Naples, the faithful continued to offer wax replicas of penises as votive offerings to St. Cosmas.[6]

If the actual belief in witchcraft causing impotence declined, the theme was still exploited by poets and novelists as, for example, by Robert Herrick in "To His Mistresses" (c. 1650):

Help me! help me! now I call
To my pretty witchcrafts all;
Old I am, and cannot do

That I was accustomed to.
Bring your magics, spells, and charms,
To enflesh my thighs and arms;
Is there no way to beget
In my limbs their former heat?
Aeson had, as poets feign,
Baths that made him young again:
Find that medicine, if you can,
For your dry, decrepit man
Who would fain his strength renew,
Were it but to pleasure you.[7]

Daniel Defoe in *Conjugal Lewdness* (1727) noted the uses of "Spells, Filtres, Charms, Witchcraft" by those seeking to ensure conceptions. As late as the 1780s references to knots were made by Robert Burns in "Address to the Deil": "Thence mystic knots mak great abuse / On young guidmen, fond, keen, an' crouse."[8]

The explanation and treatment of impotence offered by the adherents of early modern medicine did not differ all that much from that provided by the believers in magic. Maintaining the ancients' view of the power of humoral influences, the defenders of traditional medicine held that a man's virility was determined by heat. If hot and lusty, men were virile and produced sons. If cold, they lacked sexual appetite and had daughters. Levinus Lemnius referred to those who were "effeminate, nice, tender, withoyt courage and spirit, sleepy, slothfull, weaklings, meycocks, and not apt nor able to beget any children." Robert Burton parroted the line that sex and intellectual activities were incompatible. "Some are better able to sustaine, such as are hot and moist, phlegmatick, as Hippocrates insinuateth . . . others impotent, of a cold and dry constitution cannot sustaine those gymnasticks without great hurt done to their own bodies, of which number (though they be very prone to it) are melancholy men for the most part." The hot blooded man was not entirely safe. Sexual excesses could result in exhaustion. Combining religious and humoral injunctions John Downame warned in 1613 that the fornicator sinned against himself, because fornication, "disableth and weakeneth the body, turning health into sicknesse, and many lothsome and pernicious diseases, and strength into impotency and languishing faintnesse; for the flame of lust devoureth and spendeth the vitall moisture, and the unnatural fire of burning concupiscence, consumeth and extinguish the naturall heat, which is the nurse of strength, and fountaine of life."[9] The sinner not only lost his "manly courage" (that is, his potency) but was likely led on into the vices of buggery, incest, and sodomy, which brought with them the French disease and barrenness.

Moreover, early modern Europeans took as a given, as Galen had argued, that both men and women produced seed (though the woman's was not as warm or dry as the man's) and that both sexes had to be pleasured to conceive. Even Catholic writers accepted the importance of female orgasm as facilitating conception. In the sixteenth century Fallopius said it was accordingly his duty—though the prudish might object—to write about the penis. He noted ways of increasing its size to help with reproduction. His advice was for parents to rub ointment on the child's member. If the man were not big enough the woman would not be pleasured, she would not produce seed, and the conception would fail. Belief in the two seed theory was maintained even as the medical understandings of male sexual functions slowly evolved. The French anatomist Ambroise Paré set aside the possibility of impotence caused by knots, magic, and incantations. Instead he described in 1585 how the blood in the arteries and veins—"which beset by the spirit of concupiscence and agitated by the fire of love sent there, inflates and erects the said virile member"—was responsible for erection. The seed in the prostate created irritation, pleasure, an itch, and finally demanded expulsion. "Now, the yard is raised by the means of blood and flatulent spirits." [10]

Writing in 1625, Louis de Serres showed himself unusually sympathetic to women, attributing most impotence to male sexual excesses. Serres noted that the community usually held women responsible if a marriage were barren but that men were often at fault. Were they to examine themselves,

> & admit their own defects, they will find that they are impotent, either naturally, as it is found only too often in those who have abused their youth with beautiful women; or by artifice, that is to say by the pain and torment that they subject themselves to in wasting their essential baume in plowing land from which they dare not and cannot collect the crop, just as we read of Henry VIII King of England, of Alexander Medicis Duke of Florence, & several other similar fellows, who only ever approached their wives after having entirely exhausted all their good genital matter with whores. [11]

Such debauchees might also exhaust themselves in games and hunting. Men who were impatient to divorce barren wives often found themselves embarrassed when their ex-wives had children with their next husband. Serres supported the view of Diogenes the Cynic that the man who could not reproduce should be ostracized. "It is certain that there is nothing which more reduces and destroys his glory than the impossibility of producing his fellow creatures, it being very certain, according to the testimony of Aristotle, that it is the most perfect and most assured mark of his perfection. . . . those who are incapable of generation must be despised, can succeed to no office, lose the support of the powerful; and finally are regarded as imperfect and defective monsters."[12]

In the sixteenth century most medical accounts were still published in Latin; vernacular works began to appear in large numbers in the seventeenth century; especially in England after the Civil War. Texts dealing with marriage and procreation focused on women's anatomy, courses, false conceptions, and labor. For writers of such conduct books "all sex was reproductive."[13] Their popular medical tracts presented a mix of citations from rediscovered ancient authors like Galen, Aristotle, and Hippocrates along with snippets of information culled from more recent medical writers.

The traditional notions of the importance of the humors held on. Sinibaldus in *Rare Verities: The Cabinet of Venus Unlocked* (1657) asserted that a "flatulous humour or spirit" extended the yard. As the seed carried away the wind and spirits, the penis became flaccid. Impotence was due to a want of seed, coldness of the stones, or defect. Michael Ettmüller likewise held that impotence was due to relaxed muscles or "the flatness of the Seminal Liquor." The latter was associated with age, illness, bashfulness (as in youngsters' fancying themselves bewitched), hypochondria, and melancholy. Such authors recommended the usual heating potions of cantharides, rocket, spices, pepper, and civet. Philip Barrough favored heating the member by the consumption of hot meats and the application of oils and ointments.[14]

Helkiah Crooke in *Microcosmographia* (1651) rehashed the old notion that the size of a man's yard was related either to the power of his father's seed or the length of the navel string the midwife left uncut. He lauded the penis as a remarkable organ, designed by Providence to be hard, soft, and hollow, so the spirits could raise it and "of so exquisite sense beside to breed that pleasure, whereby man is provoked to rush into so obscene a piece of business." Blood, spirit, and muscles all played their role. John Pechey concurred with reports on the importance of the navel string while attributing erections to abundance of seed, wind, urine, and the heat of the reines (kidneys).[15]

Jane Sharp, one of the first English women to produce a midwifery manual, referred to the yard as the "plow wherewith the ground is tilled, and made fit for the production of fruit." While the woman was the "ground" or field, Sharp insisted that she "brings Seed also." In the popular medical texts the woman, though she was said to produce cooler and "lesser" seed, was presented as sexually active. Her clitoris was recognized as her "seat of venereal pleasure." The clitoris and womb both experienced erection "for the motion and attraction of the seed." Indeed the womb, it was stated, "seems to take hold and embrace the glans," drawing in the male seed as a magnet drew in iron filings. And if "the woman perceives little or no pleasure in the act of copulation," it was concluded, barrenness could result. The same acceptance of the two-seed theory was found in John Sadler's *The Sick Woman's Private Looking-Glasse* (1636); Sadler attributed some barrenness to the man being too quick and the woman too slow in ejaculating. A concourse of both seeds was needed for a couple to be fruitful.[16]

Male issues were marginal in most of the early texts. In *A Directory for Midwives* (1651), Nicholas Culpeper discussed briefly the male genitalia and then turned to the woman's. The opponent of Culpeper who produced the *Compleat Midwifes Practice* (1656) followed the same format, asserting that the hotter the testicles the more salacious the man, his erection resulting from the stimulation of seed, wind, urine, and heat. The best known of the sex manuals, *Aristotle's Master-Piece* (1684), appeared in countless editions between the seventeenth and on into the eighteenth and nineteenth centuries. Like Culpeper's, *Aristotle's Master-Piece* was really a midwifery text that, beginning with the menses, followed the female life cycle, dealing with such issues as green sickness in virgins, barrenness, frigidity, signs of conception, labor, delivery, and nursing. In the 1694 edition the male organs were not discussed until page 172. The 1749 edition began with the anatomy of both sexes, but if the issue of barrenness was investigated, impotence received scant attention. *Aristotle's Master-Piece* did repeat the old notion that youths were damaged by having sex too early, while mature men—needing to rid themselves of excess seed—were made healthy by it. Men were described as being able to procreate at sixteen, at their peak between forty and fifty, their heat thereafter declined, and for most after fifty-five, "the Seed by Degrees becoming unfruitful," and the yard shriveled. Sexual excesses hastened the decline. To ensure erection juicy meats, nuts, and turnips were recommended.[17]

Nicolas de Venette's *Conjugal Love*, which first appeared in French in 1696 and in English in 1703, was written by a doctor who critiqued the more outlandish notions of the popular manuals. Yet Venette warned that the man had to decide on how much marital intercourse would take place since he was the active partner and the most at risk for fatigue, whereas the woman was the more lascivious and amorous. Man owed his spouse a conjugal debt but at times had to refuse. It was more tiring for him: "She beginning to be inflamed when the man is wasted." The man's parts could turn cold and languid, and his penis become "flaggy." Tired men should wash their nostrils, wrists, and hands with wine, which Venette held to be simple but salutary.

At sixty, Venette warned, "whatsoever heat and spirits we have are required for our more immediate preservation, and too scant to suffer any dissipation."[18]

Venette also was representative of the popular writers who preceded the eighteenth-century quacks; he simply advised either moderation or a few of the traditional aphrodisiacs. Seventeenth-century authors recommended the same sorts of stimulating herbs and potions used by the ancients. Alcohol remained popular. Marriage parties in the eighteenth century provided grooms with sack to provide strength on the wedding-night. In *MacBeth* Porter, when asked by MacDuff, what drink provokes, replies: "Lechery, sir, it provokes and unprovokes; it provokes the desire, but it takes away the performance: therefore much drink may be said to be an equivocator with lechery: it makes him, and it mars him; it sets him on, and it takes him off; it persuades him, and disheartens him; makes him stand to; in conclusion, equivocates him in a sleep, and, giving him the lie, leaves him" (2.3)[19]

In 1655 John Goodyer translated Dioscorides's classic herbal. Now a popular audience was informed that a vegetable such as rocket "eaten raw in great quantitie doth provoke Venery" (2:170). Nicholas Culpeper, an important herbalist who, carrying on the of idea of humors in his *Galen's Art of Physick* (1652), asserted that hot and dry foods led to venery. In *The English Physician Enlarged* (c. 1654) Culpeper drew on Dioscorides and Galen to assert that warming foods such as prickly asparagus, earth chestnuts, Clary leaves or seeds, Heartichokes, mint, and mustard seeds "doth mightly stir up Bodily Lust."[20]

Such sexually stimulating food stuffs were humorously cited in a Civil War tract entitled *Now or Never: Or, A New Parliament of Women* (1656) in which women threatened to turn the tables on men and fatten them up. "That such men as are of ability, do feed them with Capons, Rabbits, Cawdles, Sack-Possets, and such like, for one quarter of a year, and they not come out of their Chambers, unless they please." More exotic aphrodisiacs were also touted. In Thomas Otway's *The Soldier's Fortune* (1681), Sir Jolly says "odd 'tis the root Satyrion, a very pretious plant, I gather 'em every May my self, odd they'l make an old fellow of sixty-five cut a Caper like a Dancing Master." Satyrion was still listed for venery in Elizabeth Blackwell's *A Curious Herbal* (1737). In Sir George Etherege's 1668 comedy *She Would if She Could*, the character Sir Oliver Cockwood took cantharides to perform for his demanding wife (1.1).[21]

Such restoratives and stimulants fulfilled social as well as sexual needs. The single-sex model that held that men and women were sexually similar supported the notion that men who could not perform adequately were not really men. In Western culture women's sexual reputations were always more at risk than men's, but reports of a man's sexual activity or, more importantly, *nonactivity* could also affect his status. A man was supposed to assume social and political responsibilities as a spouse, husband, father, and patriarch.[22] To be known as impotent was to be labeled as unmanly and lacking virility, power, morality, and strength. Sexual impotence was not so much a problem in itself, but in what European culture believed it represented and could inevitably lead to—the social disorder starkly represented by the woman becoming the sexually active partner and making her man a cuckold. A sense of how preoccupying men found such a scenario is indicated by the many references made to impotence in seventeenth and eighteenth-century plays, poems, ballads, and court cases.

In the early modern period humiliation and honor were gendered. It was a grave insult to call a woman a whore, whereas to say that a man was promiscuous was rarely regarded as slanderous. To claim that he was impotent was a far more serious charge as it questioned his status as husband and father. Such insults abounded. In 1637 a Cambridge stranger affronted a man coming home to his wife by telling him that "he need give her a good prick." In New France a busybody called a neighbor a "capon" as the man had been married for a dozen years and had no children. During the English Civil War similar sexual slanders were hurled. With Cavaliers gone, wives were left with boring husbands, claimed one mock anti-Puritan petition: "In the good old days 'Cavaliers alwaies stood stiffe to the City,' but now the dames only custom is from a 'mouse-hair'd fellow, with a long thing God blesse us by his side as rusty as himself.'"[23]

The charge of impotence was used by young men to disparage the power of their older and propertied rivals who controlled wealth, marriages, and inheritances. According to the poets, rustic couples were happy but the wealthy man only thought of property.

> And when in Bed he shou'd Embrace his Spouse,
> Like a Dull Ox, he's still amongst the Cows;
> Chew's all the Night upon the next fair Day,
> How much this Horse, how much that Load of Hay.[24]

In satires, one historian has found, "the potency and poverty of youth are set against the wealth, but impotence, of age." Even medical manuals mirrored such scripts. "The youthful age lies open to Cupid's dart / But the old man is valued not a ——."[25]

Older men were castigated for resorting to every means to arouse their desires. John Henry Meibomius, in *A Treatise of the Use of Flogging in Medicine and Venery* (1643), noted that the ancients, understanding that hot blood was needed to heat the kidneys and quicken the seed, recognized the use of nettles and the lash. School boys picked up the practice and prostitutes reported having clients who asked to be whipped. One seventeenth-century tract attacked the elderly who sought the help of prostitutes to raise their passions. "But what may we think of those decrepit half-pint Lechers, who being as sapless as a dry'd Fennel-stalk, yet you may dog them shuffling along with their crickling hams, till they pop into one of their old haunts of iniquity. Where they call for *Vice* to correct *Sin*, for forgetting their former Lessons of Lasciviousness. While the sturdy Quean belabours their buttocks, till their impotent wimbles peep out of their bellies to beg a reprieve for their Tayles." In *The Oeconomy of Love* (1737), a poetic treatment of sex, John Armstrong warned against excesses and hectored the old man using flagellation to "rouse the Venus loitering in his Veins."[26]

Sexual slanders provided the raw material for much crude humor. Rochester lampooned Charles II's difficulties in performing for his mistress.

> This you'd believe, had I but time to tell ye
> The pain it costs to poor, laborious Nelly,
> Whilst she employs hands, fingers, mouth, and thighs,
> Ere she can raise the member she enjoys.[27]

Impotence always posed a challenge to dynastic succession. Serres argued that Henry VIII and Alexander de Medicis had been rendered impotent by sexual excesses. Henri III of France had himself operated on in a futile attempt to produce an heir.[28] Elected politicians were not spared ridicule. When in 1784 William Pitt the younger became Prime Minister his uninterest in women was noted:

> 'Tis true, indeed, we oft abuse him,
> Because he bends to man;
> But Slander's self dares not accuse him
> Of stiffness to a woman.[29]

The Romans joked about limp swords and bent spears; the early moderns about faulty guns and inkless pens. In a 1674 tract against coffee purportedly written by women, the authors asserted that they once prided themselves on "the brisk *Activity* of our men, who in former Ages were justly esteemed the *Ablest Performers* in Chistendome; But to our unspeakable grief, we find of late a very sensible *Decay* of that Old English *Vigour*; our *Gallants* being every way so *Frenchified*, that they are become meer Cock-Sparrows." Drinking coffee, the authors argued, had emasculated them and now like poor troops, "their *Ammunition* is wanting; peradventure they *Present*, but cannot *Fire*, or at least do but flash in the *pan*, instead of doing execution." *Aristotle's Last Legacy* likewise referred to a "vanquished Bridegroom" on his wedding night, "for he must be vanquished that has in the Encounter lost his Artillery."[30]

Jests that had been once part of an oral culture entered the print world in the seventeenth and eighteenth centuries. So we find in *Polly Peachum's Jests* (1728) the joke about the gentleman who, while urinating, caught two ladies laughing at him. When asked why: "O! Lord, Sir, said one of them, a very little Thing will make us laugh." In *Joe Miller's Jests* (1739) appeared a story about a gentlewoman who accused her husband of a "defect," but was too ashamed to describe clearly the problem. The judge therefore gave her pen and ink so she could discreetly put down her complaint on paper. Without dipping the pen she began to write. When the clerk protested, "Madam, there is no ink in the pen," she replied, "Truly Sir, that's just the case and I need not explain myself further."[31]

Elite authors made similar jibes. Pope and Swift compared bad writers to impotent lovers who lacked character and will. Jokes about impotence and short noses running in the family entered the world of the novel in Laurence Sterne's *The Life and Opinions of Tristram Shandy* (1759–67). Allusions to impotence, castration, and premature ejaculation pop up everywhere in the book: Uncle Toby's groin injury received at the battle of Namur; Tristram's father's difficulty in begetting him (Mrs. Shandy interrupting her husband in midclimax to ask if the clock is wound); and (as "nothing was well hung in our family"), the accident of the sash window dropping on Tristram's penis. Even the Shandy farm animals have difficulty in reproducing.[32]

Early modern Europeans coined a variety of terms to describe the sexually incompetent male, including malkin, pillock, fumbler, fribble, bungler, bobtail, domine-do-little, weak-doing man, Goodman Do-Little, and John Cannot. "Fumbler" was perhaps the most common appellation for the incapable male. One of Samuel Pepys's chapbooks was entitled "Fumblers-Hall, kept and holden in Feeble-Court, at the sign of the Labour-in-vain, in Doe-little-lane." It presented trials in which wives testified against their husbands, one asserting that her man has only "a Fiddle-string that will make no musick to a Womans Instrument." Pepys himself, never having sired a child, was called a fumbler by his drinking friends. "Old fumblers" were treated at length in Edward Ward's *Nuptial Dialogues and Debates* (1710). In one poem, a wife intent on producing an heir berates her spouse, "an old fumbling Libertine": "I was a maid, when to your Bed I came / And may, for ought I know, be still the same."[33]

The Ten Pleasures of Marriage (1682), attributed to Aphra Behn, portrays the impatience of the frustrated young bride. After three months of marriage no conception occurs and the wife compares notes with friends, asking each if her husband "understands his work well." They give advice on the hot foods he should consume and the drying substances such as tobacco he should avoid. They also instruct the woman on "pretty Wanton postures" that will fire his passions. All this failing "then she begins to mump and maunder," and "oftentimes calling him a Fumbler, a dry-boots, and a good man Do-little, &c" or "a John Cannot." In France similar jokes abounded of "un Jean qui ne peut." In a 1733 poem coauthored with Lord Hervey, Lady Mary Wortley Montague—an equally outspoken female writer—attacked Pope as a hunchbacked impotent toad, and in "The Deans Provocation" (1734) castigated Swift as an impotent fumbler.[34]

The sting of these insults was based on the expectations that the man was supposed to have sexual power, that is, be on top. If he was not, the tables could be easily turned. A ballad like "The Cruell Shrow: or The Patient Mans Woe" reminded men that women always wanted to wear the britches. They also were sexually demanding. The popular literature was peopled with the "sexually predatory, lewdly dominating woman," and the eager bride who, once she experienced sex, was insatiable. The pornographic pamphlets that played up such notions of untrammeled female desire obviously indulged male fantasists while rationalizing any guilt the weaker man might feel. For example, in *Now or Never: Or, a New Parliament of Women* (1656) women were presented as setting up new rules in which aphrodisiacs and "'spermmakers' were to be fed to 'men of abilities.'"[35]

According to common medical beliefs, the docility of women resulted from their sexual satisfaction. But this theory had its inherent tensions. Women, though passive, were said to be naturally lascivious, and if sexually frustrated could fall ill of the greensickness. The theory more threateningly raised the specter of the insatiable female, and the awkward question of whether even the modest woman whose husband failed to satisfy her had a right to rebel. Rebellion might consist of making demands, of attempting a role reversal. Rebellion could even go so far as adultery. Young women married to old men, or "brisk widows" already accustomed to the pleasures of the marriage bed were thought to be especially demanding. On meeting an impotent man a widow's response, according to Daniel Defoe, was "I love the virtue but hate the infirmity." According to John Marten, women were naturally prone to lust and could be driven mad by excess seed. Such passions were "incident to *Virgins*, but peculiarly to young *Widows*, and such Women that have *impotent* Husbands, or Husbands that they don't affect, whereby their *Seminary* Vessels are not sufficiently disburthened, or their amorous Affections duly satisfy'd." One early-eighteenth-century author likened the frustrations of a young woman married to an old rich man to one yoked to a eunuch. "And it would be a Matter of no great Surprize, if a Woman, that does not find at Home, wherewithall to satisfy a provok'd Passion, should receive elsewhere, what may be necessary to lay and becalm its Rage and Fury." The early eighteenth-century upsurge in interest in eunuchs allowed for a reiteration of the message that the impotent were not to marry and that it was the duty of a "husband" to father children.[36]

The idea of a man unable to satisfy his exigent spouse was clearly preoccupying. It led to an outpouring of songs and ballads that played up notions of the "fumbler," the husband being tested and failing the demands of his insatiable wife. So in "The Forc'd Marriage; or, Unfortunate Celia" the woman sings:

> When my fumbler's in bed,
> & has laid down his head,
> He lies with closed eyes,
> just [as] though he was dead.[37]

Similarly in "Tom Farthing; or, The Married Woman's Complaint," the new bride laments:

> Tom Farthing, Tom Farthing, thou mak'st me mad, Tom Farthing!
> 'Twas not for this I did thee wed, nor brought thee to my marriage-bed,
> But 'twas to loose my maiden-head, *of which I'm wondrous weary;*
>
> Could'st thou once but do [what's meet], and show thy self to be no cheat,
> My heart with joy would beat, *And 'twould make me wondrous merry.*
>
> But by thy side, thou idle drone! I lie like one that lies alone;
> And remedy I can get none, *which makes me wondrous sorry, sorry.*[38]

Such songs pointed out that a great age disparity could likely lead to heartache. In "A Young Woman's Complaint; or, A Caveat to all Maids to have a Care how they be Married to Old Men," the fifteen-year-old girl who has married a seventy-two-year-old man warns her sisters to avoid her unhappy fate.

> In bed as I lye, he groaneth, he cryeth;
> Like one that is dying in sorrow he lyeth:
> Instead of Love's blisses, he scratches and grumbles,
> And all night long he tosses and tumbles.
> And [I] lying and dying, and telling the clock,

Weeping and wailing, expecting a knock,
And wiping away the tears as they ran:
What shall a young woman do with an Old Man? [39]

Elderly husbands were fair game in plays, songs and lampoons. An old man in *Jack of Dover* (1604) gives his wife fancy stockings: "Because I can't please her above the knee, I must needes please her below the knee." In reviewing the errors of marriage, *Aristotle's Master-Piece* noted a great gap in age would inevitably lead to the cuckolding of doting old husbands. The song "Cuckolds Haven" warned men of the fate that awaited them if they did not sexually subdue their wives: "Let every man who keepes a Bride / take heed hee be not hornify'd. [40]

A salacious tract entitled *Fifteen Real Comforts of Matrimony* (1683) concurred that sexual unhappiness was the bane of marriages. "But the real discomforts of Marriage then clamour loudest, and give the bitterest twinges to the heart, when the man is reproached for his Impotency, or the woman tax'd for imperfection." An old man might marry a strapping young woman, "but cannot give her the least content." Society should protest, "yet not one will open his mouth, when they know the old Dottrel to have no more pith in his back than an Elder-gun. And thus the young Gentlewoman, all fire and high-mettel'd is deluded and frustrated of all her Expectations." The inevitable result, the author warned, was a loss of offspring and violation of the marriage bed, since the wife would naturally seek ease elsewhere. "Her amorous fires kindled by the Embers of his drooping years, grow violent, and prey upon her lusty blood. And is it not time to call out for help, when hardly the spout in a Whales neck will serve to send forth streams sufficient to quench her inward fires?" The writer concluded: "If an old Hunks without life or vigour, have such an inclination to lechery, let him in imitation of the former examples, please those senses which are least defective, and not go about to make a young and better-deserving Gentlewoman's life miserable and loathsome to her, where she expects her greatest felicity and enjoyment." [41]

The unhappy women would, these accounts argued, be justified in seeking satisfaction elsewhere. Their adultery was, in short, blamed on their husband's failings. Much of early modern humor was cruel, coarse, and misogynistic. Physical imperfections were mercilessly targeted. Accordingly it is no surprise that the cuckold should have been a source of humor, especially as he was construed in the jokes, ballads, and lampoons as being the author of his own fate. A 1700 pamphlet writer stated baldly that a cuckold was a "Civilized Monster and a Rational Beast patched up between Action and Forbearance, which by his Impotence and his wife's Incontinence is soon brought to perfection." The "young clergyman" who was the supposed author of a 1735 tract defending adultery, argued that the wanderings of a sprightly girl married to a "silly, sour ill-natured fellow" unable to give her due benevolence were defensible.[42] And the woman singing "The Scolding Wives Vindication, or, An Answer to the Cuckold's Complaint" likewise asserted that her husband's passivity gave her the right to stray.

> He's lain like a Log of Wood,
> In Bed, for a year or two,
> And wont afford me any good,
> he nothing at all would do.
>
> I am in my blooming Prime,
> dear Neighbours I tell you true,
> I am lost to my Teeming Time,
> yet nothing at all he'll do.
>
> He lyes like a lump of Clay,
> such Husbands there is but few,
> 'Twould make a Woman run astray,
> When nothing at all he'll do.[43]

She fed her spouse with cock broth and egg caudles, but nothing worked. After two years of marriage she still had her maidenhead and so now felt fully justified in taking a "friend" or two.

There were men, the ballads claimed, who tolerated being cuckolded. As one writer put it, "Some men love to open their Oysters themselves; others care not for that drudgery. . . . Some men lye fumbling five or six years together, and loose all their labour."[44] So in "The Old Man's Complaint; or, the Unequal-Matcht Couple" the man confesses:

> My Wife is a neat young woman, and I am an aged man;
> I cannot tell how to please her [though] do I the best I can:
> *For ever she cryes, 'O turn, turn, and I will turn to thee';*
> *She looks for the thing that I [can] not [learn], for the cramp lies in my knee.*
>
> What had I for to wooe her? I being old and tough;
> All that I can [fetch] unto her, she thinks it not half enough.
> *For ever, etc.*[45]

In short, such a "wittol" or complacent husband would not mind being cuckolded if his wife did it discreetly. *The Wandring Whore* (1660–61) has one strumpet recalling: "I remember two lusty, strapping, bouncing Girles, whose names were *Lada* and *Lycoenium*, each of them married to a bed-full of old bones, with which they could not be satisfi'd, so that *Lada* counterfeits her self sick, the old dottard presses her to know her distemper, which she told him was occasioned for want of due benevolence, he knowing his insufficiency and impotency, grants her desires, and by the help of a well-trap't Doctor, was perfectly cured." One eighteenth-century jest book told of a parson who discovered a lady consorting with her coachman. When the parson told her husband, the latter explained she was hard to satisfy and that he paid the coachman twenty pounds a year for that service. The shocked parson protested that he should have been told; he would have done it for ten.[46]

As suggested in the Scottish ballad *The Fumbler's Rant* (1808), some men, as a sign of bravado, embraced the role of fumbler.

> Come Carls a' of Fumbler's Ha',
> and I will tell you o' our fate,
> Since we ha'e married wives that's braw,
> and canna please them when 'tis late.
>
> A pint we'll tak, out hearts to chear;
> what fauts we ha'e, our wives can tell;
> Gar bring us in baith ale and beer,
> the auldest bairn we hae's oursell.
>
> Christ'ning o' weans we are rid off,
> the parish Priest 'tis he can tell,
> We aw him nought but a gray groat,
> the off'ring for the house we dwell.[47]

In more sophisticated literary productions, libertine writers also exploited the notion of women as more sexually demanding. In Thomas Hamilton's "The Disappointment," a lad who seduces a maid by saying he can do it ten times, has to explain why he stops after five.

> "I've done but half, I must confess,
> But many are content with less,
> And I, if you'll forgive my crime,
> Will do the rest another time."[48]

Married men soon lost, claimed Robert Gould in *A Satyr Against Wooing* (1698), their sexual capabilities:

> For Women know too well the Wants of Sapless Age.
> 'Tis true, some Men t' a Vig'rous Age arrive,

But it is then too late to *Woo* and *Wive*.
Who' shake the Sands when there's so few to run?
And clap on Leeches when the Blood is gone?
Yet e'en in Impotence they're still the same,
And hold the Cards tho' they can't play the Game;
When Nature does in Opposition strive,
And the last rak't up Ember's scarce alive.[49]

In "A Satyr Against Women" Gould condemned women for being too lustful and went on in "The Step-Mother, a Satyr" to present the hideous portrait of the woman who exhausts her elderly spouse:

In her old Dotard's feeble Arms she lies,
And kindly with his *Impotence* complies;
And when his Vigor's ready to expire,
Molds his cold Clay, and warms it to *Desire*,
And blows the *Ember's* till she find the *Fire*;
At once his *Body* and his *Coffer* drains,
And leaves his *Purse* as empty as his *Veins*.[50]

The Greek and Latin playful accounts of male sexual disasters reemerged in the late seventeenth century. Rochester copied Ovid; Dryden translated Juvenal. Poems about the failures of excessive passion came into vogue. Drawing on French models, George Etherege produced "The Imperfect Enjoyment" (1672), a verse that described premature ejaculation.

But oh, strange passion! oh, abortive joy!
My zeal does my devotion quite destroy:
. . . .
She blush'd and frown'd, perceiving we had done
The sport she thought we had yet begun.[51]

Perhaps the best known of this ilk was Rochester's poem that was also called "The Imperfect Enjoyment" (1680).

Eager desires confound my first intent,
Succeeding shame does more success prevent,
And Rage at last confirms me impotent.
Even her fair hands which might bid heat return
To frozen Age, and make cold Hermits burn,
Applied to my dead Cinder warms no more,
Than Fire to Ashes could past Flames restore.

Trembling, confus'd, despairing, limber, dry,
A wishing, weak, unmoving lump I ly.[52]

William Wycherley contributed to the genre in "To a Mistress, disappointed by her Lover's Meeting her too Soon" and in "The Unperforming Lover's Apology." "The fault was not, tho' the Misfortune, mine / I was too eager, and Thou too Divine!"[53] Like Etherege, Wycherley has the man blame the woman for his shortcoming. A woman writer took much the same approach. In Aphra Behn's "The Disappointment," Lysander is described failing to pleasure Cloris:

Faintness its slack'ned Nerves invade:
In vain th' enraged Youth essay'd
To call its fleeting Vigor back,
No motion 'twill from Motion take;
Excess of Love his Love betray'd:
In vain he Toils, in vain Commands
The Insensible fell weeping in his hands.

. . . .

He curs'd his Birth, his Fate, his Stars;
But more the *Shepherdesses's* Charms,
Whose soft bewitching Influence
Had Damn'd him to the *Hell* of Impotence.[54]

In such poems the narrators sought to make up with their wit what they failed to do with their flesh. They inevitably blamed the woman's irresistible charm for the fiasco. How many were taken in by such arguments? In one French novel a frustrated lover declared that she refused to believe "that the more a man loves, the less he can show his mistress that he does."[55]

The popular assumption that woman, being naturally lascivious, would seek comfort elsewhere if not satisfied by her spouse was taken up by upper-class writers as well. In much of the bawdy poetry of the late seventeenth century, the fact that she is married to an impotent old man justifies the heroine's sexual escapades. Thomas Hamilton, the earl of Haddington, described demanding women in "The Excuse" and "The Rebuke." In "The Chaplain" he portrayed a young wife cuckolding an old husband who "was sparing of his flesh."[56] Such libertine poetry clearly aimed to shock, but such writings also reflected a self-consciousness and unease. The author of *The Whore* asked respectable women married to incapable men if they did not dream of straying.

Your spouse; perhaps, lies snoring all the night,
While you are wishing for the soft delight.
Is impotence the case?—he old, you young,
Weak in his back, while you are stout and strong;
If he can't eat, pray why should you be starv'd?
The craving Womb of Nature must be serv'd.[57]

In her play *The Royal Mischief* (1696) Mary de la Rivière Manley had a young woman castigate her elderly spouse.

Thou dotard, impotent in all but mischief,
How could'st thou hope, at such an age to keep
A handsome wife? Thy own, thy devil will
Tell thee 'tis impossible.

(5.1)[58]

Contrariwise, some playwrights recognized the comedic potential of men *pretending* to be impotent. In Ben Jonson's *Epicoene* (1609), Morose attempts to get out of his marriage by claiming to be *manifeste frigidus*. The ladies believe he is lying.

TRUEWIT: Why if you suspect that, ladies, you may have him searched.
DAW: As the custom is, by a jury of physicians.
MOROSE: O me, must I undergo that!
MRS. OTTER: No, let women search him, madam: we can do it ourselves.

(5.4, 50–56)[59]

In Wycherley's *The Country Wife* (1675), a quack is asked by the rake Horner to spread the news that he is castrated:

QUACK: I have been hired by young gallants to belie 'em t'other way; but you are the first would be thought a man unfit for women.
HORNER: Dear Master Doctor, let vain rogues be contented only to be thought abler men than they are, generally 'tis all the pleasure they have; but mine lies another way.[60]

(1.1, 34–39)

The irony is that Horner, by pretending to be impotent or castrated, is allowed access to these women (and thus their seduction); whereas the self-satisfied husbands of the "wine widows," in failing to service their spouses, are little better than eunuchs. Exploiting young men's fantasies of cuckolding their superiors, a string of seventeenth- and eighteenth-century plays presented the young gallant as seducer and the nouveau riche husband as fumbler who because of impotence, stupidity, or inattentiveness, could not control his wife.[61]

Complementing the plays, poems, and ballads that drew what humor they could from the specter of a man failing to satisfy his wife, were court reports of women's attempts to free themselves from impotent spouses. If women sought an annulment or sued for divorce on the grounds of their husband's impotence, men again risked being made laughing stocks. Such suits had their basis in the Christian concept of marriage. William Gouge devoted a portion *Of Domestical Duties: Eight Treatises* (1634) to "impotent persons that ought not to seeke after marriage," making it clear that on the one hand barrenness was not the same as impotence and children were not the sole end of marriage, but on the other hand that one should not marry if one could not perform the essential duties of marriage, which entailed giving to one's partner "sufficient satisfaction."[62]

In some American colonies unconsummated marriages were considered neither complete nor valid. And unlike Britain, the civil courts in the New England colonies of Massachusetts and Connecticut allowed divorces. Although sterility and impotence were often regarded as the same thing, married couples did not have to be fertile, but they were expected to be able to provide each other with "due benevolence." The community recognized the importance of pleasure and sexual performance. When a woman claimed that her husband was impotent an examination might take place. In a 1728 Pennsylvania case the examiners reported the following: "Being met in a proper Room for the intended Examination, the forsaid George Miller retired to a Corner of the same; and in a short space of time returned & presented himself before us; He then having a full Erection of the Penis, with some Semen virile (vel similline quid) newly emitted upon the Palm of one of his Hands, and also at the extremity of the Glans issuing out of the Urethra." A review of eighty seventeenth-century New England divorce petitions found that in fourteen references were made to male sexual incapacity. These were serious charges inasmuch as the man, if he were found impotent, could not remarry. Given that male courts regarded most female sexual claims with suspicion, it comes as no surprise that few wives won their suits.[63]

In 1635 Lady Desmond charged that Lord Desmond had an "insufficiency to please a reasonable woman." While an unhappy wife could file suit for annulment in England, few apparently did. In 1618, one did declare publicly in the court of the archdeacon of North Wiltshire that she intended to sue for nullity on the grounds of her husband's incapacity, but there is no evidence that she actually did so. Nevertheless there were a handful of sensational English cases that galvanized the public's attention. James I was himself very much interested in the famous 1613 suit of Frances Howard, countess of Essex.[64] In her deposition against the earl of Essex, Lady Frances Howard stated

> That since the *Earl of Essex* was Eighteen Years of Age, he and I have for the space of three Years diverse and sundry times lain together naked in Bed all Night. And at sundry of the said Times, the said Earl hath purposely endeavoured and attempted to consummate Marriage with me, and to have carnal Copulation with me for procreation of Children: And I have at such Times, as the said Earl hath attempted so to do, yielded my self willing to the same Purpose. All which notwithstanding, I say and affirm upon my Oath, that the said Earl never had carnal Copulation with me.

Her claim to still be a "virgo incorrupta" was confirmed by midwives or "inspectresses." The earl's response was that she was not fit: he had tried but been unable to penetrate her.[65]

The court sided with the earl and Lady Frances Howard lost her suit. The same bias was made clear in the case of George Downing who married Mary Forester but failed to consummate the marriage. When Edward Weld's wife Catherine appealed to the Court of Arches in 1727 she asserted that in three years of marriage he did not converse with her, and witnesses stated that he confessed to his "insufficiency." Weld insisted that he did succeed once or twice, but three midwives confirmed on inspection that Catherine was still a *virgo intacta*. Male solidarity was again maintained when the doctors defended Weld and the court found in his favor. In the reportage of such cases, a historian has noted, "the text almost always includes implicit attacks on women who dare to question their husband's sexual powers. Thus, after an initial shock, the masculine pride is restored by a section of the book which attempts to prove 'that there are no certain signs of virginity in women.'"[66]

Although in Catholic Europe a woman could obtain an annulment based on her spouse's impotence, the English ecclesiastical courts were less responsive. Nevertheless such trials were unsettling. First they raised the specter of female power. Essex was not examined, but midwives backed up Lady Frances Howard's claim. Such cases, even when they went against the wife, highlighted the public's acknowledgment of female sexual knowledge. Secondly, these accounts made aristocratic men look like fools. As one historian has observed, "the impotency implied was patriarchal as much as corporeal." The public was treated to the humiliating spectacle of elite males having to assert or even prove their manhood. Trials exposing the sexual failures of the elite were seized upon by the first generation of muck-raking editors. In 1710 Edmund Curll retold the sensational story of the earl of Castlehaven's

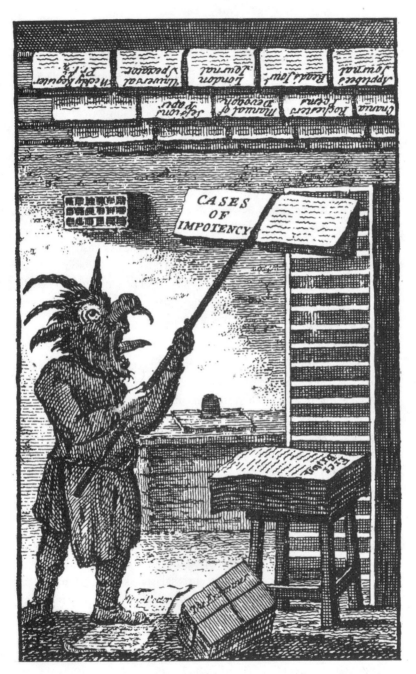

3. Edmund Curll, the notorious publisher of *The Cases of Impotency*, portrayed as a monster by the *Grub-Street Journal*, October 26, 1732, from Ralph Straus, *The Unspeakable Curll* (London: Chapman and Hall, 1927), 145.

1631 trial for rape and sodomy in *The Cases of Unnatural Lewdness.* In 1714 Curll included the account in *The Cases of Impotency as Debated in England,* a best seller that included additional scandals in each subsequent edition. In the early eighteenth-century, divorce court proceedings became a popular genre exploited by such unsavory characters.[67]

And last, but not least, such trial accounts inevitably gave rise to bawdy humor and subjected powerful men to public ridicule. Curll took advantage of the editing of these reports to add his own salacious comments on such questions as why some men's "pizzle" never stood whereas others suffered from premature ejaculation.

> There are many Men whose Penis very readily rises, nay, lifts its self up in a most proud and ostentatious Manner; but then it's [sic] Fury is soon spent; like a Fire made of Straw, the Moment it approaches its Mistress's Door, it basely falls down at the very Threshold, and piteously vomits out its frothy Soul.... For tho' he appears to be a Man, he is not presently to be concluded such, because there are some whose Ensigne of Manhood is a mere Cheat, gives mighty Hopes, but performs nothing.[68]

Jokes were made at the expense of those cited. It was said of the earl of Essex "that it was a Truth, that the Earl had no Ink in his Pen."[69] Lord Roos, caught up in his own sexual scandal was described by his wife as a "bungling base blockheaded bedfellow." When the duke of Beaufort filed for adultery in 1742, the duchess launched a countersuit for nullity. "The privy members of the Duke," she claimed, "were never to my knowledge turgid, dilated or erected in such a way as (in my opinion) may be usual and necessary to perform the act of carnal copulation." The Court of Arches found in her favor so the duke was forced to accept a test of virility and, to the surprise of many, passed. In eighteenth-century England the man was not required to provide proof of penetration or emission; only of erection. Horace Walpole laughingly furnished a correspondent with an account of the two doctors, three surgeons and the dean of Arches waiting for the duke to produce his erection: "He was some time behind the scenes: at last he knocked, and the good old folks saw what amazed them—what they had not seen in many a day! Cibber says 'His Grace's—is in everybody's mouth.'"[70] That even members of polite society exchanged such tales reflected the fact that most people in the early modern period took the view that both a man's private and public life should be open to public scrutiny.

On the continent the Catholic Church continued to hold consummation necessary for a marriage to be valid. It was considered so important to Catholic theologians that they declared that a man, though he promised his bride not to consummate their marriage (as in the case of a spiritual or Josephite marriage), was not morally bound to keep his word. Writers such as Paolo Zacchia carried into the early modern period their forebears' argument that marriage was instituted for the bearing of children and to control concupiscence. The young and healthy who could not perform were likely victims of "frigidity" or "maleficium." If after three years they had no success an annulment was allowed. Other church doctors declared point blank that impotent spouses should be separated.[71]

Complications arose when the woman insisted that she still was a virgin, and the man denied it. At this stage a visitation would be ordered and if a determination still could not be made a trial by congress might be required. In the sixteenth century there were several famous French cases of annulments sought on the basis of impotence such as that of Mlle Corby versus Debray; or the baron du Pons versus Catherine de Parthenay. There is no way of knowing how many there were in total, but their importance resided not in their number but in what they symbolized. In France from the mid-1500s to the late 1600s—and possibly in Spain and Italy as well—a determined wife could have her husband subjected to a trial of congress, in which he would have to demonstrate his ability to come erect, to penetrate, and emit. The ecclesiastical courts could find for the man and so maintain the marriage, find against him and grant the woman an annulment, or impose on the couple a three year probationary period. The woman who launched the suit understood she had to protest her desire for children, not simply her desire for sexual pleasure. The cards were initially stacked against her. For example, the church courts regarded a man's old age as "a kind of illness." According to the theologian Fevret (1654), "the cold winter of their late season has extinguished all natural vigour, and the blood, half-frozen in their veins, is no longer capable of heat."[72] Young wives—viewed as gold diggers—rarely won against such elderly spouses. And the Catholic Church, which, it will be remembered, in the Middle Ages refused to accept princes' presentation of their barren marriages as a reason for their dissolution, in the seventeenth and eighteenth centuries continued to oppose such pleas.

In being administered by men, the trials of congress were inherently misogynistic, yet could be exploited by wives. The genitals of the husband and wife would be subjected to inspection by doctors and midwives. If the examinations raised doubts, the man would have to demonstrate an erection and witnesses provide proof that congress had taken place. When a woman's suit was successful it was because the court had determined that the impotent had committed a sort of fraud in marrying or, in the words of Gayot de Pitaval, that such men "do contaminate all commerce with a coin of doubtful quality; they deceive not only the women whom they do wed, but the parents who do entrust them with their daughters." In addition such men had violated the sacraments. Some were credited with indulging in perverted desires and immodest and unnatural positions. One wife accused her husband of "employing his fists and hands rather than those natural parts that were incapable of erection."[73]

An anonymous 1735 defender of divorce argued that many impotent husbands were not content to be continent but engaged in lascivious, sinful "touchings" that put the wife's salvation at risk and had no procreative justification. Marriage, like any other contract, had to be honored and obviously was not if the woman found her spouse was only a "shadow" of a man. Her going to court could not be considered as scandalous as some claimed, given that many women now went to doctors and surgeons to be examined for a variety of complaints. And the visitation itself, the author claimed, was not as intrusive as many believed. The bed was curtained and only the vestiges of lovemaking were examined. A few simple reforms of the process were all that was needed.[74]

Not surprisingly, many men wilted under the pressure of having to perform in public. And as in England, it was almost impossible for any accused man—even the successful—to avoid becoming a laughing stock. The published accounts, such as that of a trial that took place in Rheims, made it clear that that there was nothing quite as amusing. "The experts waited around the fire. Many a time did he call out: 'Come! Come now!' But always it was a false alarm. The wife laughed and told them: 'Do not hurry so, for I know him well.' The experts said after that never had they laughed as much nor slept as little as on that night."[75]

What are to we make of all of these reports in which impotent men were mocked? A first conclusion might be that they reflected a world in which there was little embarrassment about discussing or even viewing the male genitals. We do know that before the age of seven Louis XIII of France was allowed to play with himself and had courtiers kiss his cock and caress his genitals. Indeed his father Henri IV exposed himself to his son asserting: "Behold what made you what you are."[76] Yet even such dramatic scenes contained mixed messages; reflecting the confidence of one party and the humiliation of the other.

Though it is tempting to interpret the many ribald accounts of "unperforming husbands" as evidence of women's power, the evidence suggests that they fulfilled a more conservative function. One literary critic has noted that, "Laughter often appears in libertine stories as a sign of the antierotic, the mark of something that must be overcome if erotic narrative is to proceed."[77]

Given that male performance was regarded as such a serious business, it was necessarily endangered by bursts of laughter. Yet the sharing of stories of bedroom fiascoes could serve as a male bonding experience, diminishing the shame of some and inflating the bravado of others. Such scenarios illustrated how one might best respond to a test of masculinity. The ballads and jokes were not aimed at turning the world upside down. In exposing to ridicule the few men who failed their tasks as spouses, humor's purpose was to reassert and affirm marital harmony.

Slandering a man by claiming he was impotent offered a common form of defamation, but the context always had to be taken into account. An impotent man who was a friend was not derided while an enemy was. Impotence per se was clearly not the problem that preoccupied the community. In the early modern period at least 10 percent of Europeans never married and, of those who did, almost as high a percentage had no children. Impotence and sterility were often regarded as the same thing and in theory it was considered shameful to be barren. In practice lampoons and charivaris only targeted cuckolded or henpecked husbands, rather than those who were childless.[78]

The community surveillance of marriage certainly relied on sexual gossip, slander, and jokes. Yet if a marriage were barren, the community's first response was usually to blame the woman rather than the man. Most of the recipes in the midwifery manuals to aid conception were directed at wives, not husbands. And in asserting that women had sexual appetites, the ballads and songs reinforced the notion that women depended on being serviced by men. For example, a scabrous tract entitled *The Natural History of the Arbor Vitae, or, Tree of Life* (1732) (that is, the penis) described a remarkable plant whose milky sap cured green sickness and all other female ailments.[79]

Most importantly, almost all the published accounts of impotence were written by men for men. Jokes about sexual humiliations played a vital part in a common male culture of the seventeenth century that only became more stratified in the eighteenth century. Laughter was used by some men to police the sexuality of other men. Men did not so much fear demanding women as they did the sneers and sniggering of their fellows. A man's honor was most attacked when his enemies mocked his competence as a spouse. In being dunned by a woman, he put the reputation of all men at stake and it was therefore essential that he be portrayed as a fool.

By denigrating the masculinity of others, one could laud one's own potency. Laughing at the weakling provided a cathartic release for other men who might harbor a fear of inadequacy. "The passion of laughter," Thomas Hobbes noted, "is nothing else but a sudden conception of some eminence in ourselves, by comparison with the infirmity of others." A century later Joseph Addison agreed: "Everyone diverts himself with some Person or other that is below him in Point of Understanding, and triumphs in the superiority of his Genius, whilst he has such objects of Derision before his Eyes." [80] The sexually deficient male provided a negative model against which normative males were judged.

Despite what the church might say, in the 1600s both low and high culture turned stories of impotence to comic purposes. Sometime in the early 1700s the enlightened began to voice the opinion that even the secular minded had to regard such crude accounts of man's failings as of interest to only the vulgar. The new view was that if impotence had to be discussed, it should be subjected to rational analysis rather than to religious dictates or bawdy popular beliefs. In this chapter we saw why for so long the subject was considered inherently amusing; the following will explain why it ceased to be regarded as a laughing matter.

"SHAMEFUL TO WIVES, RIDICULOUS FOR HUSBANDS, AND UNWORTHY OF TRIBUNALS"
Impotence in the Age of Reason

In 1709 John Marten enjoyed the dubious distinction of being the first man in England indicted at the Queen's Bench for pornography. His crime was to have authored *Gonosologium Novum; or, A New System of All the Secret Infirmities and Diseases, Natural, Accidental, and Venereal in Men and Women*. The indictment was in the end thrown out and whatever slight notoriety Marten enjoys today stems more from his purported authorship of *Onania* (1712), the classic text that launched the masturbation panic in eighteenth-century Europe. Historians have been understandably fascinated by the role Marten played in fanning fears of self-abuse and by his salacious accounts of female sexuality.[1] What they have failed to note is that in the first portion of *Gonosologium Novum*, he also provided an unprecedentedly detailed and exhaustive account of the causes and cures of male impotence. Succinctly portraying the continuation of old anxieties and the emergence of new worries, the *Gonosologium Novum* marked a watershed in the analysis of male sexual incapacity.

Yet, far from being an original writer, Marten was an inveterate plagiarizer. His book's interest resides in the fact that it reflects the ways in which, in the seventeenth and eighteenth centuries, the discussion of impotence went through two striking transformations. First, impotence was increasingly described by commentators as a physiological problem rather than as a consequence of sin or Satan. Such a perspective was best represented by, if not primarily due to, enlightened medical men countering theology by offering new, materialistic explanations of the workings of the body. And the western European culture was becoming more secular-minded as well as more commercially-minded. A market emerged for practitioners peddling products guaranteed to cure a range of sexual ailments. On the other hand, just when sexual dysfunctions were increasingly viewed as resulting more from physical than from moral deficiencies, the very subject came to be treated by the respectable with greater and greater reserve. In the mid-1660s, the upper classes shared the common view that impotence was inherently funny; by the mid 1700s, the elite seized on the notion that it had to be regarded as inherently tragic. It was, the elite declared, a private sorrow that only the vulgar would seek to subject to public scrutiny. These two transformations in the discussion of impotence, so apparently contradictory, were in fact intimately entwined. The linkages can be detected in a number of cultural changes: the success quacks had in attributing impotence to venereal disease and masturbation, the public's interest in embryological advances that undermined the assumption of women's desire for pleasure and their right to judge a man's performance, and in the bourgeois stress on privacy that curtailed a wife's right to have her marriage to an impotent spouse annulled. The discussion of male dysfunctions was, in short, intimately implicated in the important shifts in gender relations in the 1700s that gave rise to new models of masculinity and femininity.

In beginning with *Gonosologium Novum*, we gain a good sense of how far the popular discussion of impotence had advanced by 1709. According to Marten, male sexual failures stemmed from a variety of causes. He first listed a number of physical problems. The "stones" might not have descended into the "cod." The testicles that produced the seed could have been rendered cold by the mercury with which diseased men purged themselves. In *A Treatise of All the Degrees and Symptoms of the Venereal Disease* (1708) Marten had first broached the subject of impotence resulting from such therapies. Accidents, blows to the head, and cut blood vessels could also have serious consequences since to produce seed the testicles needed a supply of the brain's matter and spirits. Turning to the penis, Marten warned that satisfactory penetration was impossible "when the erection of the *Yard* is deprav'd or not fit for Copulation, as oftentimes it happens, as when it stands awry." The urethra might not exit at the end of the penis and the surgeon would have to deal with such cases of hypospadia. The "yard" could be too small, but stretching, he cautioned, did not work. The fraenum could break and bleed. An overlong prepuce might have to be cut. Contrariwise, if the foreskin were too tight paraphymosis would result and circumcision would be needed to free the "nut" of its prepuce. In addition warts, ruptures, obstructions, ulcers, and gleets all posed means by which "the *Venereal* edge is dull'd."[2]

Assuming that there were no physical problems, the man's duty was quite straightforward. "For as the due Erection and Stiffness of the *Yard* is

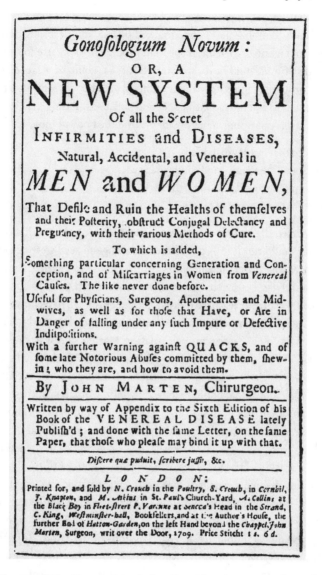

Gonoſologium Novum :

O R, A

NEW SYSTEM

Of all the Secret
INFIRMITIES and DISEASES,
Natural, Accidental, and Venereal in

MEN and WOMEN,

That Defile and Ruin the Healths of themſelves
and their Poſterity, obſtruct Conjugal Delectancy and
Pregnancy, with their various Methods of Cure.

To which is added,

Something particular concerning Generation and Conception, and of Miſcarriages in Women from *Venereal*
Cauſes. The like never done before.

Uſeful for Phyſicians, Surgeons, Apothecaries and Mid-
wives, as well as for thoſe that Have, or Are in
Danger of falling under any ſuch Impure or Defective
Indiſpoſitions.

With a further Warning againſt QU A C K S, and of
ſome late Notorious Abuſes committed by them, ſhew-
ing who they are, and how to avoid them.

By J O H N   M A R T E N, Chirurgeon.

Written by way of Appendix to the Sixth Edition of his
Book of the V E N E R E A L D I S E A S E lately
Publiſh'd ; and done with the ſame Letter, on the ſame
Paper, that thoſe who pleaſe may bind it up with that.

Diſcere quæ puduit, ſcribere juſſit, &c.

L O N D O N:

Printed for, and ſold by *N. Crouch* in the *Poultry, S. Crouch*, in *Cornbil*,
J. Knapton, and *M. Atkins* in *St. Paul's* Church-Yard, *A. Collins* at
the *Black Boy* in *Fleet-ſtreet P. Varenne* at *Seneca's* Head in the *Strand*,
C. King, Weſtminſter-hall, Bookſellers, and at the Author's Houſe, the
further Bol of *Hatton-Garden,* on the left Hand beyond the *Chappel, John
Marten,* Surgeon, writ over the Door, 1709. Price Stitcht 1 *s.* 6 *d.*

4. The title page of John Marten's *Gonosologium Novum* (London: N. Crouch, 1709), which provided the early eighteenth century's most thorough account of the causes and cures of impotence.

one main qualification for the performing the Office of a Husband, so no less is the regular ejaculation of the *Seed* thro' the *Yard* so erected." A failure of either process resulted in "no pleasing Conversation either to Man or Woman." To respond to the lack of erection due to weak muscles and inactive spirits, Marten recommended "sharp" aromatics like ginger, pepper, and cantharides. Even so a man might only have what Marten described as a "flatulent Erection," that is one marked by the "dullness" of the seminal liquor or in fact no seed at all. If the man produced "as we use to say, *but dry Stuff*," the womb would be disappointed. Fatness could be a cause of lack of seed as corpulence took away the best blood. In addition Marten attributed semen losses to idleness, abstinence, and soft beds. Indulgence in tobacco drew his ire as cramping venery by depriving the body of moisture.

> Tobacco that out-landish Weed
> Both spends the Brain, and spoils the Seed;
> Doth dull the Spirits, and dim the Sight,
> And robs the Woman of her Right.[3]

For Marten the final proof of potency was conception and that could fail if the man could not last. A good erection and good seed were not enough, as the latter was "Infertile when it is emitted in the Act with too much precipitancy or hast, before the Woman's Parts are raised, or so fit to receive it, with that Pleasure necessary to occasion Conception." The assumption here (as in the above poem) was that a woman had to be pleasured to conceive. What we would call premature ejaculation Marten said was caused by "a sharpness of the *Seed* which excites it to expulsion." Elsewhere he claimed pleasure was caused not by the salt of the seed, but by the spirits that tickled the parts. This problem could be cured by baths, opiates, and astringents. Opiates had their noxious side effects, however, and his own mixture, he promised, "causes no stupidity or sleepiness, but to the contrary, makes the Spirits Vigorous and Vigete, encreases the Desire, and causes a deliberation and prolongation of the Embrace, to a very great Satisfaction."[4]

In listing the many causes of impotence, Marten made it clear that he did not number witchcraft among them. He acknowledged, like Burton, that the mind had a role to play and that problems could ensue "when the Spirits are depressed by Trouble, Grief, Fear, Passions of the Mind, Hypochondriack Melancholy, over-Thoughtfulness, Study, &c." All the cures he offered were internals and externals aimed at recuperating the force of the seed and muscles. He drew on older authors in listing ointments of amber, rosemary, and lavender. To enrich the seed he recommended the traditional heavy diets of eggs, wine, oysters, chocolate, and rich broths, but the few recipes he provided were so elaborate and expensive that few could have afforded to employ them. Moreover Marten denigrated the old herbals for their often contradictory advice. At the same time he expressed his shock that unscrupulous quacks were now offering the public new, dangerous pills and potions. Both the old and young who abused such remedies would, Marten warned, find their health shattered. Some of the remedies on offer could even result in the patient ejaculating blood. Having sufficiently alarmed his readers, Marten presented himself as the caring practitioner, concerned for each patient's particular needs. He generously offered for sale his *Grand Aphrodisiack* or *Generative Drops* and his *Liniment Virilitatus*. They assured, he claimed,

> that the greater, more lasting and substantial Erection and Titillation is occasioned, strengthening the Seed-Vessels and all the Nervous and Musculous Parts contiguous thereto, with that Spirituous Turgescence and Magnamity, as if no such imbecility had before been; and serves for the same purpose for Women as well as Men, not giving a base stimulation or flatulent Erection and Desire as most Provocatives do, to the only irritating and forcing the parts for a while (which afterwards grow more inactive dull and flaccid, and consequently bring a perpetual *Sterilitas* or *Venus Languida* never to be recovered) but a substantial Desire and Ability.

Such help was desperately needed. A man suffering from impotence, Marten lamented, "will always till that be removed, be Unfruitful, and not able to Generate, and in that respect is a useless Member to the Commonwealth in which he lives, and One, whom the Fair Sex would avoid, unless it were to look at him, Point and Laugh with their Fans before their Faces, as not fit for that Conversation, which they are so susceptible of, and take so much Delight and Pleasure in."[5]

In acknowledging women's right to pleasure and their mocking of men who could not produce it, Marten was playing on old male anxieties. Where he struck a new note was in claiming that much impotence was due to the vice of masturbation, or what he at times simply referred to as "friction." He had earlier made the same claim in his treatise on the venereal diseases, and again, he was not particularly original. A decade earlier Michael Ettmüller had warned that semen could be ejaculated too soon, attributing such dribbling to luxury, "high feeding," abstinence, "excessive venery" and what Ettmüller called "manual violence." Marten was, however, apparently the first to use the word "masturbation" in its modern spelling and to seek to reap the rewards offered by exploiting the fears of this new vice.[6] He was soon followed by hoards of quacks.

Marten was probably the author of *Onania* (1712), which launched the eighteenth-century panic over masturbation. The book was a hodge-podge of ideas, many drawn from tracts on venereal disease, claiming that self-abuse inevitably led to a range of sufferings, including thin semen, premature ejaculation, and general weakness. Few commentators prior to the eighteenth century had regarded masturbation as worthy of note. If not required to remove excess seed, the ancients regarded it as a childish activity. Catholic scholars labeled it as a sin but devoted little attention to it. Why did such an innocuous practice suddenly come to be regarded by the intelligent as a filthy vice that could have long-term physical and psychological consequences? Much has been written on the subject and there is no need to go into the historical debates in any great detail. Roy Porter provided the most concise account in arguing that the panic "arose partly at least because it was feared that masturbation would jeopardise other cherished ideals of the Enlightenment," such as childhood innocence. Concern for the health of young men rose as they were increasingly shut up in schools. A bourgeois culture that lauded privacy and self-gratification almost immediately feared the perverse directions in which such freedoms might be pushed. Medical texts had always warned about sexual excesses yet still held that health could be jeopardized if seed were not expended. Such views were increasingly elbowed aside by a stress on the far greater danger of semen losses.[7]

Worried doctors and unscrupulous quacks agreed that the most feared symptom of masturbation was impotence, representing as it did softness and lack of manhood. "The frightful consequences of self-pollution" according to *Onania* were legend:

> In some it has been the Cause of fainting Fits and Epilepsies; in others of Consumptions; and many young Men, who were strong and lusty before they gave themselves over to this Vice, have been worn out by it, and by its robbing the Body of its balmy and vital Moisture, with Cough or Spitting, dry and emaciated, sent to their Graves. In others again, whom it has not kill'd, it has produc'd Nightly and excessive Seminal Emissions; a Weakness in the *Penis*, and Loss of Erection, as if they had been Castrated. . . . In some Men of very strong Constitutions, the Mischiefs may not be so visible, and themselves perhaps capable of Marrying; and yet the Blood and Spirits impair'd, and the Seed render'd infertile, so as to make them unfit for Procreation, by its changing the Crasis of the Spermatick Parts, making them become barren, as Land becomes poor by being over-till'd; and few of those that have been much accustom'd to this Vice in their Youth, have ever much Reason to boast of the Fruits of their Marriage-Bed; for if by Nature's extraordinary Helps, they should get any Children, which happens not often, they are commonly weakly little ones, that either die soon, or become tender, sickly People, always ailing and complaining; a Misery to themselves, a dishonour to the humane Race, and a scandal to their Parents.[8]

On the continent the subject was picked up by writers such as Louis de la Caze who asserted that "la liqueur séminale" was similar to mother's milk inasmuch as all parts of the body were involved in its elaboration. Orgasm exhausted the body; the young could recuperate quickly but the weak could not. Studding his book with religious injunctions, Jean-Philippe Dutoit-Mambrini lamented that masturbation—"the vice of colleges"—was a sort of libertinage that was reaching epidemic proportions. Worse than normal sex, it destroyed the procreative powers. The man who arrived at his marriage half-dead tempted his wife to go elsewhere as both were deprived of the legitimate pleasures of matrimony.[9]

The most influential of the attacks on masturbation was made by the famous Swiss doctor, S. A. D. Tissot in *L'Onanisme: dissertation physique et morale* (1760; translated into English in 1766). He stressed the psychological as well as physical afflictions resulting from the loss of animal spirits and genital liquor. He too cited impotence as a key symptom of the vice.

> A fourth cause why masturbators are debilitated is that, independent even of the emissions of seed, the frequency of erection, though imperfect, with which they are afflicted, greatly weakens them. Every part that is in a state of tension, exhausts the powers, and they have none to lose: the spirits are conveyed thither in greater quantities; they are dissipated, and this occasions weakness: they are wanting in the performance of other functions, which is thereby only imperfectly done: the concurrences of these two causes is attended with the most dangerous consequences. Another accident to which the fourth cause renders masturbators more liable, is a kind of palsy in the organs of generation, from whence arises impotency, through a defect of erection, and a simple gonorrhaea, because the relaxed parts suffer the real semen to escape as soon as secreted, together with an efflux of that humour which the prostatae separate: and, in a word, all the internal membrane of the urethra acquires a catarrhous disposition, which excites a running similar to the *fluor albus* in women.[10]

Here Tissot was reflecting the fact that by late eighteenth-century doctors were abandoning their belief in the humors and focusing on the "nervous" origins of illness. It was all too easy for such practitioners to attribute vague male complaints—worry, malaise, debility, exhaustion—to masturbation. Like his countryman Jean-Jacques Rousseau, Tissot believed that nervousness was spawned by the artificiality of society. To enjoy a vigorous constitution, men needed to follow a moderate, balanced regime. Simply maintaining health required energy; to squander it in sexual excesses would wear out and irritate the fibers of both the brain and body. One's physique reflected one's morals; so the abuser—pale, effeminate, exhausted—made himself known. Men were, in short, threatened with exhibiting the nervousness and feebleness usually associated with women. John Hunter was one of the few doctors who in the late eighteenth century declared that onanism did not pose a serious threat and was certainly not as harmful as "natural" sexual excesses. He found that his sentiments were immediately castigated as immoral.[11]

G. Archibald Douglas, in *The Nature and Cause of Impotence in Men, and Barrenness in Women Explained* (1758) went so far as to suggest that "a schoolboy's practice, which is but one remove from bestiality," should be criminalized. Douglas went on to observe that the point of marriage was children and if man could not give them, the woman "might as well abuse herself with those implements which they say are sold for that purpose." The general eighteenth-century belief that Europe's population was declining goes some way in explaining the exaggerated worries occasioned by masturbation and impotence. In *Domestic Medicine* (1779) William Buchan upbraided gentlemen for devoting more of their attention to the care of their dogs and horses than to their progeny. "Family constitutions are as capable of improvement as family estates; and the libertine, who impares the one, does greater injury to his posterity, than the prodigal, who squanders away the other." Most of the quacks and moralists who attacked sexual excesses began with the premise that they were living in an age of degeneracy and depopulation. No idea was more depressing, asserted Buchan than knowing one could not reproduce. It led some to contemplate suicide. Nevertheless "numbers hazard the loss of virility for a moment's gratification" in the arms of a prostitute; others lost it by "another vice incident to youth." In his classic text on aging, *The Art of Prolonging Human Life* (1797), Christopher William Hufeland preached moderation in all things as the best medicine. Accordingly he asserted that bachelors did not live as long as the married since only "a certain abundance in the power of generation is favorable to longevity." Marriage regulated and moderated sexuality. Life was shortened by "amorous indulgence," especially sex outside of marriage, which was inevitably overstimulating, and onanism, which represented a waste of "juices" as well as the "vital spark for a new being."[12]

Determining exactly how many men believed such scare tactics is obviously impossible. Many, no doubt, saw nothing wrong with the pleasures of the hand. Indeed, "May Prick nor Purse never fail you" was the motto of an eighteenth-century Scottish men's club where men "frigged" (or masturbated) together as an enrollment test. Later, to prove themselves they only had to demonstrate erection. As bizarre as such rituals were, they were safer and cheaper than consorting with prostitutes while still offering a means by which men could demonstrate their virility. We only know about such clubs in Scotland, however, and even there these forums for male sociability declined in the 1790s.[13] That they even survived in the last decades of the eighteenth century was remarkable, given the disgust with which the respectable claimed to regard self-abuse.

Quacks had an obvious commercial interest in playing up the dangers of impotence and the other doleful consequences of masturbation. New publication opportunities available in the eighteenth century allowed the enterprising to broadcast such alarms. In the seventeenth-century herbals the assumption was usually made that the reader would grow or have made up most of the concoctions recommended. An important shift occurred in the early eighteenth century with the appearance of authors who, taking advantage of an extensive print culture of handbills, pamphlets, books, newspapers, and magazines all carrying advertisements for quack remedies, raised fears of a range of sexual complaints such as syphilis, masturbation, and impotence. In response, these enterprising men offered for sale their curing pills and potions. Medical historians once labeled such practitioners quacks to set them apart from regular doctors. Given that the remedies they offered were no more effective than those of their counterparts, the distinction is not all that helpful. Claiming in 1722 that simple cold bathing could cure "the effeminacy of the virile sex," John Floyer castigated both quacks and intemperate doctors for their exaggerated claims.[14] John Marten was a case in point. He might have been a surgeon and acquainted with many of the ancient and modern writings on venereal complaints, but few early eighteenth-century practitioners were more tenacious in seeking to exploit male anxieties for their own profits.

In *Every Man His Own Doctor* (1671), John Archer was among the first to follow up a warning that too much venery dissipated natural heat and debilitated the body with a plug for his own restorative pills. Despite its title, *The Ladies Physical Directory* (1739) also was directed at men "who from some Defect of the *Semen, Imbecility* of the Genital Parts, or Weakness and Disorder of the Spermatick Vessels, find themselves incapable of propagating their Species, altho' in other respects in a Reasonable State of Health." Absolute impotence, declared the author, was rare. More common was a "languid or faint Capacity" due to a "Deficiency of the Animal Spirits, or their ceasing to flow in such abundance to the particular Muscles, and other Parts administering to Generation." Such problems could be caused by strains, excesses, self-pollution, and gleets. Other men shed their semen "almost as soon as they entertain any amorous Thoughts." Still others, given to "fast living" and drink, had infertile or effete semen or a "Want of *Animalcula.*" All would benefit from the author's Prolifick Elixir, the Powerful Confect and the Stimulating Balm that promised to "fortify the Nerves, increase the Animal Spirits, restore a juvenile Bloom, and evidently replenish the crispy Fibres of the whole Habit, with a generous Warmth and Moisture." They would moreover allow men to prolong the embrace and so provide their partners with "prior Endearments and proper Dalliance to raise their Inclination." [15]

At the end of the century Dr. Brodum offered his Nervous Cordial and Botanical Syrup to repair debility and make men ready for the married state. Ebenezer Sibley, like Brodum and other quacks, published testimonials from the supposedly happy consumers of his reanimating "Solar Tincture." So did Samuel Solomon, who followed Tissot in listing the forms of "debility arising from self-abuse" and offered his Cordial Balm of Gilead for "impotency or seminal weakness." He advised patients to take the cordial and bathe their testicles in cold water or a mix of vinegar and alcohol "until they cabbage" (grow). The cordial purportedly favored the production of semen and removed the flaccidity of the muscles. [16]

Youths who indulged too early or those of advanced age who had over indulged would, argued James Hodson, soon note a loss of "firmness and vigour." "From relaxed and debilitated constitutions, proceeding from any of the causes above alluded to, arise many disagreeable circumstances, such as impotency, barrenness, palpitation of the heart, weakness, dullness, trembling, melancholy, loss of memory, nervous affections, lowness of spirits, nocturnal and involuntary emissions, particularly in making water or upon stool, with a total disinclination as well as inability for venereal enjoyments; and in the end palsies, lethargies, or a wasting consumption, with a complication of everything destructive to the human frame." [17] Husbands were warned if their weaknesses went untreated, it could even drive their wives into adultery. Fortunately Hodson could offer to the afflicted at one guinea per bottle his Persian Restorative Drops.

Quacks kept up with the times. Once electrical experiments came into vogue it was soon asserted that electricity and magnetism could also counter flaccidity. Galvanic cures began to be offered in the 1770s by orthodox and quack practitioners. The famous Dr. James Graham touted the dangers of impotence caused by either masturbation or marital excesses, both of which could be cured by cold bathing, moderation, and his amazing electrical bed. [18] First in France and then in England, Mesmerists promised similar relief. Older, earthy notions of sexuality were thus undermined by quacks seeking to frighten men into the purchase of their wares.

The quacks' warning that masturbation could cause impotence no doubt alarmed many men, but they could find a more reassuring message in the works of medical scientists. Over the course of two centuries, anatomists and embryologists slowly transformed traditional views of the male and female roles in procreation as they advanced a more mechanistic model of reproduction that undermined the woman's contribution—and right to pleasure—while emphasizing the man's. From the sixteenth century onward, medical scientists sought to reconcile their observations with the explanations of procreation provided by Galen, Hippocrates, and Aristotle. The dominant view of embryological development was that all parts of the new creation developed out of the two parents' seeds. A rival theory—first advanced by Plato and Aeschylus—argued that a miniature embryonic life, like an egg, was already present in the parent. The problem was that the human egg had not yet been discovered. Even William Harvey, hailed as the founder of modern embryology for his study *De generatione animalium* (1651), found neither eggs nor semen in the pregnant does he dissected and so maintained the old idea that male seed acted as a force or contagion. The egg, Harvey concluded, was the first product of conception, not the cause.[19]

On the continent, the anatomist Marcello Malpighi's investigation of the development of the chick led to his belief that "the egg is weak and powerless and so requires the energy of the semen of the male to initiate growth." A real breakthrough occurred in the 1660s when Regnier de Graaf, without the aid of a microscope, observed what were to be subsequently known as the Graafian follicles that contained the mammalian egg. Graaf was primarily interested in the female organs. It says something of seventeenth-century doctors' rudimentary understanding of male anatomy that Graaf cited butchers as the experts on the subject of undescended testicles. He also lauded mothers for the interest they had in their sons' scrotums, taking the wrinkled as a sign of health and the relaxed as a sign of illness. In contrast Graaf critiqued Aristotle and Hippocrates for their many mistaken ideas, such as the right testicle being hotter than the left, the testicles serving only as counterweights, and the spermatic artery being empty. He likewise denied the popular beliefs that the size of the penis was related to the length of one's umbilical cord or nose. Semen, asserted Graaf, was concocted in the testicles from blood and "animal spirits." The semen's tickling quality itself excited one to intercourse, and it followed that having lost a quantity of one's best blood and animal spirits, one would be sad after sex. Erections, Graaf believed, were not due to muscles raising the penis but in their preventing blood from leaving it. Erections could therefore be assisted by increasing animal spirits, giving potions to increase the quantity and speed of blood, and strengthening the muscles. There was nothing much new here. Graaf's real importance lay in his believing that he had actually seen the egg and he thereby popularized the ovist theory of reproduction, the notion that the woman, like the chicken, contained within her, miniature offspring.[20]

Defenders of the importance of male seed were not slow in responding. In 1677 Leeuwenhoeck's microscope finally revealed the animalcules contained in each drop of semen. Obviously worried by the unseemly nature of the investigation, he assured his readers that the sperm he examined had been acquired, "not by sinfully defiling himself but as a natural consequence of conjugal coitus." Leeuwenhoeck subsequently defended the spermist or animalcule side in the generation debate, arguing that though the "worms" in men's seed were not children, children came from them. He was seconded by Albrecht von Haller who produced a detailed, materialistic description of male anatomy in the *First Lines of Physiology* (1747). A century earlier, he noted, Leeuwenhoeck's microscope revealed semen to be filled with "living animalcules, resembling eels, only with a thicker head." Semen in turn was produced by the blood as revealed in the "sudden alacrity to venery that happens after eating." For erection, the cavernous bodies of the penis had to fill with blood, excited by love, pleasure, irritations, seed, cantharides, or even "whipping with rods." And to keep the erection, pressure had to be maintained on the vein. The semen, having to be expended, served as a stimulus to intercourse. "Nature herself, therefore, enjoins venery," concluded Haller, "both for preserving the human race, and likewise the health of every sound man."[21]

By the late eighteenth century as a result of the anatomists' investigations, writers such as Haller and Lazzaro Spallanzani were portraying conception as a mechanistic rather than a spiritual process. One aspect of this materialist approach was doctors' dismissal of the popular beliefs in the semimagical and aphrodisiac powers of so many herbs. One compiler, for example, flagged his disbelief in the purported virtues of mandrake by flatly declaring, "I shall not trouble myself with the useless Accounts that the Ancients have given of this Root." As far as embryology was concerned, whether one stressed the importance of the egg or the sperm, the new theories undermined the two-seed Galenic notion of the basic similarity of the two sexes. Now animalculists—returning to the Aristotleian view that women were simple nests—presented women as being little more than passive partners. The "ovist" school might have been more sensitive to women's contribution to reproduction, but in fact its members presented the egg as almost inert, having to be "shaken" into life by the sperm or allowed by its intervention to "escape" into the fallopian tube. The defenders of the Galenic two-seed theory had argued that the woman had to be aroused and delighted for conception to occur. They defended the woman's right to sexual pleasure on the grounds that her genitals were very much like the man's. Men had to be aroused to ejaculate and likewise women had to be pleasured to produce seed. But by the end of the eighteenth century a new consensus was emerging that argued males and females were not on the same continuum but were "opposite" sexes. Some doctors stated categorically that the pleasure of a woman was not only unnecessary for procreation, but possibly not even attainable. A Scottish physician asserted in 1789 that few women felt pleasure. In France, F. E. Fodéré informed his female patients that in place of passion, "complaisance, tranquility, silence, and secrecy are necessary for a prolific coition." Indeed John Hunter proved this to be the case in 1776 when he instructed a man suffering from hypospadia how to use a warm syringe to impregnate his wife.[22]

Though these new scientific understandings of procreation were no doubt restricted to an intellectual elite, they nevertheless indicated the direction in which social attitudes were already moving.[23] Men, it was increasingly assumed, were by nature sexually active and women sexually passive. In literature the convention that respectable females lacked sexual desire emerged as early as the 1690s and was popularized in such maudlin novels as Samuel Richardson's *Pamela, or Virtue Rewarded* (1740) and Jean-Jacques Rousseau's *Julie, ou La Nouvelle Héloïse* (1761). Though they addressed quite different audiences, artists and the scientists were producing remarkably similar accounts of gender. Changes in the understanding of the workings of the body were not simply due to empirical advances in science, but were themselves products of a culture. These new explanations were as much interpretive "fictions" as the novels that downplayed women's sexual desires.

Banished from respectable literature, references to impotence resurfaced not only in quack handbills but in pornographic novels. Such texts typically attributed sexual dysfunctions to their least likable characters. Premature ejaculation (regarded as a type of impotence) figured in several key works. Fanny Hill survives her first sexual encounter because of a man's lack of control. "The brute had, it seems, as I afterwards understood, brought on, by his eagerness and struggle, the ultimate period of his hot fit of lust, which his power was too short liv'd to carry him through the full execution of; of which my thighs and linen received the effusion." The Marquis de Sade's Justine had a similar escape from a brothel customer: "His excesses were my salvation; less debauchery and I should have been a fallen maid. Dubourg's ardor was extinguished by the effervescence of his desires. Heaven avenged me for the offense the monster was about to commit, and the loss of his forces before the sacrifice saved me from being its victim."[24]

If the pornographic pleasures of the portrayal of premature ejaculation were exploited, so too were the appeals of flagellation. Writers portrayed eighteenth-century brothels as being patronized by the elderly, the impotent, and those suffering from premature ejaculation. Fanny Hill described her first customer. "Impotence, more than necessity, made him seek in variety the provocative that was wanting to raise him to the pitch of enjoyment, which too often he saw himself baulked of, by the failure of his powers: and this always threw him into a fit of rage, which he wreak'd, as far as he durst, on the innocent objects of his fit of momentary desire." Most of Sade's monsters are "formidably proportioned," but a cruel count who resorts to blood letting as one of his tortures is said to be, "scarcely a man. The slenderest, slightest protuberance of flesh or, more accurately, what one sees in a child of three, was at most to be found in this individual who was otherwise so enormous and corpulent. . . . His satiety and impotence were such that the greatest efforts did not succeed in wresting him from his torpor."[25] If women could not be portrayed in respectable literature as judging men's sexual capacities, it was inevitable that they would be so presented in subversive fictions.

In France the attack on the wife's right to have her marriage annulled on the basis of her husband's impotence was yet another sign of the increased distaste with which the reputable regarded manifestations of female sexual agency. In the sixteenth century Antoine Hotman argued that as impotence was the only grounds for divorce, men were forced to prove themselves in public like brutes. By the seventeenth century many protested against the improprieties of such proceedings. Serres lamented that men were obliged to shamelessly endure the shocking trials of congress. Critics claimed that such contests were inherently unfair to men. For a woman to even launch a suit was outrageous inasmuch the mere suggestion that a man was inadequate was a slander. The trials, asserted the surgeon Ambroise Paré, could not provide men with a fair hearing. He asserted that he knew, as a doctor, that a man could not perform in front of witnesses and with a woman he did not love.[26]

A thorough critique of the trials of congress was provided by Vincent Tagereau in 1612. To him it was no surprise that in front of a brutal court made up of three doctors, three surgeons, and three matrons, a man would be put off by shame and fear. The mutual hatred of the couple in any event doomed such procedures. The women, claimed Tagereau, had all the advantages. Some lied; others used astringents or fomentations to make it appear that there were still virgins. It was difficult to determine virginity, but it was obviously easier to fake it than to fake an erection. And though the inspections of women were themselves immodest and uncertain, Tagereau was more distressed to report that women happily gave the most outrageous accounts of their private lives, one asserting, for example, that her husband used his finger to deflower her. The trial by congress was the most shameful procedure imaginable; the witnesses, according to Tagereau, going so far as to check the bed partners afterwards to see if they have done anything to "advance or hinder copulation." Scandalous confrontations could ensue with the experts employing spectacles and candles while scrutinizing the genitalia in search of evidence of intromission. These trials did more than place a man's reputation in jeopardy. If the woman succeeded in her claim her dowry had to be returned and damages and interest might also be sought, leaving her spouse ruined. Critics often cited the Langey (or Langeais) case of 1659 as proof of the injustices of the system. Though found by the court to be impotent, Langey purportedly succeeded in a second marriage in fathering seven children.[27] As a result, the Parlement of Paris in 1677 decreed that though annulments for unconsummated marriages could still be sought, trials by congress were no longer to be allowed. Nevertheless the memory of these trials was kept alive by eighteenth-century enlightened thinkers who used them both to attack the Catholic Church for its meddling in marital affairs and to upbraid women for betraying their husbands.

The leading writers of the Enlightenment presented the pursuit of pleasure as good thing. At the same time they distanced themselves from the sexual excesses associated with the aristocracy and the bawdy, vulgar penchants of the lower orders. As rationalists they wanted the body to be governed by the mind and lauded moderation and self-control. The Catholic Church embraced the pessimistic notion that only because of the fury of sexual desire did men engage in such an act as ignominious as intercourse and women accept the resulting pain of travail. Eighteenth-century optimists rejected the Christian explanations of the fall and original sin, preferring to regard the sexual instincts as natural and therefore good. Sexual instincts were part of nature, and their regular expression a sign of health. Indeed sexual relations held society together. Human progress could not take place without them. Eramsus Darwin accordingly referred to the penis as "a wonderful machine." But as the *Encyclopédie* (1750–60) of Diderot and d'Alembert made clear in its articles on *indécent*, *galanterie*, and *libertinage*, when the rationalists defended sensuality and hedonism it was only the sexual prerogatives of males that it had in mind.[28]

This two-pronged campaign of defending the pleasures of sexuality while condemning dissatisfied women can be seen in the *Dictionnaire historique et critique* (1702) of Pierre Bayle. Attacking the attempts to end an unconsummated marriage, he argued that a bashful bride would not launch such an unseemly charge, though a vindictive mother-in-law might. Women were inevitably soiled by such trials. The wife who sought to dishonor her husband only dishonored herself. "It is certain, that in all times and places, processes of this nature bring very little honour to those that enter them; and whether they obtain a new husband, or not, they are always an object of raillery and contempt as long as they live, and not without reason; for the steps they take are so contrary to modesty, a virtue which is the crown and ornament of that sex, and without which they cannot share in human glory, that no body can have any respect for a woman who takes such a course." A woman who launched such a charge—though she might claim she only wanted to become a mother—thus revealed her incontinence. Bayle glee-fully cited the case of a woman who was asked how she—if a virgin—could know that her husband was defective. "If you have your maidenhead, as you pretend, you ought not to know that your husband is impotent; and if you know it, is it a sign that you have tried what another man can do?"[29]

Obviously it was wrong to allow a woman to judge a man's potency. Her body was not reliable, her tongue was deceitful. In effect, the woman who charged her husband with being sexually inadequate revealed that she knew too much. How could she make such a claim if she had no other man with whom to compare him? Her complaint revealed more about herself; in par-ticular her desires and demands for sex that eighteenth-century rationalists could only regard as unseemly. The ideal woman was to be responsive but neither demanding nor wanton.

The authors of the *Encyclopédie* (1750–60) turned the discussion of impo-tence into an attack on the unhealthy morality preached by the Church. In his article "Impuissance," Antoine Gaspard Boucher d'Argis asserted that lack of sexual exercise was for men as bad as excesses, and cited the case of a young ecclesiastic whose dried out spermatic vessels and shortened member were due to his prolonged continence. Boucher d'Argis was later to provide a review of the trials of congress in *Principes sur la nullité du mariage pour cause d'impuissance* (1756). In his *Philosophical Dictionary* (1764) Voltaire followed up this criticism of Catholics' meddling in the lives of married couples. While noting the Church's view that impotence ended a marriage, he had to laugh that celibate churchmen prided themselves on their "irreproachable manners in their development of the mysteries of sexual intercourse. There is no singularity, however strange, on which they have not treated. They have discussed at length all the cases in which capability may exist at one time or situation, and impotence in another." And having dealt with priests Voltaire turned his fire on wives. He cited as a typically duplicitous woman the wife of Alfonso of Portugal who had him declared impotent so she could marry his brother Don Pedro. Voltaire insisted that all examinations of potency should be ended: "These causes are shameful to wives, ridiculous for husbands, and unworthy of tribunals, and it would be better not to allow them at all. Yes, it may be said, but, in that case, marriage would not insure issue. A great misfortune, truly, while Europe contains three hundred thousand monks and eighty thousand nuns, who voluntarily abstain from propagating their kind."[30] Another author in 1775 agreed that the *épreuve* that previously had been required to end a marriage was shameful. When *Traité de la Dissolution de mariage pour cause d'impuissance* (1775) appeared claiming trials of congress should not have been abolished, critics attacked it on the grounds that it encouraged women's lack of modesty.[31]

Strikingly enough many of the eighteenth-century accounts that blamed bedroom fiascoes on women's lack of sensitivity, went on to discuss the parallel problem of men being overly sensitive. We know that doctors prescribed for humoral impotence "bleedings, purges, pills, aposemes, medical wines, baumes, ointments, injections, etc." Finding out what individual men thought about their sexual dysfunctions is difficult, but thanks to his extensive medical correspondence with well-known doctors such as S. A. D. Tissot in Lausanne and Antoine Petit in Paris we know a good deal about the problems of Elie-de-Beaumont. This prominent lawyer and friend of Voltaire was rendered impotent by a belly that was so big he could not even see his genitals. Tissot was convinced that doctors could help such men and quoted Boerhaave who cured the Duc de Richelieu of conjugal impotence: "Il avait déposer [sa semence] hors du mariage; je l'ai remise dedans." [He had left his seed outside of the marriage; I put it back.] Beaumont complained of the doctors' contradictory advice regarding the use of tea and white wine. In the main, his advisers were true to the old theory of compensation, which assumed that the fat body drained energy from the genitals, and gave him advice on diet, exercise, and massage. To deal with his enormous girth one doctor suggested that he stand while his wife lay on the bed with her thighs supported by his arms and her legs around his shoulders.[32] He did succeed in siring one child in 1772 which he credited to Tissot. He sought help again in 1775 while stating that he did not want to subject his respectable wife to "painful and disagreeable attempts." Referring to himself in the third person he noted the variety of stratagems he had tried:

> It must not be denied that in order to recover this faculty sometimes frolics with accommodating women are permitted that Religion would not allow to a married man if it were not for the fact that the goal legitimizes or at least excuses them, since it was to rehabilitate him to his conjugal duty. In

general in such situations he managed rather badly; and as he felt at the very moment that he was violating a duty, this idea joined to his natural contempt for these types of women instantly took possession of him, making these exercises pointless.[33]

Such reflections direct our attention to the view the enlightened took of the deflating powers of the imagination. For the eighteenth-century rationalists, sex was one part of the mechanics of society, so a failure had to be due, not to witchcraft, but to either natural causes or the powers of the imagination. The *Encylopédie*, while acknowledging that those who thought they were bewitched could not perform, went on to insist that "it would be ridiculous to attribute it [impotence] to the effects of magic or the power of the demon." Such cases simply demonstrated that the force of the imagination agitated the blood and spirits. Of course the opponents of the trials of congress had repeatedly argued that most men would find it difficult to perform before witnesses. Shame could be an inhibiting force; even libertines were constrained when in the public eye. But now it was asserted that even in the privacy of his bedroom a husband would fail with a wife who was "ugly, disgusting, licentious, spoiled, who, instead of love, will excite in him aversion, contempt or fear."[34]

It had always been recognized that woman might not enjoy sex and so fail to conceive. Men, it was generally assumed, were by nature lustful and most early modern writers on reproduction therefore focused simply on the mechanics of copulation. They took male desire as a given and said little about psychological motivations. Though earlier writers such as Burton and Culpeper were aware of the impact passions such as anger, sadness, and fear had on the body, they said little about their relation to male sexual performance. Only in the eighteenth century were male sensibilities recognized and the psychological causes of male dysfunctions paid serious attention. Observers frequently pointed to the fact that a man could be impotent with one woman, but not with others as the classic indicator of the power of the mind over the body.[35]

When James Boswell was first admitted to his mistress's chamber he could not rise to the occasion. "I was very miserable. I thought myself feeble as a gallant, although I had experienced the reverse many a time. Louisa knew not my powers. She might imagine me impotent. I sweated almost with anxiety, which made me worse." This initial setback served to highlight Boswell's boast that ten days later he demonstrated a "godlike vigor" by coming five times in one night. A less happy account of psychic impotence was provided by Jean-Jacques Rousseau in his *Confessions* (1782). Having finally been accepted by the courtesan Zulietta after whom he had long lusted, he reports that he found he was, to his dismay, rendered impotent by the unbidden and unsettling notion that, for her to be so beautiful and yet still a common prostitute, she must have some hidden flaw. "Suddenly instead of flames which were devouring me, I feel a mortal coldness running through my veins; my legs shake, and ready to faint, I sit down, and I weep like a child."[36] Shrugging off these disturbing thoughts and rallying himself for a second attempt he then noticed that she had a slightly deformed nipple. He wilted again. The flustered and frustrated young woman, having had enough, left him with the curt advice that in the future he should avoid women and study mathematics.

Doctors described similar scenarios. After having ridiculed the idea that masturbation played a major role in causing impotence, the English surgeon John Hunter asserted that men's imagination could prevent them from performing, especially when their pride was at stake. For example, the daunting prospect of sleeping with a virgin incapacitated some. When William Buchan discussed impotence he noted that, if due to sexual excesses, it could be treated with tonics and cold bathing. To protect oneself, the best remedy was for a man to marry for love. "When this is not the case, satiety and disgust will succeed, and the unhappy husband, in the vigour of life, may, by mistake, impute his want of ardour for the connubial enjoyments to his impotency."[37]

The assertion that lack of love could impede male sexual function was new. It implied new models of masculinity and femininity—the sensitive man and the chaste woman. They were to be the two chief characters in the more affectionate partnerships of the long eighteenth century, which replaced the pragmatic marriages that Western culture had traditionally lauded. Along with romantic love in marriage came a call for a separation of spheres, symbolized by the stress on the woman's domesticity. The eighteenth-century bourgeoisie aspired toward gentility, one mark of which would be the idle wife. As a result ever more rigid lines were drawn between work inside and outside of the home. Moralists declared women in the public realm a danger and with the rise of capitalism, they played a less central role in the community. On the other hand in the private realm it has been suggested that the ideal of companionate marriage increased pressure on the man to perform.[38] This would explain why the discussions of annulments reveal that by the mid-1700s, the elite regarded women's presumption to judge their husbands as scandalous.

Though trial by congress was ended in France, a woman suing for divorce on the basis of her husband's impotence could still demand a medical "visit" or examination. As in England, both spouses would be inspected and the man obliged to demonstrate his erection. Impotence could only end a marriage if it was visible and absolute and even many of these cases were unpopular and rejected. As a result of the Revolution, secular divorce was made available in France from 1792 to 1815, but it could no longer be sought on the basis of a husband's impotence. Bayle and Voltaire's argument that the public discussion of impotence was morally outrageous was finally confirmed by law. The state's purported aim was to protect the stability of the family. Indeed article 312 of the Napoleonic Code asserted that the husband was the father of his wife's child unless he could prove that from the 300th to 128th day before the birth he was absent from the home or physically incapacitated. The relation of paternity to impotence was thus covered although the law avoided mentioning the embarrassing word.[39]

In declaring that the sexually demanding woman was unnatural, the new models of acceptable masculinity and femininity indirectly spoke to male performance anxieties. Among the respectable accounts of lusty women and jokes about cuckoldry declined. In place of the disorderly and demanding virago appeared the virtuous wife. While portrayals of feminine virtue had long existed, the eighteenth century saw the rise of a cult of womanhood in which attempts were made to draw clear boundaries between the sexes. On the one hand the culture dropped the employment of the cruel misogyny of seventeenth century with its vicious attacks on shrews and scolds and adopted softer forms of disparagement. On the other hand, undisciplined female sexuality was increasingly regarded as dangerous. Doctors told women that they were by nature more passive, and as a consequence their sexual rights were diminished. The culture produced new understandings of biology that in supporting its view of gender, naturalized women's softness and men's hardness. Medical scientists shifted from talking about sexual differences in degree to differences in kind, with P. G. Cabanis and Pierre Roussel stressing the incommensurability of the sexes. Such investigators declared that, as far as reproduction was concerned, the female orgasm was not as important as once thought. Such conclusions must have allayed some male fears.[40]

The fact that the sperm could be observed and the human egg was yet to be discovered also played some role in legitimating notions of the active male and the passive female. Did that mean, as some have argued, that men felt they had to be more aggressive, and that the growth in the bastardy rate proves that penetrative sex, displacing mutual masturbation, became more common in the eighteenth century?[41] The opposite argument can just as easily be advanced: the culture provided men with rationales of why, if they chose, they could be less rather than more active and yet feel no less manly. Underlying the demand that women show a greater modesty appeared to be the concern that men were not simple animals who could perform at will. Doctors, in providing men with a conception of the body composed of nerves and fibers, assured them that health was best served by controlling rather than indulging the passions. This bourgeois ideal of rationality and self-control was always coded as male.

The term "masculinity" entered the English language in 1748, implying a new self-consciousness of what it meant to be a man. In private many men no doubt believed that their manliness was best demonstrated by their sexual abilities. In his diary William Byrd left a meticulous account of the maids he harassed and the prostitutes he slept with. He was scrupulous enough to record both his successes and failures, as with the woman who "could provoke me to do nothing because my roger would not stand with all she could do. About ten I went home and said my prayers." But in public the refined eighteenth-century individual sought to demonstrate a character marked by sentiment and virtue. In its moralism and greater concern for privacy and discretion, the bourgeoisie set itself apart in particular from effete aristocrats.[42]

The old-fashioned rake had not regarded his sexual exploitation of men as undermining his masculinity. Lord Rochester famously prided himself on ten thousand penetrations and lamented the decline of his penis, which once "Stiffly resolv'd, twould carelessly invade, / Woman or Man, nor ought its fury staid." Increasingly, however, the man attracted to members of the same sex was labeled effeminate, a "mollie." The poet Andrew Marvell, who remained a bachelor, was slandered by one rival as impotent and a sodomite and by another as a "gelding." Yet in the eighteenth century men who pursued other men were generally presumed to have an excess rather than a lack of desire and were rarely accused of being impotent. The Earl of Leicester (later the third Marquess Townshend) was left by his wife in 1808 purportedly because of his impotence—but the *Morning Herald* libeled him for his affairs with young men.[43]

Satirists spent more time castigating fops than in attacking mollies. An age that sought to make men more refined and sensitive was at the same time worried that they might become less virile. Tissot, for example, asserted that excessive study could destroy a man's sexual abilities. The beginnings of racialization can be detected in this literature, which played off the notions of the threats of nervousness and feebleness that urban living engendered to Western males against the idea of the sexual potency of less civilized races. Marten exploited such fears in reporting that Indian and Turkish women, being naturally salacious, especially prized the man's use of opium as they "do not value a Man that cannot hold out long, and accompany with them often." Marten was obviously drawing on Ettmül-ler who in discussing "the over hasty Ejaculation of the Seminal Matter" recommended the juice of the poppy. "Upon which account it is much in use among the Indians and Turks, whose Women are most delighted with deliberate and prolong'd Embraces."[44]

In the seventeenth century Europeans laughed at a man's lack of body control; in the eighteenth-century the respectable bewailed it. With the increased privatization of domestic relations impotence—like adultery—ceased to be a joke.[45] In part the increased discretion with which these topics were broached reflected their growing importance in an age in which privacy was especially prized, yet also threatened by the purveyors of the cheap press. Moreover, when marriages had been openly arranged, the old story of the elderly groom disappointing his eager bride had obvious comic possibilities. When a marriage was supposed to be based on romantic love, each partner having entered it freely, a husband's inability to perform would have to be regarded as tragic.

Public references to impotence did not, of course, disappear. Rather the eighteenth century witnessed a splitting of the discussion of the subject along class lines. We have already noted how quacks and pornographers fastened on the topic. And whereas the middle classes sought to clearly de-marcate the public and private realms, the lower orders still appreciated the subversive effects of sexual slanders. The best example of the latter was the Parisians' disparagement of the sexual inabilities of the Bourbon monarchs. In his last years Louis XIV was accused of being militarily and personally im-potent. Songs were sung about Louis XV's inability to please his mistress Ma-dame Dubarry with his "machine antique." And finally, the fact that it took the youthful Louis XVI eight years to consummate his marriage made him an obvious target for ribald humor.[46] His problem was probably due to his tight foreskin and Marie Antoinette's resistant hymen, but rumors ran rampant that he was overly timid and she was either frigid or contemptuous.

That Louis was ultimately able to perform was attributed by some to doctors' intervention, by others to the advice given by his brother-in-law, Joseph II. It was too late to spare the royal couple the jibes of the public. The irony was that the royal couple were more domestic, faithful and loving than their predecessors, but in the crowd's estimation Louis' very attempts at guarding his privacy made him all the more a figure of fun. He was called a *cocu* (cuckold) and spoofed as the *roi-sommeil* (sleep king) rather than the *roi-soleil* (sun king). A street song that could have been written a century earlier asked, "Chacun se demande tout bas: / Le Roi peut-il? ne peut-il pas?" [Everyone quietly wonders: / Can the king or can't he?"] These libels, which continued after the birth of the dauphin and peaked in 1789 when the French Revolution broke out, obviously played a role in bringing the royal family into disrepute. Cartoons harped on the notion that Louis was undersexed and Marie Antoinette oversexed. One bore the caption "Gémis, Louis, ta vigueur inactive / outrage ici ta femme trop lascive." [Groan, Louis, your lack of vigor / outrages your too lascivious wife.] The general charge was that the degenerate and exhausted aristocracy had to make way for the virile representatives of the people. Royalist troops who opposed the revolution were in turn represented in cartoons as dropping their guns—that is, losing their erections—when mooned by women.[47] The crucial point is that it was not Louis' impotence that made him unpopular; it was being unpopular that made him a target for sexual slanders.

Why was George Washington, sterile if not impotent, spared such attacks? In 1759 Washington married a twenty-seven-year-old widow. He was never to become a father, a fate he tried to blame on his wife despite the fact that with her first husband she had produced four children in eight years. As a great athlete, hailed as the "stallion of the Potomac," Washington could never accept the barren marriage as his fault and in old age mused about marrying "some girl" to produce an heir. Nevertheless Washington's sexual shortcomings never elicited the sort of slanders the Bourbons endured. Indeed, in a draft of his first inaugural (which was never given) he actually used his lack of heirs as a reason why he should be entrusted with the presidency. "It will be recollected that the Divine Providence hath not seen fit, that my blood should be transmitted or my name perpetuated by the endearing, though sometimes seducing channel of immediate offspring. I have no child for whom I could wish to make a provision—no family to build in greatness upon my country's ruins."[48] He succeeded in portraying childlessness as a strength rather than a weakness. Whereas Louis XVI's sexual failings resulted in his enemies labeling him a contemptible cuckold, Washington's were used by his friends as yet another reason to hail him as the "Father of the Country." Louis' drubbing reflected the tenacity with which the popular classes clung to the old tradition of employing wounding sexual metaphors; the discretion with which Washington was treated by his colleagues suggests that they embraced new concerns for decorum.

Male sexual dysfunctions appeared distinctly different when viewed through an eighteenth-century prism. Quacks sought to alarm men with claims that sexual dysfunctions were evidence of youthful indulgences. Discussion of such subjects in courts was denounced by the respectable

NEURASTHENIA, DECADENCE, AND NINETEENTH-CENTURY MANHOOD

When John Ruskin and Effie Gray married in 1848, the nervous Ruskin suggested on religious and practical grounds that they wait five years before having sex; he was twenty-nine and she was twenty. His trepidation later led to the rumor that this art historian who rhapsodized over the beauties of marble nymphs was shocked at the sight of a real woman's pubic hair. His bride would only say that she found her "different" from what he imagined women to be. The union was not consummated. Effie had doctors certify her virginity and the marriage was annulled in 1854. The decree noted that it had taken place "whilst the said John Ruskin was incapable of consummating the same by reason of incurable impotency."[1] Ruskin subsequently lamented the fact that by not refuting Effie's claim he appeared to admit it. He would only concede that he had been foolish to marry her.

John Ruskin's inability to consummate his marriage with Effie Gray was perhaps the nineteenth century's most famous case of marital impotence, but Ruskin was far from being the only Victorian male who had difficulties in dealing with women. William Morris, Ruskin's disciple, also idealized a sort of monastic brotherhood and in his writings portrayed women as a sexual threat. And Ruskin was not unique in suffering wedding-night jitters. Charles Kingsley was fearful that the first sight of his wife's naked body would place him under too great a strain. A few months before their wedding in 1844 he wrote Fanny, "I have been thinking over your terror at seeing me undressed, and I feel that I should have the same feeling in a minor degree to you, till I had learnt to bear the blaze of your naked beauty. You do not know how often a man is struck powerless in body and mind on his wedding night." They waited a month before consummating their marriage.

The painter John Everett Millais, Effie Gray's second husband, was, as one writer has noted, similarly anxious. "Millais's dread of the honeymoon was very understandable, for he, like Ruskin, was almost certainly a virgin, and the thought of Ruskin's failure must have increased his own nervousness a thousand fold." Even the great Victorian historian Thomas Caryle was eventually "outed" with the posthumous publication of J. A. Froude's *My Relations with Carlyle* (1903). Originally written in 1887, the work created a scandal in intimating that the writer best known for castigating flaccid sensualists and lauding a hard, heroic, muscular type of masculinity, had himself been impotent.[2]

A number of historians have pointed out that the Victorians were not nearly as sexually ignorant or repressed as twentieth-century commentators so often claimed.[3] Determining the sexual feelings of the "typical" nineteenth-century male is, of course, impossible. The discussions of impotence do tell us, however, how a man was supposed to behave. As such they performed a specific sort of "cultural work," that of maintaining boundaries. In discussing impotence one was obviously discussing masculinity but also femininity, in short, gender relations. Western culture had always stressed male and female differences, but in the 1800s gender became privileged, often eclipsing one's rank, status, profession, race, or religion as the key determinant of personality. In a little over a century a process of construction of what many in the West came to assume were natural, timeless male and female traits took place. In particular, the nineteenth century witnessed extreme claims being made for sexual incommensurability.

The model nineteenth-century man was governed by reason, the woman by sentiment. By the 1850s raffishness was no longer in vogue and it was understood that restraint was the mark of the middle-class male.[4] Both doctors and health faddists produced repressive, prescriptive accounts of sexuality that stressed the dangers of excesses. Such writers implicitly or explicitly began with the premise that a man's health was based on a spermatic economy in which dangers of depletion had to be countered by moderation, continence, and self-control. With the new masculine ideal being that of the thrifty and cautious businessman, writers of middle-class manuals popularized the notion that sexual overindulgence led to a loss of manly vigor and ultimately to impotence or physical and psychological "bankruptcy." Men had to exert their willpower to control themselves, delay gratification, and practice restraint. In addition they had to monitor women, who lacking masculine resolve, were even more at risk to succumbing to the lure of the passions.

To complicate matters, the Victorian period also witnessed the blossoming of the model of companionate marriage, which held that in this loving institution both partners would find their ultimate happiness. Middle-class marriages were more privatized and romanticized, which in turn produced higher expectations and crueler disappointments. For the affluent, the wedding tour was by the 1870s being replaced by the private honeymoon, producing its own tensions and pressures.[5] Sexual performance became more important and failures all the more tragic. Marriage evolved as did the shift in bodily experiences—plotted by sociologist Norbert Elias—from being public to private experiences. The more such acts were privatized the more humiliated one felt if they were exposed.

A culture that craved privacy found discussions of bedroom disasters especially distasteful, but given the middle-class fixation on the notion of the active male and the passive female, the issue of impotence could not be ignored. Cultural commentators attributed male sexual dysfunctions to the stresses and anxieties posed by a whole new range of issues pertaining to sex, marriage, reproduction, and modernity itself. They asserted in so many words that the main cause of a man's impotence was the woman. Joan Scott has observed that nineteenth-century men's references to sexuality "seem to be part of a more complicated process of 'class construction' in which definitions of the middle class involve notions of sexual self-control and depend on negative examples or 'social others.'" The "other" was the nonwhite or working-class man or woman. Indeed much of the exploration of male impotence took place when men were purportedly discussing the opposite sex. Male commentators who fantasized about young girls and valorized virginity, who worried about frigid brides, demanding hysterics, lustful nymphomaniacs, and sullen menopausal matrons, were by a process of displacement often talking about men's fears of performance.[6] In what follows we will trace the various ways in which writers, while acknowledging the fact that men appeared to be increasingly incapacitated, sought to reassure their readers that masculinity itself was not at risk.

Marriage, having taken on a new emotional significance in the nineteenth century, posed the inexperienced man with his first sexual test. Although marriage manuals commonly cautioned grooms not to give vent to their unbridled lusts, some men wondered if they would pass muster. William James even claimed "marriage would allay a man's fears about his sexual potency," and was thus a good reason to wed.[7] Some claimed that their religious scruples inhibited them. Others found long courtships exhausting. The sexual double-standard could incapacitate the promiscuous. If a man had used public women he might either accumulate guilt that would make it impossible to perform with an "innocent" woman or he might mistakenly expect her to be as responsive as a prostitute.

Doctors believed that it was their duty to reassure grooms that the respectable bride had no particular expectations and would accept whatever treatment was offered her. Perhaps the most famous description of the modest woman's lack of sexual needs was provided by the English doctor William Acton. In 1857 Acton reported that he was daily asked by young men worried about marriage. Foolish ideas occasionally led grooms to flee. They were relieved when told that "the well-brought-up English maiden knows absolutely little or nothing on these matters." Acton went on to assure husbands they should not worry if they were temporarily impotent and only able to have sexual relations with their wives from time to time. Most women would prefer to have no sex at all. A woman's complete lack of sexual feeling was blameworthy, but Acton stressed that many women could never be fully aroused. Men might have got the wrong idea by consorting with prostitute-like working-class girls with uncontrolled passions. "As a general rule, a modest woman seldom desires any sexual gratification for herself. She submits to her husband, but only to please him; and, but for the desire of maternity, would far rather be relieved from his attentions. No nervous or feeble young man need, therefore, be deterred from marriage by any exaggerated notion of the duties required from him. The married woman has no wish to be treated on the footing of a mistress."[8]

Almost all doctors agreed that married women were not as libidinous as their spouses. At the end of the century Acton's words were echoed by a colleague, exasperated by some men's fears of disappointing their brides: "It is difficult to impress on such minds as these with such a standard of marriage and 'its duties,' that their wives are not as educated as themselves in these matters, that they will be glad enough to be spared from excesses, and that to look upon them as being as expectant as themselves is to place them on a level but little higher than that of a harlot." According to Harry Campbell, the woman could best be considered an "undeveloped man," and therefore more prone to hysteria and lower sexual desires. Sex after pregnancy was redundant for woman but, since she was passive, it was not injurious. Indeed he reported it was not uncommon to find a happy couple in which the husband was totally impotent. Physician R. W. Shufeldt recalled that he instructed the pretty spouse of one young husband "to inform him shortly after retiring for the night, that she did not especially care whether he was ever able to do his duty or not, and that she was quite willing to remain a maid for life for all that she cared to the contrary."[9] With that calming knowledge and two and a half bottles of beer at bedtime, the husband was suitably prepared.

Men were told that they were not to be disappointed by the female who was not overly responsive. Her absolute frigidity would, however, be naturally off-putting. Acton castigated as "selfish" those women who made their distaste for intercourse known. Robert Ultzmann reported that "relative impotence" was common in arranged marriages. "Book-worms" and intellectuals, he reported, were especially sensitive and "can do it only when the woman willingly yields herself." [10] He thereby implied some were unwilling. Eugene Fuller, a New York doctor, disagreed with the psychological explanations of impotence and instead insisted that most problems were "located in the sexual apparatus." Nevertheless Fuller did concede that grooms brooded over their coming test and even married men might flop.

> This is usually the result of some incompatibility, the fault lying with the wife. The author has in mind an extreme case illustrating this condition. A very nervous man of thirty-six sought advice for sexual weakness such as has been described. He had been married about five years, and for a time had experienced no difficulty in performing the sexual act, and had, in fact, impregnated his wife. His wife, however, apparently had no feminine instincts. She experienced no pleasure from the sexual act; in fact she thought it vulgar and unbecoming, submitting to it only as being part of the marital contract. When her husband was in the midst of his sexual attempts she frequently essayed to divert her mind by reading, asking him from time to time if he were through. The result was at first a marked dampening in the sexual enthusiasm of the husband, followed later by a weakness so marked as to be little short of impotency. [11]

Doctors critiqued such untaught, thoughtless, passive, cold, and tactless wives, insisting they learn how to respond or at least pretend to respond to their partners' overtures. As early as 1841, R. J. Culverwell stated that many male patients were too respectful of their spouses and then called on the latter to be more exciting. "Many women, moving in a respectable sphere of life, have the idea that it is unbecoming and indecorous to meet the embraces of their husbands, or to shew any solicitude in the matter; thus directly opposing the dictates of nature, and setting themselves in opposition to one of the main purposes for which they were created." Suggestions that wives show more enthusiasm increased as the century wore on. A man of the world reported to U.S. physician William Hammond that once married he was incapacitated "at the thought that it was a profanation for a man like him to subject so beautiful and pure a woman to such an animal relation as sexual intercourse." He was fine with an old mistress but failed with his wife. "'She was too good, too delicate for a mere animal like him,' he told Hammond, 'he could not desecrate her beautiful body by any such vile act.'" Hammond's response was to instruct the wife to play the vamp. In another

American case Shufeldt reported that a patient was similarly rendered impotent: "At the very thought of such a dissipated reveler as he has been having intercourse with that sweet girl is sufficient to completely defeat his intentions." Shufeldt recommended that the wife act the part of the "little wicked scapegrace," who was "going to have her way, and that right now."[12] Almost without exception, Shufeldt reported, such stratagems cured husbands of their complaints. Commentators agreed that whatever a woman did or did not feel, her duty was to follow the man's lead.

Doctors were divided over the question of how sexually responsive a respectable woman should be. Pierre Garnier noted that some men mistakenly interpreted woman's "natural prudishness and reserve as indifference and frigidity." If such coolness inhibited the man he should be told that the woman "tastes the surplus voluptuous feelings more in her heart and soul. The normal role of women during copulation is much more moral than physical. Otherwise it would only be an unequal battle between unequal organs." Victorian medical texts presented women not as passionless, but as sexually dormant, needing to be aroused by a partner. Women were caught in a double bind. The respectable had been educated to believe that, no matter what they felt, they were not to be as passionate as men. If the groom feared he was insufficiently assertive, the bride dreaded humiliation by the revelation of her shameful appetite. By demanding a degree of sexual moderation, middle-class women protected their reputations without denying the importance of sex. Moreover those who wanted to limit their fertility might have been purposefully unresponsive. Some continued to believe in the old theory that mutual orgasms were needed for conception, a belief that was cited by writers such as J. Marion Sims, George Napheys, and Alice Stockham.[13]

Women's frigidity and men's impotence were believed by some to be the price to be paid for fertility control. In the eighteenth century, manhood was still inextricably linked to the ability to reproduce. This began to change in the nineteenth century, which witnessed a dramatic decline in birth rates, first in France and the United States, and then in England. Even the opponents of artificial means of family limitation recognized the disadvantages of excessively large broods. Following Malthus, many commentators recommended delaying marriage, and after marriage some form of abstinence no doubt served as birth control for numerous couples. Acton, for example, recommended that coitus be limited in married life during pregnancies and while the wife was nursing. Seeking to spare women unwanted pregnancies, the first feminists also played a significant role in calling for sexual moderation. The fertility decline was due in short, not to mechanical methods of contraception but to either coitus interruptus and/or abstinence, both of which required a good deal of male self-control. Because rubber goods were expensive, regarded as disreputable, and not mentioned in respectable public discourse, they were not widely used.

The older model of masculinity that held virility measurable by procreation was now challenged by one that esteemed restraint, willpower, and a reasonable number of offspring. As early as the 1820s a few public defenders of contraception, including Richard Carlile and Francis Place, appeared in England. They argued that a real man could control himself. Sexuality and reproduction were split. The notion that manhood was proven by siring children did not, of course, disappear. Impotence at the beginning of century was still associated with failure to reproduce. According to William Buchan, "there is no idea more depressing to the human mind than that of not being able to propagate the species." Indeed the appearance of small families could also be taken as a sign that husbands were losing power. Many doctors pointed to declining fertility as an indication that men were bowing to women's desires. Louis Seraine noted in 1865 that the purpose of marrying had always been to have children, but in an age of decadence and corruption women no longer wanted to be mothers. Given that so many tried to avoid children, one had to honor those who still wanted to follow nature's law. The birth rate dropped most dramatically in France and resulted in an outpouring of books on possible causes. Was the drop in fertility voluntary? Pessimists insisted on attributing the fall—which became so preoccupying after 1870—to declining potency. This was a circular argument because the same people also insisted that attempts at contraception caused impotency. In the United States Hammond noted that some women, as a contraceptive practice, "press during the act of sexual intercourse upon the urethra of the male just in front of the vera montanum in such a manner as to prevent the passage of semen through the canal, and cause it to be directed backward into the bladder." Eventually the man's body was broken to the habit and he was rendered both impotent and sterile. Even worse, some men wore "an India-rubber ring around the penis" to similarly prevent ejaculation.[14] Hammond said he knew of three cases in which the result was sterility. Cassandras thus sought to frighten men with reports that any attempt to limit fertility could undermine their virility.

The most widely employed method of birth control was withdrawal or coitus interruptus. Commonly known as conjugal onanism, its detractors claimed it would have the same debilitating effects as masturbation. Indeed in the United States, Charles Knowlton provided both birth control information and suggestions on how to counter impotency. As sedentary habits and sexual excesses led to exhaustion, he recommended "tincture of flies, bark, preparations of iron, cold bath, exercise, and employment that will, if possible, divert the mind, &c." Critics claimed that the chief danger of birth control was that it led to sexual excesses. The health reformer Sylvester Graham noted the spread of "works pretending to teach how pregnancy may be avoided, and thus encouraging illicit commerce." The fact that quacks included on their list of dangerous excesses those made possible by employing coitus interruptus, indicates how common the practice was. The French translation of R. and L. Perry and Company's *Silent Friend* (1847) singled out excesses due to conjugal onanism. Of all forms of unnatural coitus, withdrawal was, for George M. Beard, the worse. F. R. Sturgis in *Sexual Debility in Men* (1901) stated that though the condom did not pose a problem, impotence could be caused by excesses allowed by coitus interruptus. And after noting that masturbation was a primary cause of neurasthenia, Richard Ebbard stated that the exhaustion from the excesses of coitus interruptus could lead to impotence, irritations, and premature ejaculation. One failure then sowed doubts that led to future bedroom fiascoes.[15] In a variety of ways the notion of restricting family size posed men with new and possibly daunting challenges. They were lauded for their self control, but warned that the very form of contraception that demanded it the most—coitus interruptus—could cause impotence.

While women's revulsion of male desire was blamed for impotence, women's sexual demand was, interestingly, just as culpable for destroying a man's virility. The same doctors who bewailed women's apathy went on to say that men were even more threatened if the woman was overdemanding. Popular culture was a repository of old tales of sexually insatiable women and exhausted men. Although in the middle classes a new prudery emerged in the nineteenth century, there was still evidence of strong folk beliefs in the need for sexual release. Jokes continued to be told about aged lechers. For example, "piss-proud" was defined by an early nineteenth-century dictionary of "buckish slang" as "having a false erection," so said of any old fellow who married a young woman. Class differences in attitudes toward sexuality were sustained. The essayist William Hazlitt was shocked to hear his landlady talking to her daughter about penis size. In the working class, charges of impotence were flung as sexual insults as in the case of a man who screamed at his neighbor "I have bull'd thy wife. . . . Yes, damn thee I've fucked her scores of times, and she's fetched me to fuck her when thy pillock wouldn't stand."[16] The slandering of a man by claiming he was impotent was a common strategy of defamation in England. Until the elimination of the ecclesiastical courts in 1855 such insults were officially reported.

The provocative figure of the sexually demanding woman appeared in off-color songs. *The Ri-tum Ti-Tum Songster* (1837) contained a number of smutty tunes including "The Blue Bells of Ireland," which concerned a woman wanting beet root, "nine inches & no more." Many of the other songs were about women's desire for a penis as in "The New Rolling Pin," while "He'll No More Grind Again" portrayed the fate of the man who was past it. The same publisher brought out in 1865 *The Rambler's Flash Songster* with suggestive ditties about the butcher's cock, Rory's shillelagh, and so on. In such pieces as "The Female Tobacconist; or, You Will Come for Some Shagg," the women were always presented as eager. Indeed in "John Anderson, My Jo" (a bawdy version of the Burns classic) the woman laments her man's decline, warning that if he doesn't act he will have horns. A physical problem like impotence was even thought fit for comic turns in the late nineteenth-century British music hall. As in seventeenth-century ballads, in the music hall songs women were often presented as sexually active, singing about men failing to satisfy their desires and using the possibility of cuckoldry (with a lodger or cousin) to deflate and debunk authority. Across the channel, saucy French songs also revealed a world of male sociability and bawdy humor. Their stock figures included masturbating priests, licentious nuns, and incompetent men seeking any form of arousal. Clear concerns for impotence were reflected in the songs' exaggerated machismo. Such proverbs as "One cock satisfies ten chickens, but ten men don't satisfy one woman" revealed that in the French countryside, women's desires were still recognized.[17]

Though medical literature failed to acknowledge women's sexual needs in the early nineteenth century, the topic surreptitiously reemerged in discussions of impotence. By 1857 Acton even worried that the mother-in-law would tell the bride what she should expect on her wedding night. With the passing of the decades, impotence was increasingly attributed to demanding women. Doctors warned men that a hypersexual woman could exhaust them. A man's single failure could psychologically wound him. The frustrated woman might mock her spouse, which, protested Auguste Debay, was a terrible offense. The man's health was also at risk. John Cowan warned that there were some passionate and diseased women with lustful natures who reduced men to the status of brutes and eventually destroyed them. He accordingly warned against marrying widows whose spouses had died mysteriously, darkly suggesting that "these sensualists were murderers." Léon Roger-Milès in 1893 compared the woman who had lived on her own and was experienced to the virgin. The former physically and morally was just like a man. She was not surprised by marriage, while the latter was dazzled when exposed to "the great mystery." She is "amazed; the other compares. This one loves; the other judges." Robert Taylor singled out American women as especially demanding. "In America the unnatural prolongation of coitus (for the alleged reason of greater gratification to the female) is very often the cause of a more or less persistent form of atonic impotence, and also of neurasthenia."[18]

The overly demanding woman not only harmed her husband, she failed to be fertile. Sexual excesses caused sterility, thus the newly married were, said many doctors, necessarily barren. Debay asserted that sterile women, known by their long clitoris and large pupils, seemed to devour men with their eyes and invite them to "erotic combats." The numerous late nineteenth-century horror stories of Stoker, Kipling, and Haggard which presented women as vampires—the mouth replacing the genitals—clearly tapped into these fears of men being drained of their vital fluids.[19]

The husband, as the rational partner, had the responsibility to determine how often conjugal intercourse would occur, rationing resources according to his health and happiness. But what of the woman's happiness? Prudish doctors carefully avoided the old notion that the unsatisfied wife might take a lover, a troubling prospect that quacks, who hoped to profit by the creation of anxieties, happily played up. Dr. Kahn warned "no woman is so likely to go astray as one who is tantalized by the abortive toying of an impotent husband." In Kahn's scenario the husband, though injured, was the actual guilty party. For William H. Parker as well, a woman was necessarily scornful of the impotent man. According to Albert Hayes, the nuptial bed of the impotent man was "a scene of blended mortification, disgust, disappointment, and suppressed anger; and it is now that the mistaken bride is made to feel herself the victim of previous sensuality,—the poor, deceived last hope of vigor,—anxious for offspring, yet baffled from day to day, in the arms of the man she has vowed at the altar to love and honor." If she fell for a seducer, Hayes warned, "her offence is not altogether without palliation."[20]

The seducer could even be another woman. In his discussion of inversion in women, Richard von Krafft-Ebing, the Austrian psychiatrist, noted it could be situational as in cases of "wives of impotent husbands who can only sexually excite, but not satisfy, woman, thus producing in her *libido insatiata* [unsatisfied desire], recourse to masturbation, *pollutiones feminae* [pollutions of a woman], neurasthenia, nausea for coitus and ultimately disgust with the male sex in general." Prostitutes disgusted by demands of their impotent customers were, investigators claimed, also led on to same sex desires. The obvious intent of such claims was to insist that women were not led into same-sex relations as a result of any positive desire, but rather driven into them by incompetent men.[21]

Medical reports reveal that, in addition to their passions, women's very physicality could incapacitate some middle-class men. One is reminded that John Ruskin, Lewis Carroll, and J. M. Barrie represented the sort of Victorians who had a marked penchant for prepubescent girls but were frightened by grown women. Sensitive men, stated Frederick Hollick, were rendered impotent because they were too idealistic: "They are ignorant of the real physical and moral nature of the being they take to their bosoms, and have formed a picture of her in the imagination very different from the reality, so that when the truth is known their feelings undergo a complete revulsion. This ignorance sometimes extends to the most ordinary functional phenomena of the female system, and the first knowledge even of that has, to my own knowledge, produced a very disagreeable and lasting effect."[22] The privacy that the Victorians so treasured made it quite likely that the sexual ignorance of both middle-class men and women was greater in the 1800s than it had been in the 1700s.

One can appreciate that poor hygiene, filthy clothing, and rudimentary sanitary facilities might well have also acted as a brake on lust. What is striking is that though in previous centuries the occasional claim was made that a man was put off by his partner's appearance, in the nineteenth century when standards of cleanliness were raised, so too were the numbers of references to men who claimed to be nauseated by the smelly, ugly or unclean female body. Such assertions in part reflected the internalization of new notions of sexual hygiene, an example of what Foucault referred to as one of the bodily forms of discipline. Doctors assured nervous men that normal women would not find their sexual requests disgusting, but they conceded that many men would be incapacitated by slovenly females. Women were thus again blamed for men's impotence. Frederick Hollick noted the newly married man could be disgusted at discovering his spouse's false hair or false teeth. Ryan asserted that a man could be hindered in his sexual activities by an "aversion from filth, odour, and preoccupations of the mind." The Italian physician Paolo Mantegazza conceded that hypochondriacs were put off by smells. According to Thomas Laycock, the "abhorrence of sexual union" was the result of sexual excesses, felt especially by the man and less often by the woman. Such revulsion frequently led to the breakup of older marriages.[23]

Doctors went further. Taylor noted one could be put off by the woman's discharges or a "flabby vulva, or a very large vagina." A French physician warned women that with age came the man's disgust for fat, fetid genitals: "Now, women whose body demands so much attention for cleanliness, must ceaselessly sustain a rose-like freshness with which to decorate the portal of the temple of pleasure." A colleague seconded this demand for feminine hygiene, asserting that marriages could be blighted by "woman's bed-bugginess."[24]

Indulging in the crudest misogyny, Shufeldt claimed that middle-class men would be rendered impotent by the sort of woman whom working men might accept.

> A woman may be as pubescent as a Macaque ape, or forever giving way to her auto-erotic desires, or her vaginal secretions might be as acid as aquaregia, or she might when passionately excited have the odor of a long defunct equus, or she might be as passionless as a sack of sand, or she might be as debauched and foul-mouthed as the most abandoned grisette in Paris, and it would be all one to any representative of the last-named class. Not so, however, with the more sensitive and refined among us, for in them any one of these peculiarities, even in their milder manifestations, becomes intolerable, and when confronted upon the nuptial bed with his life-chosen partner in whom any one or several of them may be discovered to be present, an instantaneous revolution of the emotion first takes place, and is promptly followed by a revolt of the powers of virility.[25]

Few nineteenth-century doctors were as misogynistic as Shufeldt. He claimed that often women had acidic secretions (usually due to prolonged masturbation) that caused men's impotency. If these men were middle aged, their impotency could become permanent. "Divorce frequently follows such mismatings, and then comes the breaking up of the home, the *persecution of the man*, and the acceptance of perjured testimony on the part of the ignorant courts to 'settle the case.'" Shufeldt lamented that lawyers were generally unaware of the difference between sterility and impotency and of "the extent to which autoeroticism is practiced by old maids, much less do they know anything of its consequences."[26]

In hindsight, the inability of some men to perform sexually with women might be read as an indication of male homosexuality. Such linkages were not explicitly made until the late nineteenth century. The discussion of impotence nevertheless played a key role in sorting out men into different sexual camps. Doctors began to attribute similar features to both the homosexual and the impotent. They noted some men were so effeminate that their impotence was impossible to cure. James Richard Smyth, gave an account of such a type in 1841.

> The body is generally delicate, rounded, and rather feminine in form; the muscles and cellular structure are soft, weak, and lax, and the gait in conse-

quence wants the firmness and elasticity which are the accompaniments of strength and vigour. The hair is soft and fine, and deficient on the face and pubes; the voice is weak, sharp and shrill; the eyes are dull, watery, of a light colour, and devoid of fire and animation; the manners are capricious and boyish; the circulation is weak and languid, and the secretions scanty and imperfect; the testicles are small and soft, and sometimes retracted towards the abdominal ring, showing a disposition to return to their primitive foetal position in the abdomen, and the scrotum pendulous.[27]

The phrenologist O. S. Fowler asserted that "light-built, fine-skinned, fine-haired, spare-built, sharp-featured, light-eyed persons" were most at risk from sexual excesses. Loss of vitality resulted, which "impares the manliness of the male and the femineness of the female." In France Debay agreed that the stigmata of the impotent male was light blond hair, a hairless body, soft flesh, and lack of energy.[28]

With other patients the inability to copulate with a woman was not a physical but a psychological problem. Absence of heterosexual desire was not uncommonly reported. James G. Kiernan described how disappointment in normal love could lead first to impotence and then to inversion. "If this disappointment should produce, as it often does, a shock causing nervous prostration, the stability of the 'ego' would be upset and the foundation laid for the creation of a parasitic 'ego.'" At the same time, if the circumstances of the disappointment not only created the belief of the worthlessness of one woman, but of women in general, "a repugnance would be created which would materially aid in development of the parasitic ego." In contrast to such acquired inversion, came reports of more deep-seated forms. Hammond described a patient who wanted to marry yet found intercourse impossible. "I saw no way of doing this, however, unless it might be possible for him to accomplish the sexual act notwithstanding the disgust, the faintness, the nausea and vomiting." One of Hammond's patients assiduously attempted to find women arousing, reading pornographic novels, buying obscene paintings, and visiting prostitutes. Nothing worked. Indeed in the midst of his therapy he confessed to having "committed pederasty eleven times before morning" with a hotel bell-boy. He was so ashamed of his actions that he contemplated suicide. In Jean Lorrain's novel *Monsieur de Phocas* (1901), the central character is impotent with women but highly aroused when gazing on the marble statue of Antinoüs in the Louvre. Exactly the same scenario was described by Hammond, who treated a patient sexually excited by nude male statues but repelled by women. "He was advised to make the intellectual effort of substituting a woman for a man in the crises to which he was subject." Though cold showers and bromides helped diminish his patient's desires, Hammond had to conclude that this was "a true instance of sexual perversion, and of consequent impotence so far as concerns the female sex." Amongst the impotent F. R. Sturgis also included those with a distaste for women and a liking for males. He noted these "perverts" were not lacking in intelligence. Their mores had been accepted in the ancient world but were no longer. He had to admit it was hard to cure such men's preferences for males; they were wedded to their idols.[29]

The apparent entanglement of impotence and same-sex desires drew the attention of late nineteenth-century psychiatrists. Alfred Binet coined the term "fetish" to describe the fact that in an age of enfeeblement, some individuals needed special types of excitation if they were to be able to perform sexually. A sort of "psychic impotence" was reflected in such individuals' obsession with a particular article of clothing or style of shoe they found arousing. Hammond reported a number of patients who required a certain type of woman or fetish to be fully potent. Some trifle could likewise instantly render such men impotent. Binet regarded inversion as a form of fetishism, which resulted from the imprinting of an early sexual experience. In his eyes fetishists and homosexuals were not truly impotent since they did have orgasms, albeit from abnormal acts. Paolo Mantegazza agreed, playfully likening homosexuality to a grammatical fault: "Because you are putting in the masculine / What should only be put in the feminine. (Car vous mettez au masculin / Ce qu'on ne met qu'au féminin)."[30]

Jean-Martin Charcot, Valentin Magnan, Richard Krafft-Ebing and the other early catalogers of deviance tended to target homosexuality as the most obvious evidence of a weakened male sex drive. "Manliness and self reliance are not," asserted Krafft-Ebing in his classic *Psychopathia Sexualis* (1885), the qualities which adorn the impotent onanist." He went on to state that "the sudden loss of virile powers often produces melancholia, or is the cause of suicide when life without love is a mere blank. In cases where the reaction is less pronounced, the victim is morose, peevish, egotistical, jealous, narrow-minded, cowardly, devoid of energy, self-respect and honour."[31]

A number of doctors claimed that impotence and homosexuality—both symptoms of a failure of the will—could be treated by hypnotism. Some cases of perversion and erotic excesses, Kiernan stated, were controllable by autosuggestion and by the other treatments offered for neurasthenia. He commonly encountered men who, as a consequence of living in an overcivilized world plagued with a surfeit of sexually suspect books and plays, suffered from defective willpower. The doctor had to harp on the morbidity of the patient's perverted ideas, prohibit him from reading arousing literature, and subject him to psychic therapy and anaphrodisiacs. Hippolyte Bernheim was unusually sympathetic, to "genital inversion," which, along with impotence, he linked to autosuggestion. He believed the invert's "ideas against nature" were instinctive and said he knew of many examples of moral, honorable people who had such obsessions since childhood. These people could not be cured, but suggestion could help them to resist their obsession. He added that instincts "against nature" were not always indicative of a perverse nature; they could be independent of the will and compatible with a perfect moral sense.[32] Those most hostile to homosexuality assumed that it was the last resort of the weak or impotent; investigators like Bernheim held just the opposite view, that because a man was homosexual, he could not be potent with women.

If more men had trouble in dealing with women's sexual demands, argued late nineteenth-century commentators, it was because many had already been exhausted by the stresses of modern life. Doctors had long labeled as hysterics women who were incapacitated by their nervous preoccupations. In the late nineteenth century, men who suffered from psychological and physical breakdowns were said to be suffering from neurasthenia. George M. Beard, an American doctor, first began speaking on the nervousness brought on by the demands of the urban world in the late 1860s. Neurasthenia was a vague malady with range of symptoms, the most important being a loss of nervous energy accompanied by somatic consequences. Nervousness in the eighteenth century had been attributed to physical causes. Neurasthenia was said to be due to psychological pressures and was a socially acceptable diagnosis inasmuch as it was gender and class specific. Doctors labeled women and working-class men as hysterics, middle-class men as neurasthenics. And to make the diagnosis even more palatable doctors claimed that many geniuses, like Herbert Spencer and Jean-Jacques Rousseau, were irritable neurasthenics.[33]

Doctors asserted that neurasthenia was a symptom of overcivilization. White middle-class men were challenged by the unremitting demands of urban life and heady, bourgeois occupations. Romanticizing a lost artisanal world, writers like Beard lamented the rise of an impersonal bureaucratic society. Its chief victim was the "brain worker" as distinguished from the "muscle worker." The former, ground down by mental strain and overwork, needed help. With higher professional standards and greater pressure in schools, nervousness, brain diseases, and insanity, the doctors argued, were bound to increase . The moralistic bewailed the emasculating effects of urban life with its stresses, perversions, and degeneration. And yet as Georg Simmel noted in *Philosophy of Money* (1900), many individuals found such forbidden fruit irresistible. In the modern city the individual experienced tensions and longings, restlessness and urgency. Such unsatisfied desires, he argued, were due to the artificiality of a society based on a money economy, its extreme objectification, and its incitement of desires for ever new attractions. Overexcited nerves were a cause and effect of the modern world. The popularizers of neurasthenia stressed the psychological basis of exhaustion. Overcivilization was the predisposing cause, but the precipitating shock that toppled a man could be an accident, the reception of bad news, a sexual fiasco. One American doctor attributed diminished excitability to masturbation, sexual excesses, spinal diseases and drugs, and added "the constant jarring of railway trains (of which I have seen several examples in railway employés and travelling men) probably belongs in this category."[34]

Freud would later claim that he had been the first to attribute neurasthenia to repression of sexual life, but the linkage of nervousness with impotence and other male sexual problems was made much earlier. In *American Nervousness* (1881) Beard said of nervous men that "there is no force enough left in them to reproduce the species or go through the process of reproducing the species." What had been earlier regarded as signs of white, manly self-restraint were now taken as signs of exhaustion and effeminacy. In his posthumously published *Sexual Neurasthenia* (1884), Beard presented sexual lassitude as a key form of exhaustion. The wide variety of male genital debilities—impotence, spermatorrhoea, and prostrate problems—were due to a complex mix of evil habits, alcohol, tobacco, and worry, according to Beard. An American doctor noted in 1894 that terror could cause impotence. "A matter of fact bearing on this point is the experience of army officers, who have observed that a man of weak sexual instinct is always a poor soldier." Curiously enough, a World War I text on malingering asserted that "some men allege falsely loss of sexual power" (or perhaps thought they had) as a result of industrial accidents. The authors concluded that most were in fact neurasthenics and that mental weakness was the main factor in their impotence.[35]

Beard noted that doctors usually did not take the sexual histories of their male patients and those who had worries were often as not dismissed as hypochondriacs. Women used to be fobbed off as hysterics, but now gynecologists recognized that they had real complaints. Similarly Beard argued that male sexual symptoms warranted serious investigation. The importance of neurasthenia was that in attributing impotence to the stresses of the modern world, it allowed middle-class men a legitimate way to admit to their sexual problems. According to C. H. F. Routh, "loss of virile power" was an "ugly symptom" of decay. In counseling against late marriages and men attempting to become fathers after fifty, S. A. K. Strahan warned that the modern artificial, feverish life aided disease and degeneration. Ludwig Biswanger reported that his male patients loved "to observe their sexual emotions and sexual life meticulously, to brood about it, and then to ask their doctors whether or not their sexual functions conformed to the norm." Although such self-absorption obviously irritated Biswanger, he instructed his students that their first duty was to calm and reassure those who sought medical treatment. The doctors' chief advice to neurasthenics was to lead more balanced lives. One American physician complained: "There is a good deal of sexual indifference, and consequently of impotence, existing among men whose whole heart and soul are in exciting business occupations requiring all their mental energy and consequently leaving nothing for the mere animal passions." They only turned to their doctor when their businesses failed and then it was too late. A French doctor reported that hyperexcitability was often followed by impotence, but only the latter was complained of.[36]

Impotence, most commentators assumed, was a Western menace. "A sensitive sexual organization is part of the price man has paid for civilization," wrote Chicago doctor G. Frank Lydston. "The more refined the organization of the human rule, the more likely he is to suffer from impotence due to psychic impressions. Laying aside organic causes, the savage and lower animals do not experience impotence. The human male who can perform the sexual act under any and all environmental conditions probably is an example of atavism, where—exceptionally—it does not prove neuropychic degeneracy. The commission of rape, in the author's opinion, is sure evidence of atavism." The intertwining of sexual and racial preoccupations was to be expected in an age of imperialism. In the United States racial anxieties increasingly framed sexual discussions following the Civil War. Fear of their own incompetence led whites to portray blacks as hypersexual. "Stronger pigmentation in the sexual organs is generally accompanied by greater capacity in venery, which in fact is seen in Negroes, who are, as a rule, endowed with large genitals," claimed Victor Vecki. "The well-known rule that brown-haired men usually have more sexual power than light-haired ones is admissible only in the comparison of men of the same race."[37]

In Europe neurasthenia and impotence were said to be caused by the stresses of civilization, but in colonies by the distance of whites *from* civilization. To justify the imperial ambitions of the virile West, Europeans frequently portrayed the Orient as sexually exhausted. Doctors warned Americans and Europeans that only through their willpower could they avoid the fate of the East. On the one hand, pornographic classics such as *The Lustful*

Turk (1829) asserted that in the Levant men were allowed to give vent to every passion. On the other hand, a literature that began with Montesquieu's *Lettres persanes* (1721) held that the hotter climate and the availability of compliant harem girls ultimately rendered the men of the Middle East impotent. One medical dictionary gave an example of sexual exhaustion from excess specific to "the despotic countries of the East." Hayes insisted every loss of sperm led to enervation, citing the decline of the Ottoman Empire as proof. Shifting the focus to South Asia, Taylor agreed "that in the East Indies there is scarcely a virile man over twenty-five years of age. The sexual decay in these men is due to the practice of long-protracted coitus." "The sexual preoccupations [of individuals] are often in inverse ratio to their sexual powers," asserted Charles Féré. "Nations that perish through sterility are remarkable for their licentiousness." In the East, opium was believed to exacerbate fatigue. "The slow weakening of the genesic functions, both from the psychic point of view—desire, sensibility, sensual pleasures—and from the physical point of view—physiology and sensations—leads inevitably to impotence. . . . This genital degradation [lack of erection and inability to ejaculate] has been preceded by the disappearance of sexual desires." [38] This observer's fear was that French colonialists, weakened by climate and drugs, their passions declining and their desire for women curbed, could end up as impotent sodomites.

Doctors noted that in cases of psychological impotence suffered by white middle-class men, the mind inhibited the body. Patients reported feeling irritable, timid, fearful, sad, dejected, and exhausted. Some men were simply apathetic, others were out of practice. Kindly advice and encouragement sufficed with some, for others attempts had to be made to strengthen their will. Rest was prescribed as the main cure though some doctors offered tonics, electrotherapy, and hydrotherapy. [39] The importance of neurasthenia lay in it offering weak men a new language, a new way of framing their suffering, and a new way of exculpating themselves. It held that rather than being ridiculed, they deserved care and sympathy.

Obviously only a small proportion of the population read medical texts. Would readers of fiction find similar discussions? Among respectable Victorians, impotence was supposedly a tabooed, unmentionable subject. For that very reason, in France at least, the issue was broached by self-consciously daring writers of fiction. It provided yet another means to prove one was not bourgeois. Just when George M. Beard was lamenting the emergence of the overcivilized neurasthenic urban male, French decadents from Baudelaire to Huysmans perversely embraced impotence as a metaphor for both sensitivity and cultural exhaustion. Neurasthenia itself was not always viewed completely negatively; some saw it as a price paid for creativity and refinement. Impotence likewise came to be viewed ambivalently. In the last decades of the nineteenth century the themes of real and metaphorical impotence, along with nervousness and irritability were intertwined by the masters of decadent art.

In England and America, a few authors dealt obliquely with the issue of impotence by portraying villains as unmanly—and therefore unsympathetic—characters. In *The Scarlet Letter* (1850) Hawthorne presents the aptly named Roger Chillingworth as an impotent, old cuckolded spouse. In *Middlemarch* (1872) George Eliot implies that Causabon and Dorothea's marriage is barren as the unlikable Casaubon is a dried up, impotent chronicler of the past. In *Bleak House* (1852) Charles Dickens similarly portrayed Sir Leicester Dedlock—twenty years older than his bored, childless wife. Writers were more daring in France where the pessimistic and morbid Baudelaire was frequently credited with having turned literature toward the discussion of perverse sexualities. In fact, even earlier romantic writers had shifted attention away from the eighteenth-century libertine to the nineteenth-century man of sentiment and then to the melancholic. Women readers came to find the sensitive, moody male character more seductive than his boisterous competitors. Provocative writers saw how impotence could be portrayed as a symptom of the sensitive youth out of place in a philistine world.[40]

Olivier ou le secret (1822), the first nineteenth-century novel that tackled the issue of marital impotence, was written by a woman, Claire de Duras, and based on fact. In 1818 the marriage of the marquis de Custine to the youngest daughter of Claire de Duras was broken off when it was revealed that he was impotent. In the brief novel, Olivier adores but cannot possess Louise; honor prevents him from revealing the secret that he hopes she will discover. The story concludes with Olivier conveniently dying of fever.[41] The significance of Duras's novel was that it inspired Stendhal to produced the most famous nineteenth-century literary account of impotence—*Armance* (1827). In that novel, Octave successfully frequents prostitutes, but with his bride Armance he finds himself incapable. Though they have a few weeks of happiness, Octave worries that Armance's pleasure is feigned. He leaves for Greece, pretends to fall ill, and commits suicide.

Stendhal was so cautious in telling his tale that many did not understand what it was about. In a letter to Prosper Mérimée dated December 23, 1826, he crudely explained why Armance could be happy with such a spouse: "Olivier, like all Babilans, is quite an expert on the auxiliary methods in which *le Président* glories. A deft hand and an officious tongue would have given Armance keen sensations of pleasure. I am sure many girls have no precise notion what physical marriage consists of. I am equally certain about this second and much more frequent case: *the consummation of marriage is repulsive to them for three or four years*, particularly when they are tall, pale, slim, and blessed with a fashionable waistline." Stendhal went on to say he felt he had no option but to kill off his fictional hero. "The genuine Babilan must kill himself in order to avoid the embarrassment of making a confession. As for me (but at the age of forty-three years eleven months), I should make a beautiful confession, and I should be told: *What of it?* I should take my wife to Rome. There a handsome countryman, at a cost of one sequin, would pay her three compliments in one night." Stendhal looked forward to the day when such scenarios could be openly described. "In 2826, if civilization continues and I come back to the Rue Duphot, I shall relate how Olivier bought himself a fine Portuguese *dildo* made of Indian rubber, which he attached to his own belt, and with which, after giving his wife one complete ecstasy, and another almost *complete* ecstasy, he bravely consummated his marriage in the Rue du Paradis, Marseilles."[42]

Stendhal might not have been joking since while frequenting brothels he had experienced his own bouts of impotence; the notion that he would exhaust himself became a fixation. A small and sickly man, he claimed to have "compensated" women he failed to pleasure in the expected manner. In 1819–1820 he produced a short chapter on "fiascoes" for his study *De l'amour*. The gist of his argument was that the more excessive a man's love, the more likely he would be to fail on the first occasion.[43]

For many nineteenth-century writers, potency was still equated to creativity. Prosper Mérimée, who had a fiasco with George Sand, fearing his weakness would be discovered, paraded his mistresses and his visits to brothels. Balzac portrayed inventiveness as a masculine prerogative reflective of man's virility, and thus in his *Massimilla Doni* (1837) the hero's impotence—referred to as "noble malady which strikes only the very young and the old"—results in the loss of his artistic abilities. Fifty years later, Emile Zola in *La Bête humaine* (1890) has the old roué and rapist Grandmorin reduced to having young girls service him, whereas in *Germinal* (1885) the middle class marvel at the fecundity of the workers. Even a decadent like Jean Lorrain would disparage his rival Paul Bourget by calling him "impotent."[44]

Yet reacting against what they took to be the crassness of contemporary mass democratic society, a number of late nineteenth-century French writers were drawn to the themes of ineptitude, decadence, and failure. Their novels were studded with references to the pathological, the psychosomatic, and the sterile. Many were impressed by the earlier investigations of such themes by Edgar Allan Poe. According to the psychoanalyst Marie

Bonaparte, Poe—because he was impotent—had a penchant for littering his morbid tales with "impotence nightmares" in which the main character cannot succeed in what he attempts. Some said Poe was incapacitated by his opium habit; Bonaparte attributed his problem to his "necrophilist psyche."[45]

In France, the fin de siècle saw the emergence of what have been called "bachelor novels," works focusing on the solitary, sterile individual. The central character's lack of productivity was the key to the genre. The heroes of such decadent novels were usually thinkers or intellectuals, and therefore by definition not people of action. Authors such as Flaubert, Goncourt, Proust, and Barrès were all fixated on the literal and metaphoric impotence of such characters.

The curious embrace of impotence by the experimental as almost a badge of honor can be seen in the works of Gustave Flaubert. He reported that like many young Frenchmen he had to endure the voyeuristic and exhibitionistic rite of passage of being sexually initiated in a brothel. Such disgusting experiences with prostitutes and the incapacitating diseases they carried incited a generation of artists to pathologize female sexuality. Flaubert went on to produce *Sentimental Education* (1869), a novel of impotence that he described as an account of inactive passion. In exalting the strange and rare, vampires and hashish, poet Charles Baudelaire most popularized the notion of the artist's flight from a banal existence in *Fleurs du mal* (1861). For his lauding of sterile pleasures critics attacked him as impotent. Baudelaire was following a line set by the poet Théophile Gautier who had claimed that if Romeo had had access to hashish he would have forgotten Juliette, for the addict would not lift a finger for the most beautiful maiden in Verona. The decadents were interested in sexuality but refused its normal forms. Their antinaturalism led to their antifeminism, especially in the case of Baudelaire for whom woman represented animality, the body, and its demands. According to him man should only use woman or seek refuge in art. "The more a man cultivates the arts," he wrote, "the fewer erections he has." The old notion that the life of mind countered the demands of body was given new life. Thus Eugène Delacroix wrote Baudelaire that his sole mistresses were his paintings.[46]

Caught in the dilemma of being drawn irresistibly to women, but finding them contemptible, decadents could logically regard impotence as one solution. As Europeans were no longer living in a robust age, the poet Paul Verlaine thought it natural that decadence and impotence were inextricably linked. The hero of Jean Lorrain's *Monsieur de Phocas*—an opium user, homosexual, and sadist—is the model decadent, an impotent, only moved by the atrocious and monstrous. Even doctors contributed to the genre. The neurotic hero of Dr. Jacques de Nittis's *Vénus ennemie* (1900) is unable to love. He becomes a laughing stock, having desires but unable to act on them. By 1900 French publishers so expected to have tales of impotence submitted to them that when Alfred Vallette tried to publish his novel Monsieur Babylas—a story of an ordinary boring fellow—they imposed upon him the title *Le Vierge* (The male virgin).[47]

The decadents' interest in the flaccid penis could also at times take a comic turn. Frédéric Auguste Cazals had success with a satirical poem that portrayed exhausted poets seeking rejuvenation by consuming quack remedies. In *A Rebours* (1884), Joris-Karl Huysmans presented the hero giving a party for his defunct organ. And noting in his Paris diary his occasional bouts of impotence, the German playwright Frank Wedekind expressed a similar concern for his little friend. "Piccolo is docile as if he didn't exist," he wrote in July, 1889. "I can't think what's the matter with him. Whether he's reached the ultimate stage of development, or whether he will some time or other rise up in hitherto unsuspected glory." The fact that in youth a man's genitals resembled a "6" but in middle age a "9" was, according to Joseph Gérard, an unsolvable mathematical problem.[48]

If readers failed to miss the references to impotence in poems and novels, they were directed to them by reviewers. In his *Essais de psychologie contemporaine* Paul Bourget was extremely attentive to the evolution of what he called "la maladie du siècle." He cited Flaubert as having launched the chronicling of nervousness, impotence, and the growing debility of will in the civilized world. Octave Mirbeau, who purportedly hated both art nouveau and women, presents in *Dans le ciel* (1890) a character based on Van Gogh and Pissarro who says hideous shapes in painting are a sign of the current crisis of masculinity: "It's in order to mask my own impotence that I go looking for crazy forms that kill me, and you know, my young friend, they do kill me!" Hostile critics responded by asserting that if the decadents spoke so much about impotence it was in order to hide their lack of creativity behind a curtain of pretentious ideas and bizarre references. Some castigated them as boneless or "impuissants." In his assault on degenerate writers Max Nordau cited the English psychiatrist Maudsley in likening such artists to "borderland dwellers" who suffered from "moral insanity" driven by egoism and impulsiveness. Their emotionalism, their incapacity for action, was their stigmata. There is in fact ample evidence that the misogyny of many of the decadents was not a pose; Huysman was the classic example of a writer whose disparagement of sex with women is only fully understandable when seen in the context of the syphilis and impotence from which he suffered.[49]

Scathing denunciations of bourgeois marriage were followed by artists' exploration of a new range of sexual types—the lesbian, the androgyne, the invert. It has been noted that in England as in France a number of homosexual writers peopled their tales with heroes who, if they were not literally impotent, were haunted by a lack of fulfillment. "Many homosexual men of the time were so accustomed to frustration, through their own reticence or others', that they habitually valued contemplation (e.g., of the beloved) above activity, which was often associated with sex with a woman." One thinks of Henry James's chronicling of disappointments, of John Addington Symonds writing of his disillusionment after his wedding, and Oscar Wilde jesting about the "importance of doing nothing." Literary accounts lauding same-sex relations could not yet be produced, but portrayals of weak men and powerful women were acceptable. A number of decadents went on from flaunting their indifference toward women to portraying them as a frightening lower species. Edmond de Goncourt confided to his journal in 1883 that he had dreamt of a dancer who "took steps that showed her private parts armed with the most terrible jaws one could imagine, opening and closing, exposing a set of teeth."[50]

In her study of early nineteenth-century French literature Margaret Waller raises an important question: "When are men's claims to feminization and their complaints of impotence a ruse that helps maintain male power?" She deals only with the French romantics, but the question could be asked of the French and English decadents of the fin de siècle as well. Striking the pose of the aesthete and expressing their distaste for both the materialistic bourgeois and the reproductive woman obviously allowed such artists to turn their avowals of impotence to the purposes of narcissism and self-aggrandizement. They flaunted the power of the supposedly weak. Accordingly there were clearly "positive and assertive aspects in these fictions of impotence."[51]

One might have expected the depiction of male incapacities to have diminished masculinity, but one finds that in fictional as in medical works it was often exploited for the old purpose of denigrating woman (representing the body) and lauding man (representing the mind). Investigating the fantasies of creative artists perhaps draws one away from the experiences of real people yet private experiences were culturally scripted. The "text-like" and constructed nature of sexual humiliations as portrayed in the medical tracts was often only too obvious. The ways in which masculinity was portrayed in contemporary poems, plays, and novels, clearly did have some bearing on how readers could perceive and describe their sexual failings.

Before concluding this review of the nineteenth-century discussion of impotence it is important to recall that this literature was produced primarily to reassure what most believed to be a small portion of the male population. The assumption was still commonly made that the healthy man's sense of self was necessarily based on his potency. In his journal George Bernard Shaw coded his sexual performances (0), (1), or (2) with (0) indicating impotence. A man's honor for many continued to be first and foremost established by his virility, and accordingly a husband whose wife duped him would be punished by ridicule. Alexandre Dumas's play *La femme de Claude* (1873) was the most famous example of a work in which the cuckolded husband could reestablish his manhood only by murdering his wife or by dueling with her seducer. Cowardice was in effect equated with impotency. Proofs of potency were so esteemed that the seriousness of sexual crimes such as rape were difficult for some magistrates to comprehend. In the 1890s one English magistrate protested: "Virility seems necessary to give a man that consciousness of his dignity, of his character as lord and ruler, of his importance. . . . It is a power, a privilege of which the man is, and should be proud."[52]

Moreover, as was noted in the opening pages of this chapter, a woman married to an impotent man could sue for annulment. In the Anglo-Saxon world, divorce and annulment cases based on incapacity could still entail humiliating physical inspections but were, because of Victorian concerns for decorum, increasingly held *in camera*. Propriety similarly demanded that the woman who sought to free herself from an incompetent spouse had to argue that she was motivated by her desire for children rather than for sexual pleasure. To obtain an annulment her counsel would have to prove that the husband's physical or psychological defect existed before marriage, that it had not been revealed to the wife, and that it was incurable. The law in Germany followed a similar line but in addition allowed the dissolution of a marriage when an infirmity of one partner so disgusted the other that the performance of conjugal duties was made impossible. France was unusual inasmuch as after the revolution it did not accept impotence as a reason for the nullification of a marriage, even if it predated the marriage. On the other hand a French husband could not disavow any child born by his wife. Voluntary or involuntary nonconsummation of marriage could only provide the grounds for nullification once divorce was reestablished in 1884.[53]

It has become a commonplace to refer to the ways in which the Victorians sought to stifle female desire. In *Nymphomania: A History* (2000), Carol

Groneman demonstrated why the image of the sexually demanding woman was regarded as so disturbing, violating as it did nineteenth-century gender norms. Groneman mistakenly assumes that the overly lustful male was the culture's equivalent of the nymphomaniac and then asks why so few men were treated for the condition. The fact is that if the nymphomaniac represented for the Victorians all that was unwomanly, it was the impotent rather than the oversexed male who represented all that was unmanly. Only by taking him into account could commentators conceptualize the full spectrum of healthy and unhealthy masculinities. The discussion of impotence was central to the maintaining of nineteenth-century gender boundaries. Instead of taking male potency for granted, the authors of sex manuals, novels, plays, and poems saw the need to devote an enormous amount of attention to something that always had to be proven, something that was always problematical.

MARKETING MANLY VIGOR
Victorian Medicine versus Quackery

Some time in the 1890s a sixty-three-year-old American merchant married an active twenty-two-year-old woman and, to his horror, found that he could not perform. "Ashamed to consult a home physician," we are told, "he flew to the different 'lost manhood restored' advertisements and tried some of the most glaring and reassuring, and was swindled alternately. Then he went to some distant sanitarium and was treated some time with no better results. He was next worked by some medical company who sold him some sort of a suction apparatus for 'restoring weak and flabby erections in men with waning power and resultant impotence.'"[1] As a last resort, he turned to a skilled surgeon and, thanks to a minor operation, his potency was fully restored. We know about this patient because in 1897, J. A. Murray, the surgeon in question, proudly reported the case to the American Medical Association. This was the sort of story that the medical profession hoped would encapsulate the history of the treatment of impotence, the eventual triumph of doctors over their commercial competitors. The reality was that another century would pass before most men would believe that doctors could provide them with effective assistance.

Yet, in the very decades when surgeons working on male sexual dysfunctions failed to establish a specialty, their colleagues who dealt with female reproductive complaints were successful in winning public recognition. In 1885 the British Gynaecological Society was founded. Why did one specialty emerge but not another? The reasons for gynecologists winning recognition seem obvious enough. They could play up the necessity of surgical intervention to safeguard the health of childbearing women. More generally, they exploited the commonplace assumption that, unlike men, women were governed by their sex organs. "A deeply entrenched belief in our culture," argues Ornella Moscucci, "holds that sex and reproduction are more fundamental to woman's than to man's nature." Many gynecologists assumed that the fact that a woman had a uterus sexed the entire female body. Contrariwise Western culture held that though men did have diseases specific to their sex, these were not defining. Accordingly, gynecology emerged in the late nineteenth century but "was not paralleled by the evolution of a complementary 'science of masculinity' or 'andrology.'"[2]

Disparagingly referred to as "clap doctors," surgeons who tended to men's health worked on infections of the urinary tract and bladder stones. Urology as a specialty, distinct from general surgery, dates from 1890, when in Paris it became a separate course of study and Félix Guyon was named the first professor of urology. If gynecology basked in the importance Western societies attributed to motherhood, urology was tainted by its association with venereal disease and impotence. Doctors who discussed such issues were acutely aware of their apparent unseemliness. Moreover, the terrain was already occupied by quacks.

In the previous chapter we surveyed the Victorians' views of impotence. This chapter focuses on medical professionals' attempts to treat the ailment. Adventurous doctors hoped that in so doing they could create a new specialty. The problem was that in competing with quacks, doctors found it difficult to distinguish themselves from their opponents. For most of the century physicians attributed impotence to sexual excesses and the advice they offered was more moral than medical in nature. And though they attacked quacks as mere purveyors of purported aphrodisiacs representing the "manly vigor" school, doctors provided similar tonics and restoratives when pressed to. Those who turned to the psychological causes of dysfunctions showed some originality, but only in the last decades of the nineteenth century when antisepsis made surgery relatively safe could doctors finally lay claim to curative methods that they alone could provide. But even the employment of scalpels and sounds were often as not framed by moral considerations. In providing at times unnecessarily severe therapies, medical men appear to have been as much interested in assuring the public of their professional respectability, as in offering their patients effective care.

Let us first turn to the quacks. Feminist historians have argued that nineteenth-century doctors did not subject their male patients to the sort of interference that was the lot of female patients. Although these claims are well substantiated one could come away from such accounts with the impression that Victorian men were not also the targets of a barrage of quasi-medical advice. Yet a glance at the back pages of almost any nineteenth-century newspaper reveals a host of quack advertisements that sought to exploit men's sexual anxieties. In the emerging mass society, the entrepreneurial employed the new cheap press both to create worries and to sell nostrums to cure "lost manhood." "Victims of abuse and excess, reclaim your manhood!" proclaimed the Erie Medical Company of Buffalo, New York. "Sufferers from folly, overwork, ill health regain your vigour!" Its countless competitors included the producers of Therapion, Dr. McLaughan's Electric Belt, and Wood's Phosphodine for sexual weaknesses. Such publicity appeared in the cheaper daily papers and in a crop of new publications meant specifically for men. In the United States the back page of the *National Police Gazette*, the crime and sporting tabloid founded in 1845, always had its full complement of advertisements for restoratives. The turn-of-the-century self-help publications like *Physical Culture* trumpeted a range of cures and exercises. "Lionel Strongfort" promised to "aid in restoring the impotent. . . . I can give you new courage, increased vigor, more pep." In England, the *Illustrated Police News*, which began appearing in 1867, listed advertisements like "Manhood Restored" or "Nervous Debility" that offered consultations and guides for the self-cure of spermatorrhoea, the wasting of the nervous tissues, lowness of spirits, and premature decline. French comic magazines like *Le Sourire* alternated pornographic stories about artists and their models or wives and their complacent husbands with advertisement for injections and pills to counter pollutions and impotence. Business must have been good because firms were willing to pay huge sums to publicize such speedy cures for "secret diseases."[3]

The quacks attributed impotence to masturbation, spermatorrhoea, sexual excesses, and venereal diseases. Sterility and impotence, asserted Goss and Company, resulted from self-abuse: "As in man, so in woman, this pernicious habit takes away the *inclination* for those pleasures with which the multiplication of the species is connected, sometimes it destroys the actual *power* of effectual communion." The same argument was made by Sylvester Graham, the American health reformer. Onanism resulted in the genitals suffering from ulcers, burning sores, bloody semen, and dribbling sperm. "In other cases, a general withering, and impotence, and decay of the parts, commences and continues on, with the continuing vice, till almost every vestige of the *insignia,* and all the power of virility, are gone." The loss of "invigorating fluid"—equal to loss of forty times as much blood—resulted in "funeral effects" including impotence. With excesses a man's organ diminished in size. Erections become impossible. Night time emissions, warned the quacks, were harbingers of impotence. Samuel La'Mert's many publications contained garishly colored illustrations of the ulcerated faces, blistered penises, and syphilitic testicles of men whose vital fluids had drained away. The symptoms of debility were so vaguely defined—loss of brightness of the eye, hesitation, stuttering, palpitations, awkward gait, poor complexion, and general torpor—as to alarm any reader. Worse would follow. The genitals withered; one's thoughts wandered. Desires cruelly increased as one's ability decreased. The end of the story was predictable enough. Several tracts carried the classic account of the suicide victim who left the chilling note: "I am impotent and unfit to live."[4]

Perhaps the most enterprising of publicists was the famous Dr. Kahn. In 1857 he appeared in a London court charged with attempting to extort money from a man he promised to cure of spermatorrhoea. In addition to newspaper advertising, Kahn opened on Tichborne Street a medical museum where he titillated his male customers with scandalous displays including those of the breasts, buttocks, and sex organs of a virgin (showing her hymen and uterus) preserved in spirits, and the model of a clitoris enlarged by masturbation. Another exhibit graphically portraying the process of erection, was followed with a display of venereally diseased penises, syphilic eruptions, and genital ulcerations. Kahn offered his nervous clients in person or by mail his *Treatise on the Philosophy of Marriage* and the assurance that his lozenges and diet drinks could better restore virility than the painful cauterizations offered by doctors. In the 1870s the similar establishment that he opened in New York City also offered men the microscopic examination of their semen to test their suitability for marriage.[5] That the gullible availed themselves of such dubious services was in part due to the fact the medical profession did not provide them.

What did doctors do? In the nineteenth century most were clearly wary of the public discussion of sexual matters and afraid that the exploration of such issues could undermine the young profession. In the 1840s contributors to the *Lancet*, Britain's leading medical journal, reported that both patients and doctors were usually too self-conscious to broach such topics. Nevertheless a number of physicians seriously attempted to medicalize impotence by wresting its treatment from the quacks. They directed appeals to their colleagues, insisting that they could not leave such an important field of practice to the irresponsible. Quackery fueled immorality, argued John Corry, in promising easy cures. "Dissolute young men are induced to continue in the practice of their pernicious habits of wantonness and excess, from their mistaken idea that a nostrum will operate as an effective restorative." Quacks not only failed to help their clients; they actually harmed them. Asserting that physical injuries resulted from the publicity given to "secret diseases," Golding Bird cited the case of a man about to marry who, having read a quack advertisement, convinced himself that he was impotent, applied caustics to his penis and did serious damage to himself. Reginald Harrison referred to the "mental demoralization" of a thirty-five-year-old man who was certain that his hair was turning gray due to spermatorrhoea. In England, medical journals reported that it was not impotence itself, but the quacks' anxiety-producing tracts that drove some impressionable young men to suicide. It was reported in 1860 that the Staffordshire coroner had killed himself, believing his hernia had rendered him unable to consummate his marriage.[6]

Every doctor, Harrison noted, met patients demoralized by symptoms they blew out of proportion. "It is impossible for anyone to be brought in contact with cases of this kind without being struck with the pernicious effect which is caused by advertising and the gratuitous circulation of a certain kind of literature upon the minds of sensitive individuals who may feel conscious of having committed, perhaps at early periods in their lives, some sexual indiscretion." Henry Bostwick, an American physician, challenged his colleagues to overcome the false delicacy that prevented them from discussing sexual issues such as masturbation, venereal disease, and impotence. "The ignorant and the wicked, seeking only gain, have strangely been permitted almost a monopoly of subjects of transcendent interest and importance." Lamenting the sight of the ignorant throwing themselves to harpies, William Acton reported some firms went so far as to dabble in blackmail by threatening to expose the compromising letters of their clients. A Cambridge student, having already paid £40 in fees was asked for a further £300. A gang purportedly extorted £1,000 from another victim.[7]

To displace the quacks, doctors called for the creation of a science of man. Michael Ryan protested that women's genitals were no more complicated than men's, but there were far more authors writing on female complaints. For the man intercourse entailed a complicated physical and moral process of arousal, penetration, and emission. For women the process was much simpler "as the organs have little to do in the act of copulation, they being merely auxiliary to it." Ryan argued that the "whole economy" of the man was affected by his sexual sentiments. Since there was as yet no reliable work on impotence, Ryan produced his own in 1831. R. J. Culverwell also saw the need for a popular account and his study boasted of ten editions in seven years. Beginning with the observation that there was too much shyness regarding sex complaints, he set out to provide gentlemen with an understanding of the dangers of venereal disease, masturbation, and too early indulgence. William Acton asserted that one should be surprised, not by failures, but by successes of erection when "the variety of ways in which it is liable to be excited, thwarted, arrested, abused, interfered with, repeated, or exhausted, are taken into consideration." In the United States Frederick Hollick asserted in 1851 that many struck down by sterility or impotence simply suffered in silence, a silence he intended to break. A man's lack of virility could pose a public as well as a private problem. James Beaney, an Australian doctor, pointed out that because charges of impotence could end marriage, doctors had to discuss it. "The relationship of families; the peace of individuals; the life-long happiness of the two parties most concerned; their status in society; the conditions of property; and the hopes of family descent, are all involved in this great question; hence, it is imperative on the professional man, when writing on kindred subjects affecting the sexual relations of men and women, to give as much prominence as possible to impotence in man."[8]

Doctors saw the need to discuss impotence. How could they do so and yet clearly distinguish themselves from the quacks? One obvious way was to devote far more attention to types of impotence that had a physical basis. First in importance would come simple old age. Augustus Gardner noted male deficiencies could be due to the size and condition of penis; and the spermatic fluid could be weak due to disease, drugs, or simply aging. Acton, like Gardner stated that older men (that is, those over fifty) had to be careful to harbor their energies. Excesses were often due to vanity, especially in the case of an older husband who did not want to be considered a "Joseph." Félix Roubaud warned that it was dangerous to overindulge or try—like King David—to seek renewal in the arms of a young woman. Men had to accept the natural decline in their powers. Certainly in the first half of the nineteenth century doctors portrayed impotence as an inevitable consequence of aging and condemned those who sought arousal by the shameful methods offered by quacks. "Each age has its prerogatives," Louis Seraine reminded his readers, "as each season has its flowers."[9]

Doctors were also far more likely than quacks to acknowledge forms of organic impotence due to structural defects—malformations, hypospadias, cancers, elephantitis, syphilic nodes, and even fractures of the penis. Impotence was, of course, also the most worrying consequence of the venereal diseases. Dr. Rauland (Félix Roubaud) in *Le livre des époux* (1852), for example, said impotence could be due to heredity, illness, imagination, onanism, excess coition, and venereal disease. And as always doctors noted the debilitating effects of obesity and the enervating influences of opiates, alcohol, tobacco, coffee, absinthe, and hashish. Mumps were reported as rendering adult males both impotent and sterile. By the 1870s diabetes was also known to result in impotence, especially in older men. Though doctors concerned themselves chiefly with the health threats facing the middle class, R. W. Shufeldt recognized that factory workers could be rendered impotent by exposure to certain materials or drugs. He gave the example of India-rubber factories, where the inhalation of sulphuret of carbon had deleterious effects.[10]

Having reviewed the organic causes of impotence, doctors still found it impossible not to revert back to the commonplace notion that most male sexual dysfunctions had to be related to sexual excesses. This was hardly a new idea but obviously enjoyed a greater purchase in a bourgeois culture that prized savings. Doctors translated into medical language the fantasies of the age. From the 1830s on, medical texts contained sharper attacks on overindulging, even in marriage, warning that nervous debility could result. According to Acton the male body, like the penis, was supposed to be hard, firm, and erect. As the genitals in effect mirrored the character of the individual, the Christian gentleman had to demonstrate his self-control by limiting his indulgences. Hammond asserted that to give way more than once a week was excessive. A French doctor like Debay held that excesses, though common to civilized life, were the main causes of male decline. An English colleague felt that especially arousing sexual practices such as "coitus ab ore" (oral sex) were particularly damaging. Health faddists preached a similarly moralistic line. Thomas Low Nichols asserted that excesses led, like castration, to "feebleness, coldness, selfishness, cowardice, and a general lack of all we convey by the word manhood." In the United States popular medical tracts warned that "vital power" had been drained away by sexual excesses leading to a loss of energy in men and "their powers of application, as business men, students, and ministers, had declined, as also their enterprise, fervor, and kindliness. They had become irritable, dull, and complaining."[11]

If marital intercourse posed dangers, extramarital sex was said to be even more risky. Impotence, claimed James Dunn, could be caused by excessive venery, especially multiple repetitions during a single night. "The liability to such oft-repeated intercourse within a short time, is the chief reason why illicit intercourse is so much more destructive to the generative organs than legitimate cohabitation." Even Walter, the pseudonymous author of the pornographic classic *My Secret Life*, was warned that "unlimited indulgence would lead to impotence and perhaps worse," and considered moderating his activities. Pursuing the question further, the French physician Félix Roubaud shockingly admitted that he had experimented with loose women and found that it was soon the case that his flaccid penis could not be aroused by either their kisses or touch. He stoutly defended himself against having any ulterior motive, reminding his readers that science like art was always "chaste and discreet."[12]

The premise that sexual excesses could eventually result in impotence led physicians to show a new concern for the role played by youthful indiscretions, in particular masturbation. A common "vice" was thus reconfigured as a loathsome disease. Ryan noted that Jonathan Swift and Jean-Jacques Rousseau were victims of bad habits picked up in school, an institution viewed suspiciously by many authors. Leopold of Belgium wrote to Queen Victoria in 1853 that he wanted to marry off his son as soon as possible as "young men often fall into a habit destructive of health, mind, spirit, in short everything." Masturbation fears were particularly preoccupying in the middle and upper classes, associated as the indulgence was with youth, secrecy, and individualism.[13]

Doctors linked masturbation circularly to impotence, the logic being that masturbation caused impotence, and those who were impotent had no other option than to resort to masturbation. The general notion was that if a patient had sexual problems and was otherwise young and in good health, they were likely due to self-abuse. Either he confessed or his statements were ignored. With exhausted patients, American surgeon Samuel W. Gross recommended the doctor not believe them, but examine the urethra. Ryan held that masturbation and venery were the main of causes of impotence and sterility and he accordingly criticized Hunter for slighting the subject. James Richard Smyth, in reviewing his list of sluggish, woebegone patients, argued that nine-tenths of impotence was due to venereal disease and masturbation. He had extorted from one patient the confession of how by accident, at the age of twenty-one, while washing, he "became acquainted with the error of the second son of Judah, which folly I practised, more or less, until the age of twenty-five." Even a progressive physician like Frederick Hollick devoted a long section of his study of male health to the evils of masturbation, holding it responsible for baldness, epilepsy, and impotence. Hammond summed up the view of most doctors: "It is a law of the organism that any function which is over-exerted before the organs producing it are fully matured is certain to lead to the derangement or even to the extinction of that function." The habit once acquired had horrific consequences including, according to Gross, strictures, inflamed prostate, sensitive urethra, enlarged prepuce, and ugly discharges. As late as the 1890s doctors were still referring to a paralytic form of impotence found amongst many "masturbators and profligates." Of the inability to produce future citizens, a Southern doctor wrote in 1892, "it is therefore the duty of the physicians of the world to recognize the enormity of the injury done by masturbation, and set to work to educate the male youth so that they would avoid early abuse of the sexual functions with the same care that they would a murder or a theft."[14]

In 1836 the French physician Claude-Françoise Lallemand declared he had discovered yet another cause of impotence—spermatorrhoea. He asserted that sperm found in a man's urine was evidence of his suffering from a sexual complaint caused by some sort of sexual excess. Seminal fluid was supposed to be reabsorbed, not involuntarily discharged. If "pollutions" occurred—involuntary emissions of semen when either awake or asleep—action had to be taken. Such losses were symptoms of a serious problem that, if not treated, could result in dangerous complications. Lallemand's message was quickly broadcast in the English-speaking world. Uncontrolled pollutions were, doctors claimed, primarily caused by masturbation, but all sexual excesses and venereal diseases, as well as rich food, heat, soft beds, spices, drink, and unremitting brain work could contribute to the syndrome. Men were informed their semen was not supposed to dribble but come out in an explosive jet. Patients suffering from discharges displayed a variety of symptoms—stuttering, deafness, epilepsy, constipation, and finally impotence. This new disease was described as the most fatal enemy of marriage. Even a mid-Victorian sex radical like George Drysdale followed Lallemand's line on spermatorrhoea in heralding it as more dangerous than simple emission since it could occur at any time.[15] Though continuing to exploit masturbation fears, quacks after 1850 added spermatorrhoea to their stock of nightmarish threats.

At the beginning of the century Buchan asserted, "for the cure of unnatural pollutions, I always recommended matrimony." Some suggested cooling the privates by sitting on cane bottomed chairs and by eating moderate diets. At midcentury far more drastic remedies were employed. John L. Milton, noting the linkage of impotence and spermatorrhoea, praised Lallemand for his recommending painful cauterizations and blisterings of the penis.[16] Strictures due to excitement or excesses were removed by applying camphor to the genitals, and inserting bougies (thin, flexible surgical instruments) and catheters up the urethra. In the latter part of the century arsenic and electricity were employed as well.

The quack remedies in contrast were fairly benign. Samuel Solomon's advice for "impotency or seminal weakness" was consumption of his Cordial Balm of Gilead—a mixture of cardamom, brandy, and cantharides, which supposedly favored the production of semen and removed the flaccidity of the muscles. On analysis Brodum's Nervous Cordial was revealed to consist of gentian, calumbo, and cardamom. Though such concoctions were unlikely to have fortified the constitution as promised, they probably did little harm. The same was likely true of Dr. Senate's Steel Lozenges and Balm of Mecca, R. and L. Perry's Cordial Balm of Syriacum, Blake and Company's Neurosian Extract, and de Roos's concentrated Guttae Vitae.[17] Nevertheless, Sylvester Graham warned that men who turned to quack remedies eventually met a direful fate.

> The instances are not unfrequent in which the offender receives, as he supposes, entire relief from the hands of the calomel, or cantharides, or balm of Gilead doctor, and, in the *feeling* of his strength and health, enters into wedlock, and by the help of high-seasoned food, and wine, and brandy, and perhaps occasionally iron, and quinine, and cantharides, &c., sustains himself in the function of virility for several months, and it may be, for some years,—begetting puny offspring, which either fall abortive to the grave or come forth to individual existence, weak, delicate, and full of predisposition to disease. . . . But they receive not all the penalty; for the time soon comes when the unhappy transgressor himself is plunged into the depths of calamity! And by so much the more as he has used violent and unnatural means to elevate and sustain himself, by so much the deeper and remedilessly will he sink![18]

Graham argued that sexual health could only be restored by restraint, good plain vegetable food, exercise, and cold bathing.

In the last decades of the century the enterprising also offered electrical cures for a wide range of male problems. Dr. Hammond sold a "curative belt" that, when connected to an electrical source, supposedly infused manly vigor. The claim was that such contraptions in supporting the testicles and providing warmth would aid sperm production and guarantee "vitality" and "renewed life." Patients also had to purchase THE RESTORATIVE POWDERS and SEMINAL REPLENISHER." "Those unable to cohabit satisfactorily, from whatever cause, should never be without a supply, as they not only create erectile power and brain matter, but likewise replenishes [sic] the seminal fluid, lost by too frequent cohabitation." In Montreal, M. H. Utley similarly praised the benefits of galvanism.[19]

Regular doctors repeatedly exposed the futility of pills, potions, and electric belts. Did physicians have anything to offer that would distinguish them from their commercial competitors? Marriage was recommended by some doctors as a cure for impotence, but their opponents were more likely to rush into print. Ryan felt incapacitated males should not marry. Acton claimed ill-planned nuptials led to suicidal grooms and humiliated brides. "Who has the right to regard her as a therapeutic agent, and

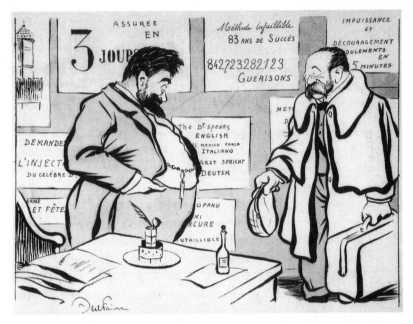

5. As this cartoon indicates, nineteenth-century quacks promised speedy cures for sexual complaints. To the traveler's protest, "But I only have three minutes until my train leaves," the practitioner replies, "Three minutes! . . . You will be cured all the same." Abel Faivre, "Mais, je n'ai que trois minutes" in "Les médecins," *L'Assiette au beurre* 51 (March 22, 1902): 832, by permission of the National Library of Medicine.

to stake thus lightly her future prospects, her repose, and the happiness of the remainder of her life?" Others agreed that such marriages could lead the husband to engage in perverse acts, leaving the wife inflamed with desires that could not be quenched. Such discussions were tinged with eugenic and racial overtones. Those rendered impotent, Dawson insisted, should not marry, and he cited one colleague as saying, "he would as soon have thought of passing a recruit with a broken arm into her Majesty's service, as he would have advised the gentleman whose case we were investigating, to marry, had all the facts been laid before him." Impregnation by some weak men was possible but was unwise as "the offspring will bear enstamped upon it the physical characters derivable from parental debility." Nichols agreed that women had a duty to reject unfit fathers for "the good of the race." Just as twentieth-century doctors held that homosexuals should not marry in hopes of curing their perversion, so nineteenth-century psychiatrists like Henry Maudsley warned the impotent masturbator that marriage would offer him no hope. "For natural intercourse, he has little power or no desire, and finds no pleasure in it; the indulgence of a depraved appetite has destroyed the natural appetite. Besides if he be not entirely impotent, what an outlook for any child begotten of such degenerate stock! Has a being so degraded any right to curse a child with the inheritance of such a wretched descent? Far better that the vice and its consequences should die out with him." [20] Doctors were clearly most preoccupied by the alarming notion of couples engaging in anything but penetrative intercourse; but in opposing the marriage of the impotent, they presented themselves as thinking first and foremost of the women and children.

For impotent men already married doctors first called for rest. "In the curable cases," argued Acton, "it is probable that the nervous system has been over-excited beyond the natural limits which a phlegmatic constitution imposes. The one object is to restore the nervous power, or rather to allow it to restore itself—not to excite or exhaust it still further." Some suggested a cessation of sexual relations for up to a year. If attempts were made too soon a failure could simply confirm one's worst fears. Next, doctors called for lifestyle changes. W. Frank Glenn recommended healthy living and restricting oneself to the company of virtuous ladies. Culverwell reported on cases of "incipient impuissance" cured by change of regime, diet, and exercise. Seraine agreed that repose and healthy food were crucial. He particularly vaunted the value of milk—be it from a cow, goat, ass, or woman—but wisely cautioned that the latter source could be dangerously arousing. Dr. Belliol in his 975-page tome touted his own "methode vegetale" consisting of calming, "anti-nervous" tonics. Taking the opposite tack, Debay's suggestion for exhausted men over forty was a fortifying diet of hot chocolate for breakfast, steak for lunch, bloody roast beef for dinner accompanied by rocket, artichokes, and bottles of burgundy. [21]

American health faddists called for moderation. They recommended an avoidance of coffee, tea, brandy, and tobacco, and encouraged a wholesome diet of "rye, corn, graham bread, oatmeal, cracked wheat, plenty of fruit." Nichols opposed the eating of meat and pushed water cures. John Cowan called for a plain, simple life and the avoidance of feather beds. Sexual power, argued Bernarr Macfadden, the turn of the century fitness advocate, indicated overall health. "Impotence sexually means impotence in everything, impotence mentally, physically, socially, etc." [22] He went on to warn his male readers against employing drugs, tonics, electricity, and the dangerous air pump. The cure resided in diet, cold air exercises, and clean water. Such advice obviously reflected the wistful belief of city inhabitants in the health-giving properties of the "natural," rural life.

Quacks were best known for peddling pills and potions. Did doctors differ? Frederick Hollick, though a marginal medical practitioner, typified doctors' responses to quacks. He attacked them for claiming that there were specifics that targeted genital complaints. He pointed out that most drugs had complicated effects. Tobacco, like opium, first stimulated and then depressed, cantharides did not work; camphor was actually a sedative; ergot, though a stimulant was dangerous; coffee caused "priapism, lascivious dreams, and involuntary emissions." Yet after condemning the search for a drug that would cure impotence, Hollick concluded by asserting that there was one substance that, in causing warmth, cheerfulness, and leaving no depressive aftereffect, did restore sexual power and desire—cannabis. Like Hollick, most doctors did provided tonics and stimulants, if only to counter their competitors. A 1830 French work recommended ginseng. Acton prescribed strychnine and phosphoric acid with either syrup of orange-peel or syrup of ginger. Nux vomica (strychnine), yohimbe, and damiana were especially popular. Glenn claimed damiana to be the most effective medicine. In cases of complete inability to produce an erection, he employed a combination of phosphide of zinc, damiana, aresenious acide, and cocaine.[23]

By the 1880s, few doctors claimed there was a totally reliable aphrodisiac, and turned to the question of the external stimulation of the genitals by frictions, flagellations, and galvanism. A handful of doctors such as Roubaud and William Belfield discussed the massage of the scrotal and surrounding areas as treatment for impotence. Flagellation had, of course, been long regarded as a perverted form of arousal. William Stead in his famous 1885 exposure of child prostitution referred to the floggings sought by jaded old men "who by riot and excess had impaired [their] vitality." Nevertheless in France a number of doctors dared to recommend percussion, urtication (the use of stinging nettles), and flagellation. Roubaud listed "mechanical means" of arousal including massage, percussion with elastic batons, flagellation, and frictions. Should these be condemned as means of debauchery? Roubaud replied that "science is like a fire; it purifies all that it touches." Every means to draw blood to the trunk and so aid in circulation was useful, though he did warn that urtication and bleedings were dangerous. He employed a metallic brush to provide a mild form of flagellation.[24]

When Roubaud had earlier written under the pseudonym of "Dr. Rauland" he had described flagellations and massage as shameful and called for the therapeutic use of electricity. He was followed by a number of English-speaking physicians. If excessive sensitivity prevented successful coition, Hollick advised penis washes, astringents, and doses of galvanism in order to render the penis less tender. For most practitioners electrotherapy was used for arousal as in effect a modern form of flagellation. Caldwell described in detail the composition and function of the erectile tissue and how an erection was produced by nervous force. If it was impaired he called for electricity—"either static, dynamic or interrupted"—to stimulate the production of nerve force. Damiana in combination with electricity was used, he claimed, in "many cases of partial loss of virility with marked success." Robert Ultzmann recommended faradization to contract the musculus bulbo-cavernosus. Hammond explained how galvanism could be applied with electrodes attached to the spine, perineum, testicles and penis, though he described the effect as "rather unpleasant." To distinguish themselves from quacks, doctors disparaged all belts, disks, and other apparatuses. Nevertheless Vincent Marie Mondat—a distinguished French physician—was credited with the most outlandish of the various external appliances. He invented the "congestor," a vacuum pump or "exhausting apparatus," which in drawing blood into the penis was designed to promote erection.[25]

As the preceding discussion indicates, nineteenth-century doctors were not as prudish as they have sometimes been portrayed. T. B. Curling argued that it was "injurious and immoral" to claim that abstinence led to impotence, but many of his colleagues regarded extended continence as posing almost as dangerous a threat to a man's health as sexual excess. Ryan felt both abstinence and debauchery led to decline. Culverwell noted premature debility resulted from onanism; yet complete continence was perilous too. Sex radicals like George Drysdale argued for the need to exercise the genitals like any other organ; abstinence could lead to abuses and nocturnal emissions. With no normal exercise, Drysdale reported, the penis became "shrunk and flabby, the testicles soft . . . the erections have in great part disappeared." The moral was that modern men needed less study and more indulgence. Paolo Mantegazza saw continence as a problem, and referred to intercourse as a sort of hygienic gymnastics. In discussing continence, Dr. Joseph W. Howe concluded, "The genital organs are not exempted from the general law, viz: that their neglect to fulfill a function may be followed by a loss of power to perform that function in a natural manner." Gross gave the case of a young man who was sexually exhausted because he had not had sex. Yet "during his engagement which preceded his marriage by seven months, his genitalia were kept in a constant state of excitement by fondling the object of his affections, and he did not have illicit intercourse to relieve his passions."[26]

Doctors' discussions moreover made it clear that, despite what moralists and fear mongers might say, their patients were not all terrorized by masturbation fears. Dawson reported that some men actually believed that masturbation was "a manly habit." "In very young infants," reported Hammond, "it is sometimes the case that in order to soothe them nurses titillate the genital organs and thus produce sensations which are agreeable and which are subsequently desired." "I regret to say," reported another American author in 1899, "that I have known some fathers to tickle the genital organs of their infant boys until a complete erection of the little penis ensued, which effect pleases the father as an evidence of a robust boy." In the later 1800s doctors themselves shifted the discussion of masturbation from its moral to its psychological effects, increasingly linking it to nervousness rather than dementia. By the late nineteenth century the psychological impact of self-abuse was noted by Hammond. Its chief danger, he held, was that ordinary sex would never be as enchanting as a man's fantasies. "He is, in fact, impotent to women; he no longer desires intercourse, but abandons himself to his fatal habit, knowing the almost limitless resources of his imagination in providing excitations to his desires. Such persons shun the society of women, become often true misogynists, and suffer an entire extinction of the sexual feeling." [27]

Some doctors pooh-poohed such sexual fears. In England, James Paget in his 1870 clinical lecture "Sexual Hypochondriasis"—the problem of male patients exaggerating trivial maladies—observed that far too many men believed an innocuous nocturnal emission was a sign of impotence. Though quacks spread a fear of masturbation, Paget assured his audience that the practice was neither better nor worse than intercourse. It might be nasty and unclean, if overdone at an early age it could cause exhaustion, nervousness, and "effeminacy," but it was not dangerous if only indulged occasionally. Gross agreed with Paget that masturbation was no worse than intercourse, but noted it could be started earlier. [28] Ultzmann followed Paget in holding that the fear of masturbation could be as be as bad as masturbation itself in causing impotence.

Paget also held Lallemand responsible for fanning fears of spermatorrhoea. George Gascoyen agreed that spermatorrhoea was an ugly subject, likening it to venereal disease and baby farming. Though he doubted there were many real cases, he knew that quacks exploited such fears and ignored the fact that the presence of semen in the urine was a sign of health, not disease. Even so Gascoyen recommended for the incontinent a restriction of sexual activity, a change in sleeping postures, calming drugs, and circumcision if necessary. William A. Roberts went further, arguing that most patients' worries about spermatorrhoea were simply due to reading the works of alarmists. Roberts gave the case of man of sixty so concerned that his virility was declining that he insisted on sending in for analysis over a hundred specimens of his urine. Such worries indicated a mental rather than a physical problem. Roberts conceded that venereal diseases, pornography, and masturbation contributed to sexual overexcitement, but protested that Lallemand and his followers went too far in cauterizing penises.[29]

Americans were more outspoken. In the *Northwest Lancet* of 1885, Dunn reported that masturbation injured the generative organs "not nearly so much more than an equal amount of natural sexual indulgence as is commonly supposed," and that he had never observed a permanent injury to the organs following "moderate" masturbation. Though it took some time for masturbators to become accustomed to "natural connection," "the man of sense who quits the unnatural methods of gratification and takes up the natural one, always in my experience gradually acquires a taste for nature's way and loses his bestial appetites, and when he has reached a stage in which onanism is disgusting and devoid of pleasure, he has fully recovered." In 1892, E. R. Palmer, professor of physiology and pathological histology at the University of Louisville, boldly asserted that the normal male began his sexual life as a masturbator and accordingly the medical profession had made an egregious error in teaching men that they had a limited amount of semen, which their early solitary indulgences largely expended. Was it not the case that the regular use of the testicles (like glands and organs generally) developed and strengthened them? If impotence occurred in youth it was due to inexperience rather than to incapacity. "As the single julep or the first cigar turns his stomach or splits his head throughout the restless night, so the early copulation, imperfectly performed, surrounded as it is by such unnerving phases, drags his loins and runs riot his heart for more than a day after the indulgence." Palmer would say to such a young man: "My dear boy, you have not lost your manhood; you rather have not found it." Just as their other physical powers had to be exercised and strengthened, young men had to learn to properly use and develop their sexual powers. Overuse of the sexual organs did not produce as many negative effects as abstinence. "Recognizing the high order of office allotted to the seminiferous organs and the consequent complex nervous relationship that they possess, I yet maintain that continence means atrophy, that disuse means decay; and not only this, but that the influence of persistent continence upon the individual, whether male or female, is to dwarf and in many respects destroy the breadth and fullness of physical and intellectual individuality."[30]

The downplaying of the role of sexual excesses in causing impotence could lead to two quite different responses. Doctors who believed that the complaint had a psychological basis would likely view it as susceptible to some sort of counseling, whereas their colleagues who felt they were dealing with an organic problem might suggest some sort of surgical intervention.

From the nineteenth-century discussions of the psychological causes of impotence it is clear that many old beliefs lingered on. In 1841 James Richard Smyth noted in the *Lancet*, "We have within the last few months prescribed with success for an impotent patient, who was fully impressed with the belief that his infirmity was the result of some spell or enchantment." Hammond reported that American physicians often met with cases in which men believed women had "laid a spell" on them. A French marriage manual published in the 1880s reported that some villagers still feared the knot tier, and that such beliefs had a noxious effect even in the cities.

Doctors were happier viewing sexual dysfunctions as a result of overexcitement, drawing on Albert von Haller and William Cullen's notions of nerve force that too much tone resulted in spasms and too little in atony. Acton held that the causes of impotence were "abuse of the generative organs, aggravated in most instances by alarm, a guilty conscience, fear of not succeeding, habits of intemperance, too free use of tobacco, from timidity, or from too frequent excitement without gratification." The way in which these causes produced impotence was not known for certain, but Acton believed they were most probably due to "lesions of the nervous system, and most especially that of the portion of it which is under the influence of the sympathetic nerve or the excito-motory system." The classic case of the overexcitement would be that of the man who was only impotent with his beloved. In addition, French doctors listed fear, disgust, shame, excessive study, and lengthy continence as all potentially playing a role. Félix Roubaud gave as examples of psychic impotence the incapacitation of one man who won a lottery and another who survived a rail crash. English physicians spoke of imaginary impotence due to fears and idle fancies.[31]

Roubaud asserted that a man's performance could additionally be influenced by climate, season, and the time of day. He asserted that the liberal professions sustained sexual health since they instilled a "délicatesse de sensibilité," but most doctors noted the baleful influences of heredity, habit, and profession, especially for the middle class. "A man studies hard, his health fails and semen is not secreted." Acton said that such men mainly needed rest. Physicians supported Herbert Spencer's claim that there was inverse ratio between the nervous and generative system. Glenn gave as an example a mathematician who was unable to keep his mind concentrated during the act: "His erections and desire were perfectly normal, yet when in the midst of the sexual act, just at the moment when the orgasm was approaching, his mind would instantly be directed to some mathematical problem upon which he had been engaged during the day, and immediately all sexual desire would be extinguished and the act never completed."

Accidents to the head, shocks, and business losses, claimed Frederick Hollick, all had a deleterious effect.[32]

Not surprisingly, late nineteenth-century doctors used the metaphors of the railway and telegraph networks to explain how impaired nerves could result in sexual fiascoes. According to Bransford Lewis, the prostatic urethra was "the focal point of nervous impressions on the genital system." In "the crisis of intercourse," he wrote, it is "intensely congested and its nerves are at a high state of tension. . . . It is, moreover, a kind of way-station, a junction for all of the nerve-telegraph lines connecting the various parts of the uro-genital system with one another; and, consequently, it bears the brunt of the injurious nervous impressions reflected from these various parts." Accordingly, excesses of any kind could derange the "spinal genital center, interfering with its control over erections; impotence is the result." [33]

Some in the medical profession had little time for men whose impotence was apparently due to lack of self-confidence. Hammond disdainfully referred to the "hypochondriac" whose whole attention "is concentrated upon his generative organs. He examines them many times a day, measures them, and is constantly applying lotions and running from one physician to the other with stories of their deficient power, the shrinkage of his penis, the gradual disappearance of his testicles, etc., etc." Such a patient soon convinced himself he was impotent. Gilbert Ballet noted "those affected with comparative impotence believe themselves threatened with irremediable loss of their virility." He had little sympathy for those given to morbid meditations. Most of his colleagues, however, saw the need to reassure their patients and tell them that they only had to deal with the fear of failure. As quacks were always attempting to exacerbate want of self-confidence, the doctor should never denigrate his patient's concerns. "Every physician who had much experience in this department of medicine knows how many cases there are in which the patient fails to perform the act merely from lack of confidence," wrote Henry Lyman, "and how many instances occur in which the use of some mysterious remedy, or the application of instruments in parts of the body which are to the patient mysterious, results in perfect cures of impotency, even though these medicines and these instruments have really not affected the individual in the least." [34]

To combat hypochondria, Ultzmann suggested that patients be shown that they could have erections. "For in fact it is possible to excite erection in these patients by applying either the continuous or the faradic current according to Duchenne's method (one of the poles being placed in the rectum, the other applied over the bulb of the urethra)." Doctors publicly agreed that the worried young man should not be advised to reassure himself by experimenting with a prostitute before marrying, but Ryan noted that it was done so generally that one could not "censure the faculty for occasionally proposing it." Somewhat similarly, a doctor advised a man to fantasize about his ex-mistress when he had had sexual difficulties with his beloved wife.[35]

If physical potency problems had a psychological basis, they could presumably be cured by psychological means. Auguste Forel, the Swiss psychiatrist, employed hypnotism. Hippolyte Bernheim, professor of the faculty of medicine at Nancy, confessed he had only a few successes, as described in his book *Hypnotisme, suggestion, psychothérapie*, and many more failures. In the latter cases a physical problem usually existed. Nevertheless impotence brought on by autosuggestion, Bernheim believed, could be alleviated by a doctor's useful suggestions.[36]

Even before hypnotic suggestion was discussed, a number of doctors had noted the role placebos could play. A man's fear of failure was, Ryan reported, the greatest threat to his potency. Ryan went on to wonder: "How many impotent persons of this class were cured by bread pills, by Hunter; and how many are annually cured by mere placebos?" French doctors, remembering Montaigne's observations, similarly admitted that talismans might have an effect. Viewed in this context it is quite possible that some of the quack remedies actually "worked," at least in the psychological sense. And since quacks sold pills, patients would feel fobbed off if their physicians did not offer them some potion or tonic. Doctors responded by doling out remedies that were aimed more at building up confidence than in having any direct physiological effect. Citing Astley Cooper's comment that if man had "any development of sexual power in the morning" he was fit to marry, Ryan advised his colleagues to give sugar pills to the nervous newly married and the assurance that all would be fine.[37]

The first extensive nineteenth-century discussions of the placebo were thus sparked by doctors' use of inactive pills to "cure" sexual problems. Austin Flint told his colleagues that many men had been simply spooked by quacks' talk of the effects of masturbation. The doctor's chief task was accordingly to convince his patient that a proposed course of treatment would work. "A remedy prescribed with an assurance of a cure, doubtless sometimes proves curative by a moral effect." Gross likewise recommended giving a placebo with the "assurance that it will afford relief." If the patient demanded more action one could always remove a "tight or redundant prepuce," galvanize him, faradize him, and prescribe a range of tonics, baths, and exercises. Since he probably had also heard of phosphorus or damiana, these too could be prescribed for "the mind is open to persuasion in this way, but not by mere assurances, or by making light of the fancied disorder." An

American doctor reported the case of fifty-two-year-old widower daunted by a new marriage. The physician told him he had "many cases of a similar nature, and that they always yielded readily to teaspoonful doses of a fluid extract of damiana taken every eight hours for three days before marriage. As a result of this ruse, he subsequently wrote me that the remedy had acted like a charm." George M. Beard, the father of neurasthenia, also experimented with use of placebos and found they worked for both functional and organic problems. The point was to treat the individual, not the complaint, so it was essential not to belittle the patient's concerns.[38]

Sharply contrasting with the calming assurances for the nervous were the often hurtful and intrusive remedies doctors inflicted on the dissolute. When dealing with cases of impotence they attributed to masturbation or venereal diseases, moralizing doctors were not averse to employing severe therapies. Described in eye-watering detail, such painful procedures were partly punitive in nature, the sufferer thereby being taught the need for self-control. Bird explicitly argued that bad habits could be countered with blistering agents and circumcisions. The assumption was that a contraction or stricture of the penis caused by excesses had to be burnt away. Doctors began with the scalding and cauterization of the penis, and insertion of catheters to irrigate the urethra. Gross described sticking "explorers"— acorn-headed bougies—up the urethra in search of blockages. Cauterization consisted of employing a syringe to force into the urethra a painful caustic solution. After experiencing such a scalding, Acton's patients often could not walk for three or four days and rarely asked for a second treatment. Ultzmann, who employed sounds, astringents, douches, and tannin suppositories to excite the prostate via the urethra noted that many patients exhibited a "dread and fear of catheterism." "When they have unfastened their clothes and have stretched themselves on the table the penis is seen gradually to shrink, grow smaller, and to move in a worm-like manner." When the sound was inserted past the prostate they were likely to cry out. Some fainted. Lewis, who recommended the injection of the entire urethra with progressively increasing strengths of silver-nitrate solutions conceded that "perhaps" bromides could be prescribed for the patient who suffered from hyperesthesia.[39]

Approaching the problem from a different angle, one French physician suggested the insertion into the rectum of a wooden cylinder to compress the prostate and so prevent emissions. The enlargement of the prostate posed many men with a serious health threat. Impotence was one symptom. Here again doctors insisted on attributing many cases to sexual excesses. Some believed that the prostate controlled male sexuality and that its enlargement—like that of any muscle—was due to its overuse. We know now that enlargement is usually due to either aging or infection. The treatments on offer in the 1890s ran from injections and cauterizations to surgical removal. Some of the first vasectomies in the United States were carried out at the turn of the century with the intention of causing the prostate to atrophy.[40]

In an 1894 lecture to the New York State Medical Society, F. R. Sturgis argued that surgeons dealing with impotence had long erred "in laying too much stress on the nervous part and too little on the physical," and that this "has worked to the detriment of both patient and surgeon, and has driven the former into the hands of the charlatan, when the surgeon could have given better and more permanent relief." The majority of cases of sexual debility were, he claimed, completely curable by application of the sound. Advances in antisepsis in the last decades of the century allowed surgeons to begin to move into the field of male sexual dysfunctions and claim that cutting could cure. The surgical revolution saw doctors shift from inserting bougies up the urethra and blistering penises to more radical interventions. Surgeons were already turning their skills to resolve issues of "ambiguous" genitalia. In a like manner they claimed to be able to restore normally endowed men's manhood. Eugene Fuller was of the opinion that most impotence was due to "seminal vesiculitis," which could be dealt with by stripping the vessels and restoring tone. Others held that restricting the flow of blood out of the penis by ligating the dorsal vein of the penis made the most sense. Most histories of surgery credit J. S. Wooten, a Texas surgeon, with pioneering the operation. In fact, an account of the procedure was first provided in 1897 by J. A. Murray whose activities we noted in the first lines of this chapter. He reported to the forty-eighth annual meeting of the American Medical Association on five cases of impotence on which he had operated, four of which he claimed were permanently cured. He claimed that all the men's problems were associated with self abuse. In cases where "imperfect erections are due to the too rapid emptying of the veins of the erectile tissue," he argued, "ligation offers good prospects for a permanent cure. This operation, is, however, of little use in neurasthenic cases."[41] Yet Murray conceded that in those cases in which patients left the surgical theater convinced that they were cured the mental effect of the operation must have been more important that its physiological consequences. It is difficult to imagine how such surgery could have had anything but a placebo effect.

In the last decades of the nineteenth century doctors launched the campaign to popularize what was to become the most common form of male genital surgery—circumcision. In North America and England the argument was made that a simple snip would prevent both masturbation and impotence. The logic of the argument was that having to draw the fore-skin back and forth gave rise to masturbation which in turn led to impotence. "The most effective preventative to the curse of prevalent self-abuse amongst the male youth of our land," argued Glenn, "would be thorough circumcision at the time of birth." Gross asserted that the circumcision of the "redundant prepuce" would help cure adult sexual dysfunctions. To improve potency Beard recommended both circumcision and the "stretching" of the penis. The English surgeon Robert Taylor was somewhat less enthusiastic, only suggesting that if the prepuce was so tight as to impede erection it should be removed. Americans were far more optimistic. The most extensive defense of the operation was provided by P. C. Remondino in his *History of Circumcision* (1900). In a chapter provocatively entitled "The Prepuce as an Outlaw, and Its Effects on the Glans," Remondino held the lowly foreskin responsible for a host of evils including onanism, syphilis, nocturnal emissions, and cancer. At the very least constriction of the pre-puce caused irritations and sufferings. Phimosis (an over tight foreskin), argued Remondino, resulted in impotence, a term which he used in the old-fashioned sense of meaning the inability to inseminate. He imagined that with evolution this redundant, restricting flap of skin might disappear. In the meantime surgery could provide relief. Citing the prophet Abraham as an example Remondino even suggested that circumcision could restore the virility of the aged. The operation was an aesthetic as well as a medical ne-cessity. Remondino disparagingly described the glans of the uncircumcised man as looking like the head of a forlorn field mouse. The circumscribed penis looked "more natural."[42]

Talk of having recourse to surgery to cure impotence or to make the pe-nis look "more natural" signaled the dawning of a brave new world of medi-cal intervention. And yet it was a false dawn. The vast majority of men were not attracted by the cures offered by medicine. Doctors remained caught in a dilemma. How could they assure their male patients they could save them from the consequences of sexual excesses without appearing to be sanctioning such behavior? One way was in wielding disease sanctions to assert that vice was inevitably punished by nature. Immorality led to ill-ness. Early twentieth-century moralists like G. Frank Lydston asserted that quacks actually provided a service in frightening the young; doctors too often downplayed the dangers of sexual experimentation.[43] He dedicated his book on impotence to the American Urological Association, stressing doctors' duties to raise society's moral tone. But this very stress on morality continually blurred the line purportedly separating quackery and medicine. Indeed nineteenth-century quackery thrived by exploiting many of the very anxieties—such as that of over spermatorrhoea—that had been first raised by doctors.

In practical terms doctors tending to male sexual problems accomplished relatively little in the course of the nineteenth century. Some progress was made in problematizing masculinity. Gross, for example, reported that whereas it was generally believed that only in 1 in 10 barren marriages was the man was at fault, he found that in his sample of 192 couples the man was responsible in 1 of 6 cases. In 1890 Ultzmann noted the microscope had revealed a new male problem that was very difficult to cure—aspermia or abnormal sperm. But few therapeutic advances were made. Paolo Mantegazza proudly announced in 1887 his "dynamomètre génital" or scale running from zero, meaning no desire or erection to ten, meaning erections at will and multiple acts many times in a night. But in asserting that morning erections were a sign of health and that extended continence could pose problems, Mantegazza was more or less repeating what Hunter had stated a century before.[44] Given such limited advances it was no surprise that in the years that gynecology emerged, a complementary specialty in male medicine failed to appear. Few patients dared to disagree with doctors' moralizing assertions but naturally enough boycotted medical therapies that were often more painful and rarely any more effective than the remedies sold by quacks. In the twentieth century doctors would continue to complain that medicine had still not established its authority in the field of male sexual ailments. Indeed, in the early 1900s psychoanalysts and the writers of sex manuals emerged and presented startling new narratives that further detracted from the urologists' organic accounts of the cause of impotence.

SIGMUND FREUD, MARIE STOPES, AND "THE LOVE OF CIVILIZED MAN"

In *The Sun Also Rises* (1926) Ernest Hemingway memorably portrayed a cast of sexual types, each representing some facet of a perceived crisis in early twentieth-century masculinity. We experience Jake's confused feelings aroused by the smoking, dancing, and drinking flappers led by the androgynous and promiscuous Brett. We witness his disdain for both simpering "faggots" and soft, self-indulgent men frittering their life away on credit. Only when we leave the city and follow Jake and his friends to primitive Pamploma do we meet real men, courageous bull fighters and honest peasants. Hemingway's master stroke is to give his macho clichés tragic weight by having them voiced by a man who is impotent yet still the most masculine of men. The novel opens with Jake's encounter with a prostitute.

> She touched me with one hand and I put her hand away.
> "Never mind."
> "What's the matter? You sick?"
> "Yes."

When she asks what happened he replies, "I got hurt in the war." Later, distraught at losing Brett, he wonders why his tragic condition "is supposed to be funny." Though Hemingway never allows his hero to refer explicitly to his impotence, his unnamed, irreparable problem casts its shadow over every scene in the novel.[1] Hemingway was not alone in tapping into the fear that the recent conflict had undermined masculinity. In France, Gabriel Chevallier lashed out at the war hospital nurses who treated their castrated patients like babies. In Germany, Ernst Toller made his point all too clear in his play

Hinkemann (1923) by cruelly presenting a wife cuckolding her emasculated war hero husband with his best friend Paul Grosshahn (Big Cock). Such a scenario had a particular resonance in the defeated nations of central Europe in which nationalists regarded their states as crippled as their veterans. Weimar filmmakers proceeded in the 1920s to mine male insecurities by producing movie after movie in which powerful women humiliated weak men. The most explicit was the Czech film *Ecstasy* (1933), in which Hedy Lamarr's spouse—shamefully exposed as sexually incompetent—sees himself as having no other recourse than to commit suicide.[2]

Many worried that World War I had created a generation of shell-shocked and physically incapacitated males whose fate was uncertain. Obviously the war focused an unprecedented amount of attention on the sexually disabled. Nevertheless the conflict exacerbated rather than created a preoccupation with Western men's declining virility. As the discussions of neurasthenia revealed, the concern that masculinity was undermined by the stresses of the modern world preceded the war by several decades. One response to this perceived threat was the displacement at the turn of the century of the Victorian restrained model of masculinity by a new ideal of aggressive masculinity—tanned, muscular, youthful, and virile. Countering older messages that manliness was manifested by postponement of gratification, a new consumer-oriented culture lauded arousal and fulfillment. Given the emergence of the "new woman"—be she suffragette or flapper—the arrival of a new complementary type of man was to be expected. A generation of novelists goaded hen-pecked males to stand up to cock-sure feminists. And as the Victorian model of masculinity that valorized restraint was displaced by a more relaxed ideal, the early twentieth century witnessed a shift from moral to psychological explanations of impotence. When nineteenth-century writers noted male sex problems, they tended to attribute them to sexual excesses; in contrast in, twentieth-century writers increasingly traced them back to a lack or a loss of desire. In James Joyce's *Ulysses* (completed in 1922) Leopold Bloom has been impotent with Molly for the past decade and kissing her rump gives him only "a proximate erection." D. H. Lawrence most famously argued in *Lady Chatterley's Lover* (1928) that modern men lacked ardor.[3] Most commentators' warnings that the stresses of the overcivilized postwar world—of work, exams, automobile riding, and demanding women—could result in male flops were not terribly original. Nevertheless two charismatic figures—Sigmund Freud and Marie Stopes—drew on their own life experiences to reconfigure the meaning of male sexual dysfunctions. Though their conclusions radically differed, they both began with the premise that impotence was a symptom of masculinity in crisis.

* * *

In 1906 the British medical journal *Lancet* carried an evocative account of forensic sleuthing penned by Dr. Charles A. Mercier, physician for mental diseases at Charing Cross Hospital. The two-page article read more like a Sherlock Holmes story than a medical report. Mercier had been asked to see a gentleman in a midland city who was said to be "a chronic, quiet, steady alcoholic." The man had a broken leg, having been "recently knocked down by an omnibus." His wife provided very little information to Mercier, seeming "to have an air of weary resignation, as if she had borne for a long time a burden almost beyond her strength," but the doctor learnt that the patient was "a man of independent means and of no occupation, a scholar of a celebrated college at Cambridge, and a man of great intelligence and culture." He took no interest in anything, although he had spent nearly two years in a slum in Birmingham, helping the poor with "energy and zeal," and had traveled to dangerous regions on the west coast of Africa and to Manchuria. His vital organs were sound; his digestion good; his urine was normal. He was not depressed. He had been examined by many physicians, yet no definite diagnosis had been made. Mercier sensed that there was some important information that both the man and his wife were withholding. After going through many possible diagnoses, Mercier reached his conclusion. The man must be impotent or at least think he was. "Such a belief [in his own impotence] would account for the shunning of society; for the solitary days, locked in his room, and brooding over his trouble; for the craving of oblivion in drink; and for the attempts at suicide. Moreover, it would account for the peculiarity, otherwise inexplicable, the devotion to slumming. The deprivation or the renunciation of sexual life is always closely connected with the display of self-sacrifice and self-renunciation in other respects."[4] Convinced that he had solved the "mystery," Mercier confronted the patient. Bursting into tears, he admitted that he was indeed impotent and that his voyages abroad were made with suicidal intent.

Mercier's self-congratulatory account tells us a good deal about turn-of-the-century English society—in particular the belief held by some that a gentleman who engaged in charity work would likely have a sexual kink—but what is most interesting in the report is that Mercier appeared to be stumbling toward the sort of psychoanalytic explanation of the impotent man's behavior that Sigmund Freud was in the very process of elaborating in Vienna. Freud's method of analysis was only to be made known to the general public following the World War I, but Mercier's article suggests there already existed a demand for a psychic understanding of sexual dysfunctions.

Freud was ready to respond. "If the practising psychoanalyst asks himself on account of what disorder people most often come to him for help," he wrote in 1912, "he is bound to reply—disregarding the many forms of anxiety—that it is psychical impotence."[5] Curiously enough this assertion has never been fully investigated. Many works have been devoted to Freud's treatment of hysteria and other female complaints, but remarkably little has been written about his view of male sexual incompetence. Given the importance Freud and his followers attributed to the phallus, the oversight is surprising. Impotence helped launched Freud's explorations of the mind/body relationship and subsequent generations of psychoanalysts built careers on the claim that they could cure impotence. The belief that anxieties impeded sexual performance had, of course, a long history. The originality of the Freudians lay in their popularizing the notion that such problems could be traced back to specific sorts of psychic causes. But on what basis did Freud made make his discoveries? And armed with his insights, did psychoanalysts actually have effective remedies to offer anxious males, or did therapists, as a cynic like Karl Kraus suggested, help create many of the very complaints they professed to combat?

In his history of the psychoanalytic movement Freud complained that at the beginning of his career he had been ostracized for arguing for the sexual aetiology of the neuroses, but that his own mentors had suggested just that. Joseph Breuer once said to him that his patients' hysteria were always due to the "secrets d'alcôve." In Paris Freud heard Jean-Martin Charcot attribute a suffering wife's ailments to her husband's impotence. And when Freud began his practice in Vienna, Rudolf Chrobak told him about a female patient suffering from anxiety attacks due to fact that her marriage had never been consummated. "The sole prescription for such a malady, he added [Freud recalled] is familiar enough to us, but we cannot order it. It runs: Rx Penis normalis dosim repetatur [repeated doses of a normal penis]."[6]

According to Freud, his mentors simply joked about sex; he set out to make sexuality an object of scientific investigation. The world in which he lived legitimated such an undertaking. In past generations, if one's sex life was not all that one might have wished, the failing could be dismissed as only another of a man's many minor disappointments. At the turn of the century, as increasing numbers of commentators claimed that any normal person should expect to experience sensual bliss, the pursuit of sexual satisfaction took on an unprecedented importance. "Sexual love," Freud asserted, "is undoubtedly one of the chief things in life, and the union of mental and bodily satisfaction in the enjoyment of love is one of its culminating peaks. Apart from a few queer fanatics, all the world knows this and conducts its life accordingly; science alone is too delicate to admit it."[7] That sex should be granted ever increasing importance was understandable given the fact that with modernization, public life was becoming more bureaucratized and the division of labor was making work less fulfilling. The middle classes, able to separate work from family, similarly split their public and private worlds. They increasingly compensated for the humdrum routine of their professional lives by embracing the romantic notion that only in the private realm was the authentic self fully revealed. Accordingly a successful sex and family life on which one's identity was based and confirmed became, so sex experts claimed, the new criteria of status and well-being.

By explaining that all neuroses had a sexual origin, Freud sought to give order to a disorderly world and provide a modern, natural, and scientific explanation of human unhappiness. A generation of researchers were talking about sexual problems; Freud's originality lay in erecting an entire explanation of civilization based on the centrality of sex.[8] He moved from first believing that adult neuroses were due to the shameful memories of actual assaults individuals had experienced as children to the idea that they were the remnants of infantile sexual fantasies. He set out to map the "unconscious," where such troubling thoughts lay buried. His message, as spread by generations of therapists, centered on the notion that infantile sexuality existed, that the neuroses were caused by sexual repression, and that the sexual drives influenced all of human history. Most readers had only a shaky understanding of the scenario that held that the id demanded gratification, the ego judiciously regulated the promptings of the unconscious, and the superego internalized the restraints of society. What the public believed Freud to argue was that if the sexual drives were frustrated illness would result.

In building up the theory that sexual frustrations underlay neuroses Freud necessarily investigated male impotence. As he made clear in his preface to Maxim Steiner's *The Psychical Disorders of Male Potency* (1913), he believed that organic and neurotic elements reinforced each other. The growing male child took on board a number of inhibitions; some could become pathological.

> The sexual function is liable to a great number of disturbances, most of which exhibit the characteristics of simple inhibitions. They are classed together as psychical impotence. . . . In men the chief stages at which the inhibition

occurs are shown by: a turning away of the libido at the very beginning of the process (psychical-unpleasure); an absence of the physical preparation for it (lack of erection); an abridgement of the sexual act (*ejaculatio praecox*), an occurrence which might equally well be regarded as a symptom; an arrest of the act before it has reached its natural conclusion (absence of ejaculation); or a non-appearance of the psychical outcome (lack of the feeling of pleasure in orgasm). Other disturbances arise from the sexual function becoming dependent on special conditions of a perverse or fetishist nature.[9]

Why were civilized men plagued by such a range of potency problems? In his early works, Freud at first carried on the old argument that excesses led to impotence. Masturbation, he claimed, was the cause of neurasthenia in youths and led to the impairing of their potency at maturity. Such weaknesses could later in married life be exacerbated by coitus interruptus. He wrote to his colleague Wilhelm Fliess of cases in which the use of the condom also resulted in weak potency.[10]

In his mature writings Freud attributed impotence to deeper seated causes, that is unresolved Oedipal urges. Why did the organs refuse to perform despite desire and ability and only with certain persons? Such problems, Freud insisted, were not just accidents, but due to the patient's incestuous fixation on his mother and associated memories of childhood sexual activity. Psychical impotence prevented men from having sex with anyone who conjured up images of affectionate family members. A woman who elicited their "high psychical estimation" could not be a sensual object. "Where they love they do not desire and where they desire they cannot love."[11] To be free and happy a man had to understand and deal with his repressed desires. "Normal termination" of a male's sexual development began with giving up such thoughts and an acceptance of new objects of desire—eligible sex partners, new objects of desire, in which were combined affectionate and sensual currents.

Problems arose for those men whose fantasies retained incestuous fixations. "The result is then total impotence, which is perhaps further ensured by the simultaneous onset of an actual weakening of the organs that perform the sexual act." For other men sexual pleasure was only possible with a "debased and despised sexual object" because a middle-class man was commonly shackled in his relations with a respectable woman: "He is assured of complete sexual pleasure only when he can devote himself unreservedly to obtaining satisfaction, which with his well-brought-up wife, for instance, he does not dare to do." This split in libidinous desires, observed a disciple of Freud's, was "most obvious in cases of facultative impotence, where, for example, the patient is always unable to have intercourse with his own wife but never fails with a prostitute."[12]

This madonna/whore dichotomy had, of course, been central to Western culture's sexual double standard for centuries and Freud himself had to admit that since all respectable men faced the same dilemma they logically should all be impotent. "We should be justified in expecting psychical impotence to be a universal affliction and not a disorder confined to some individuals." Having apparently painted himself into a corner, Freud faced down potential critics by boldly asserting that a degree of impotence "does in fact characterize the love of civilized man." He thus stretched the definition of impotence to include the failure to find pleasure. Just as there were frigid women, there were some men who were "psychanaesthetic: men who never fail in the act but who carry it out without getting any particular pleasure from it—a state of affairs that is more common than one would think." In short all men, according to Freud, were to some degree or another impotent. Substitutes would never fully replace mother. Civilization therefore had to be based on a degree of renunciation and suffering. "We must reckon with the possibility that something in the nature of the sexual instinct itself is unfavourable to the realization of complete satisfaction."[13] Well-balanced males learned how to respond creatively to such challenges, whereas the weak succumbed to their neuroses.

The central male neurosis was fear of castration. Freud believed the male child—ashamed of his guilty desires—feared being punished by losing his penis, which led to the grown man's self-consciousness and incapacitating fear of using it, which could result finally in impotence. As feminists later complained, Freud credited women with "penis envy" and based his understanding of both sexes on the examination of male patients. He presented the penis as the only genital worth noticing. The penis was so important not because of the pleasure it could give, according to Freud, but because of "its organic significance for the propagation of the species." It represented a victory of the needs of the race over those of the individual. He asserted that men found women's genitals disgusting. "Probably no male human being is spared the fright of castration at the sight of a female genital." This revulsion was hardly surprising, as he was sure that men's conviction that women did not have a penis led "them to an enduringly low opinion of the other sex." Psychic impotence was one symptom of the castration complex. The child's discovery of the mother's lack of a penis "gives place to a feeling of disgust which in the years of puberty can become the cause of psychical impotence, misogyny and permanent homosexuality."[14]

Where did Freud get his information on impotence? Surprisingly enough, he based much of his discussion of male sexuality on the second hand reports of his women patients. For example, Freud gave an account of one woman's description of her disastrous honeymoon: "On the wedding night her husband had met with a not unusual mishap. He found himself impotent, and many times in the course of the night he came hurrying from his room into hers to try once more whether he could succeed. In the morning he said he would feel ashamed in front of the hotel maid who made the beds, and he took a bottle of red ink, and poured its contents over the sheet; but he did it so clumsily that the red stain came in a place that was very unsuitable for his purpose." The compulsive woman patient now had a mania of repeatedly arranging her table cloth and calling in the maid for useless errands. Freud concluded that her unconscious desire was for the servant to see that the cloth was stained, a symptom of her fixation on the unhappy memory. In another case a young woman dreamt of having a candle that would not stand up properly. The symbolism here, declared Freud, was "obvious enough." He was equally categorical in dealing with an aggressive female patient who had been so enraged by her husband that she had the wish of telling him, "Go and hang yourself." "It turned out," reported Freud, "that a few hours earlier she had read somewhere or other that when a man is hanged he gets a powerful erection. The wish for an erection had emerged from repression in this horrifying disguise." In such cases Freud implicitly began with the basic premise that civilized man would likely be undersexed. Freud posited the notion that in turn the poorer the man's potency the more hysterical his wife would be. Freud clearly knew what he was looking for—the weak male—which made it highly likely that he would eventually find him. His motto might well have been "Cherchez l'homme!" The notion that a woman's distress might be due to a sexually overdemanding husband never seems to have occurred to Freud.[15]

Freud's reports of unhappy women patients have to be regarded with some suspicion as they were based on his often convoluted interpretations of chance remarks. His famous analysis of Dora is a case in point: "She had once again been insisting that Frau K. only loved her father because he was 'ein vermögender Mann' [a man of means]. Certain details of the way in which she expressed herself (which I pass over here, like most of the other purely technical parts of the analysis) led me to see that behind this phrase its opposite lay concealed, namely, that her father was 'ein unvermögender Mann' [a man without means]. This could only be meant in a sexual sense—that her father, as a man, was without means, was impotent."[16]

Freud was so taken by this inversion of meaning that he cited the same play on words in yet another essay:

I also know of an elderly man who married a very young girl and who decided to spend the wedding night in a hotel in town instead of on the honeymoon journey. Hardly had they reached the hotel when he noticed in alarm that he was without his wallet, which contained all the money for the honeymoon; he had either mislaid it or lost it. He was still able to reach his servant by telephone; the latter found the missing wallet in the discarded wedding suit and brought it to the hotel to the waiting bridegroom who had accordingly entered upon his marriage without means [*ohne Vermögen*]. He was thus able to start his journey with his young bride next morning. In the night, however, he had, as he had apprehensively foreseen, proved "incapable [*unverögend*]."[17]

That is, impotent. While there is no denying that Freud was always the master storyteller, there remains the nagging question of what one was to make of such carefully crafted tales. Freud's failure to explain the provenance of this particular story makes it difficult not to suspect that he was attempting to pass off an old joke as a serious psychoanalytic finding.

Did Freud actually see many males who admitted to suffering from impotence? In his most famous essays there are only occasional references to men who explicitly referred to performance problems. A young man, for example, is reported as having dreamt of a limp balloon that Freud had him recognize as symbolizing his penis. In a more extensive report Freud gave an account of an older man who had dreamt of laughing about his inability to turn off the light no matter how hard he tried, even with his wife's help. By the process of reversal, argued Freud, the dream revealed itself as really being about the man not being able to turn the light on, that is, his being unable to perform sexually. Such a dream was not a joking matter, but a sad contemplation of impotence and death. To protect himself, declared Freud, the man had turned his sobs into chuckles.[18] Here again the analysand did not himself mention impotence; Freud took the liberty of attributing to the patient a fear of failure.

As his male patients did not provide as much material on impotence as one might have expected, Freud supplemented their accounts with his own insights. For example, in reporting on his self-analysis to Fliess, he referred to a dream he had of his old nurse. "She was my teacher in sexual matters and scolded me for being clumsy and not being able to do anything. (This is always how neurotic impotence comes about; it is thus that fear of incapacity at school obtains its sexual substratum.)" Ernest Jones, Freud's biographer, discreetly noted, "the more passionate side of married life subsided earlier with him that it does with many men." Freud was more open. He wrote Fliess in 1897, "Sexual excitation is of no more use to a person like me." He even discussed with Emma Jung the ending of his sex life, for in 1911 she reminded him of a conversation they had had: "You told me about your family. You said then that your marriage had long been 'amortized,' now there was nothing to do except—die." [19] Freud sketched out the same pessimistic account of married life in "'Civilized' Sexual Morality."

> A marriage begun with reduced capacity to love on both sides succumbs to the process of dissolution even more quickly than others. As a result of the man's weak potency, the woman is not satisfied, and she remains anaesthetic even in cases where her disposition to frigidity, derived from her education, could have been overcome by a powerful sexual experience. A couple like this finds more difficulties, too, in the prevention of children than a healthy one, since the husband's diminished potency tolerates the use of contraceptives badly. In this perplexity, sexual intercourse, as being the source of all their embarrassments, is soon given up, and with this the basis of married life is abandoned. [20]

On the basis of his self-analysis, Freud argued that haunting vestiges of infantile desires lurking in the unconscious led to some form of impotence. He then proceeded to collect the evidence to support his hypothesis. Some patients might have found the analysis helpful. Those who did not could find themselves being chastised for their "resistance." Unlike scientific hypotheses, Freud's argument could not be disproved.

Freud's followers and the refractory post-Freudians, if less gloomy, carried on the essence of the master's message. Though they differed between themselves in many ways, in general they agreed with the founder of their discipline that much psychic impotence resulted from childhood fantasies. Haunted by incestuous desires for the mother, the patient's unresolved guilt manifested itself in self-punishment, piety, overestimation of the sexual object, fear of castration, and homosexual desires. Widening the net of psychic causes of sexual incapacity, post-Freudian psychoanalysts also included a range of forbidden acts indulged in later in life—including adolescents' mutual masturbation, the petting of servants, and married men's hankering after younger women—all of which could lead to transitory impotence. Sexual weaklings and the semi-impotent were declared to be common. Wilhelm Reich reported that 28 of his 30 private patients and 164 of 175 patients seen at the Vienna Psychoanalytic Outpatient Clinic in 1923–24 were suffering from impotence. [21] Some incapacitated themselves by the process of autosuggestion. It was not sufficient for the therapist simply to reassure the patient, however, as it was not just his fear of failure but his unconscious desires that had to be addressed.

Like Freud, the first generation of the psychoanalytically inclined held that impotence was one of the prices one paid for a civilized society. Unlike primitives, modern men had inhibitions. "In men love-inadequacy is increasing to an alarming degree, and impotence has come to be a disorder associated with modern civilization. . . . The percentage of relatively impotent men cannot be placed too high. In my experience, hardly half of all civilized men enjoy normal potency." With these alarming words Wilhelm Stekel began his two volume study *Impotence in the Male*, the most extensive of the interwar psychoanalytic accounts of the problem. For the Freudians the modern world placed more pressures on men and impotence was one of the side effects of progress. Peasants and laborers were spared the burden of the nervousness and inhibitions of the more cultivated.[22] And man more than woman bore the brunt of such psychic costs because he had the task of policing himself.

For all their purported radicalism, Freud's popularizers presented a fairly traditional model of sexual relations in which the man had to be dominant and the woman subservient. In their discussion of impotence they implied that the struggle between the sexes was more acute than ever, with rising rates of impotence a symptom of men feeling themselves under siege. Some might regard their fiascoes as a joking matter, but the experts warned they not infrequently led to suicide. No frigid woman ever thought of killing herself, unlike the deficient man who could not hide his condition.

Moving away from the notion that all problems stemmed from infantile issues, Alfred Adler argued that psychic impotence originated in a "repressed recollection of aggression associated with intercourse." Organ inferiority, he asserted, led to neurosis. The underendowed man, in seeking to prove his masculinity, disastrously sought compensation in masturbation and fantasies. Adler presented the case of a man so fearful of women that he safeguarded himself from marriage with "massive pollutions, premature ejaculations and impotence." Such behavior Adler construed as part of a "masculine protest." Henry Dicks, an adherent of Adler, suggested that the impotent patient unconsciously sought to punish the female partner who made him feel inferior. At the same time one failure wounded the vanity of the narcissistic type, who in worrying about it, failed again. "He must 'exert control'—it is intolerable that such a one as he had failed in so essential a task of masculinity and power. . . . It is not altogether surprising that members of the military profession are quite prone to this type of impotence."[23]

According to Otto Fenichel some men found the loss of control in orgasm created anxiety. "Impotence is a physical alteration arising from a defensive action by the ego which prevents the carrying out of an instinctual activity regarded as dangerous. The part of the ego that exerts this action is certainly an unconscious one; it is the part in which castration anxiety is operative and which has at its disposal pathways that are not subject to voluntary control." In severe *ejaculatio praecox*, wrote Fenichel, there were three major determinants: a feminine orientation, a sadistic orientation "which has as its aim to soil and to injure the woman," and "an intensified urethral eroticism which makes the individual unconsciously regard semen in the same way as he regarded urine as a child." [24]

It was impossible, argued Freud's biographer, Ernest Jones, for a man to suffer impotence and not lose his sense of worth. The mere suspicion was terrible. The furtive, suspicious, phobic victim, plagued by both neurotic fears and "sexual hunger" soon found he had "a total inability to hold his head erect and look the whole world in the face." Frigid women did not suffer a sense of inferiority; in fact they were likely narcissistic man-haters. Theodore Reik agreed. Why did the impotent man feel ashamed and guilty? He has not done anything wrong. His guilt, Reik insisted, was really an aspect of his anger at those who prevented him from realizing his incestuous desires. And women who pretended to console the impotent were in fact revealing their "unconscious hostility" in pardoning their man in an insultingly maternal fashion. Thus a woman who dreamt of tripping her partner, claimed Reik, really wanted to cause his impotence. Such a desire, he claimed, "expresses itself not only in [a woman's] lack of sexual response, but in some inappropriate behavior during sexual intercourse. In a case known to me the woman laughingly said to her husband near the climax: 'You looked so funny just now!' The sobering effect of this remark can well be imagined. It is remarkable how rarely a woman feels guilty about such cruelly frustrating behavior." [25]

Frigidity in women was common because they were narcissistic, claimed the Freudians; they overvalued foreplay. Women, Reik pointed out, did not feel guilty about their own frigidity since they were largely passive, though in the last few years the "modern woman sometimes feels that her cooperation in sex is necessary." Yet most still felt no responsibility. According to Adler the frigid made up one third to one half of all women. An American expert concluded that the therapist confronted with "true frigidity in women, which is undoubtedly homosexually determined, is almost helpless." [26]

Though Freud and his followers critiqued some aspects of the older moral code, they continued to perpetuate constrained notions of gender roles and sexual relationships. Freud spoke in an old-fashioned way of maleness being "activity" and femaleness "passivity"; of a "brake" necessarily being put on young women's sexuality while young men's libido had to be released; of women stoically accepting the prohibitions on sexual activity that men were supposed to happily violate.[27] Readers of the psychoanalytic texts found repeated references to what made a healthy man "normal" or "manly." Homosexuality and effeminacy emerged from such psychoanalytic discussions clearly suspect.

It was important for modern man to be reassured that his failures might be due to the unresponsive women, because impotence was frequently taken as a symptom of homosexuality. In 1915 a contributor to the *Practitioner* wrote that some impotence was due to "psychological abnormalities indicative of a neuropathic strain of heredity." Treatment was difficult, but psychoanalysis could be used, as "it can be shown that the sexual inversion and consequent impotence is due to a definite psychical trauma in the past history, the very fact of its discussion during psychanalysis [sic] may be sufficient to dissipate its influence, and allow of a return to more normal sexual habits." Homosexuals, according to the Freudians, had failed to resolve their Oedipal desires and even the most active could ipso facto be declared "impotent." Israel S. Wechsler, professor of clinical neurology at Columbia University, asserted that, "it is notorious that sons excessively devoted to their mothers make poor husbands, and not a few actually are impotent." Ernest Jones defined potency as the ability to carry out vaginal intercourse satisfactorily. "It will be noticed that homosexuals would by this definition be regarded as impotent (except in so far as they are ambisexual), and I think rightly so, however potent they may be with members of their own sex; it must be admitted, however, that both the genesis and the results of the impotence here are in many respects different from those of the other, heterosexual type." The American writer John F. W. Meagher, warned that the homosexual who married would suffer from impotence or premature ejaculation. An English psychiatrist similarly attributed such complaints to a man's latent bisexuality or homosexuality.[28] It had long been a commonplace that a homosexual could not be potent with a woman. The Freudians reversed the argument, asserting that homosexuality was really a cover adopted by a man who was afraid he would be exposed as impotent.

Stekel claimed that hundreds of thousands of men had been made impotent as a result of the war, many of whom he referred to as "war-impotent homosexuals" who had embarked on a "flight from womanhood." He had a number of homosexual patients and held contradictory views on the subject. He argued that all heterosexuals could at times have homosexual urges and that accordingly such desires could be "cured." Key to the analyst's success would be making the patient admit to his sadistic hatred of women. Stekel had grave doubts that such patients could successfully change. Such analyses were often broken off, which Stekel recognized as a protective tactic on the patient's part.[29] He, like most psychoanalysts, recognized the futility of criminalizing same-sex relations, while still regarding homosexuals as neurotic.

The sort of treatment patients received depended very much on the type of therapist they saw. The popularizers of psychoanalysis tended to be far more optimistic than Freud. Adler, for example, was convinced that straightforward man to man chats could lead to commonsense solutions. Whereas Freud regarded impotence as a classic symptom of the impossibility of reconciling culture and instinct, many of his followers stressed the possibility of adjustment and cures. Sandor Ferenczi believed that incestuous fixations on mothers, sisters, nurses and servants were common causes of impotence though the censor made the patient's recall of such desires difficult. At a 1908 conference in Budapest Ferenczi presented a case in which he attributed his patient's impotence to the man's desire for his fat, older sister with whom he had played as a child. As an adolescent he fantasized about her when masturbating with the result that sex became disgusting to him. Once the patient accepted this interpretation, so Ferenczi claimed, he was miraculously cured, and proved it by having intercourse with three women in one day.[30]

Stekel, a prolific writer and innovative therapist, claimed to have been cured of his own impotence by Freud. Stekel placed much of the blame for his condition on his unsympathetic wife. "One day I was no longer a man. I tried everything to overcome my weakness, but I failed. This period lasted two years." Stekel did not believe that all sexual dysfunctions were a result of the incest complex, but he did view impotence as a way a man sought to protect himself against his asocial tendencies. In his own work Stekel broke Freud's "rigid rules" that forbade the patient from posing questions and relied on free association in treatments that could take years. Stekel preferred a short intuitive and intrusive "active method," convinced that he could tell within an hour the patient's basic problem. He claimed that he had "almost always" cured cases over which other therapists had ineffectively labored. Yet Stekel, like Freud, believed his task was to trace nervous problems to the underlying repressions, release them, and so affect a cure via "mental orthopedics." He reported that much psychic impotence was due to the fear of failing, so that simply recommending a few months abstinence often resulted in the patient soon returning to say he was cured. He admitted that in some cases therapy only worked as a result of suggestion. He boasted that he cured "almost all" the impotent men who came to him and gave their "life" back to them. Stekel sounded most like a huckster in asserting that even the elderly could have their sexual powers restored. "A *man only becomes old when he feels old! And only he becomes impotent who gives up his potency*" (author's emphasis). Any decline of potency from the fifties onward he attributed to psychic causes.[31]

Psychoanalysts revolutionized the study of male sexual disabilities in declaring that almost everything that nineteenth-century doctors had targeted as the causes of impotence—masturbation, sexual excesses, addiction to drugs, drink and tobacco, and even the lessening of desire associated with old age—might only be symptoms of deep seated psychic traumas. Some like Stekel even argued that the absence of morning erections was not a sign of organic problems. Indeed most asserted that it was not possible to draw a sharp line between incurable and acquired forms of impotence. Stekel acknowledged that medical writers of marriage manuals such as Theodoor Hendrik van de Velde were making useful contributions to the discussion of marital sex, while insisting that they had no insights into the psychic basis of aversion and lacked the "profound knowledge which we [psychoanalysts] have gained." The denigration of the role of organic causes served the interest of a profession in which lay practitioners increasingly displaced the medically trained. At the same time it is no doubt true that their downplaying of the significance of self-abuse and sexual excesses was a step forward. Stekel was especially outspoken in declaring that masturbation was harmless in and of itself. In his eyes it was not the cause, but a symptom of man's fear of women.[32]

This reappraisal of self-abuse launched by the psychoanalysts seeped into texts meant for general readers. In 1927 R. G. Gordon reported that it was not masturbation, but the fear of the ravages that the vice purportedly caused that led to impotence. He noted that fatigue, pain, failure, surgery, and fear of venereal disease all played a role, "but by far the commonest cause is the dread of the results of masturbation as portrayed by quack literature and even in would-be moral homilies. If punishment should fit the crime, then, in view of the mental torture they inflict on their victims, there is no depth of the inferno sufficiently terrible to house the authors of these publications." Yet a 1937 study of the neuroses meant for general practitioners reported that fears of masturbation were still common and that impotence could be caused by listening to such scare stories. The author recommended doctors try to have a reasonable chat with their patient, warning him against quack remedies and experimenting with prostitutes.[33]

The psychoanalysts obviously turned the discussion of impotence in a new direction, shifting the focus from the organic to the psychic causes. Who benefited from such an undertaking? Freud did help break the conspiracy of silence about many sexual issues, and thanks to his work, repression was increasingly recognized as a cause of crippling inhibitions. The popularization of a more relaxed, less moralistic view of a range of sexual practices must have relieved some anxieties and cured some forms of impotence. Such successes were proudly chronicled by the psychoanalysts. They saved some patients from the quacks. Stekel noted that one of his clients had previously been subjected to the "suction of the penis with a vacuum-margonal apparatus of Professor Bier," electric shocks, and doses of muriacetin.[34] Yet psychoanalysts primarily opposed such medical and hormonal therapies because they might conceal the psychic causes of the disorder, not because they were actually harmful to the patient. What the analysts failed to mention—indeed what their training prevented them from recognizing—were the patients whose sexual problems did not have a psychic basis and who found themselves subjected to useless if not damaging injunctions to confront their incestuous desires or other purported traumatic memories.

Love played a greater role in the life of modern man, and according to the psychoanalysts, so too did inhibitions. They exalted the importance of problems they said they could solve, focusing unprecedented attention on the genitals as the synecdoche of the individual. "The penis," boldly declared Stekel, "is an image of the entire man." If it failed, to whom did the despondent turn? Ironically many men looked for help from those experts—the "anxiety-makers" some would later call them—who were undertaking the problematizing of sexuality. Psychic impotence, they asserted, obviously manifested itself in lack of erections, premature ejaculation and absence of orgasms, but any phenomenon that impeded heterosexual coitus also had to be included—from fetishes, phobias, and homosexual desires to the most innocent bouts of forgetfulness or bashfulness. A majority of men could thus be construed as suffering from some form of impotence, therapists asserted, but at the same time they refused to view such behavior as "normal." Impotence was only a symptom of a deeper-seated problem. Patients, the analysts noted, might seek to defend themselves by lies and subterfuges from the charge of harboring shameful secrets, but most would eventually be unmasked. Those who refused to acknowledge the psychic basis of their problem could not be cured, because they chose to remain ill. In this catch-22, the man who had no reason to believe that his sexual problems had a psychic cause was clearly the most disturbed and would require extended care. The evidence suggests that there was more than a grain of truth in Karl Kraus's observation: "Before Freud, doctors cautioned that the cure may be worse than the disease; now they ought to caution that there is a cure which is a disease—namely, psychoanalysis."[35]

* * *

For Freud, the possibility of achieving complete sexual happiness was slim at best. As such his writings appeared to run counter to the optimistic cultural currents reflected in the marriage manuals of the interwar years. If their authors never rivaled Freud in intellectual sophistication, they nevertheless reached a far larger readership and introduced the notion of modern impotence. By "modern impotence" I am pointing to the fact that middle-class commentators set out to establish new standards of what constituted normal and healthy masculinity. Self-consciously contrasting themselves with the purportedly repressed Victorians, the advocates of companionate marriage explicitly argued that its foundation was the sexual satisfaction of both partners. When it was assumed that the woman was sexually passive, it was largely left to the man to grade his own competence. In the last decades of the nineteenth century the critique made of unresponsive wives signaled the emergence of a new model of marriage in which it was expected that women could be both respectable and passionate. Marriages were eroticized, even in Europe where the elite continue to arrange them. The sexualization of marriage was pushed furthest in the United States as indicated by the arrival of texts with titles like *Sex Happiness* (1922), *Marriage in the Modern Manner* (1929), and *Married Sweethearts* (1933). This recognition or rediscovery of female desire in the early twentieth century led commentators to argue that the woman's erotic needs had to be satisfied. "Accepting that women had sexual desires of their own ultimately meant the extension of the performance principle to the realm of sexuality." [36] An unanticipated result was that the men who failed to please could find their manhood in doubt. The question was then posed: who or what was responsible for such tragedies? Amongst the first to answer was Marie Stopes. Her disastrous first marriage offers a unique perspective on both the private and public discussions of male sexual performance. She ultimately won fame by forging an impressive career as a birth control advocate. Less well known is the key role she played in recasting the discussion of impotence.

Raised in an enlightened upper middle-class family, Marie Stopes was a first rate scientist (the first Englishwoman to receive a doctorate in paleobotany), and claimed to be a late learner in sexual matters. Recently evidence has turned up that undermines her protestations of sexual naiveté. Though in later life she attacked the evil of girls' crushes on teachers and homosexuality, in her twenties Stopes was passionately attracted to a number of women and was so intent on marriage that she pursued a male scientist all the way to Japan. It was just after these hopes were dashed that

she met the Canadian botanist Reginald Ruggles Gates. Gates proposed after they had known each other for little more than a week. Three months
later in March 1911 they were married in Montreal. She was thirty-one, he
was twenty-nine. The marriage, entered in haste, proved to be a failure. She
overshadowed her younger spouse. He became ill-tempered. The relationship degenerated to such an extent that Stopes claimed that Gates tried to
stab her with a butter knife; he reported that she put poison in his coffee.

Stopes harped repeatedly on her innocence and alleged that only by reading up on sex in the main reading room of the British Museum did she finally
discover that her marriage was incomplete. However June Rose has argued
that Stopes was more sexually experienced than she let on. In the very year
she had married she began a study of sexual relationships, and in 1913, when
casting about for a way to sever her tie with Gates, she asked her solicitors
if a divorce could be obtained if a wife were adulterous. In the end she decided to argue that the marriage had never been consummated and that she
had remained a virgin. She told her lawyers that though Gates indulged for
hours in foreplay he had been only partially rigid on three occasions. He was,
she graphically asserted, "so limp as he struggled to enter that he pushed it
in with his fingers." Though she obtained from her doctor only a curiously
qualified certificate of being an intact virgin, in October 1914 she filed a nullity petition.[37] As Gates did not oppose it, the marriage was dissolved.

The story might have ended there. Every year a few English marriages
were annulled on the grounds of nonconsummation.[38] The couples involved
in such unhappy events naturally sought anonymity. Marie Stopes, who
had a pronounced exhibitionist streak, did not. She attributed her own purported ignorance to a lack of sex education. To spare other women a similar
fate, she felt the need to broadcast her ex-husband's failings. She was thus
led to write books on marriage and—after realizing the disastrous threat
posed women by unwanted pregnancies—on birth control.

The first fruit of Stopes's research was her book *Married Love: A New Contribution to the Solution of Sex Difficulties*. Appearing in 1918, it was an overnight sensation, going through seven printings and eventually selling more
than a million copies. "In my first marriage," she began, "I paid such a terrible price for sex-ignorance that I feel that knowledge gained at such a cost
should be placed at the service of humanity. . . . I hope (this book) will save
some others years of heartache and blind questioning in the dark." Stopes
proceeded to provide the public with an even fuller account of her blighted
marriage in a 1923 play entitled *Vectia*. The heroine (obviously Stopes), un-
happily married for three years until rescued from her impotent husband
by a neighbor who informs her of the facts of life, is presented as finally

winning a nullity suit. As the Lord Chamberlain refused to grant the play a license, Stopes in 1926 wrote *A Banned Play*, a book containing the script and calling for the reform of theater censorship. In correspondence she openly admitted the drama was based on her own experiences and its purpose was to end what she regarded as a protective code of male silence.[39]

Gates provided a markedly different account of the marriage, but he is a man both difficult to like and to believe. When Stopes met him he was a bright, if stuffy, young Chicago-trained scientist. In England he quickly established himself as an expert in cytology and genetics. He was awarded the prestigious Mendal Medal in 1911, the Huxley Gold Medal in 1914, and in 1915 brought out his first book. Made a Fellow of the Royal Society in 1931, he worked on the issue of mutation and chromosomal changes and eventually drifted into the controversial field of racial genetics. He was almost alone among twentieth-century scientists in holding a "polyphyletic origin for mankind," believing that race crossings had harmful effects. He was certainly a eugenicist; some regarded him as a fascist. When Julian Huxley and Alfred Court Haddon sought to counter Nazi race propaganda in *We Europeans* (1936), Gates violently criticized it. One of Gates's friends congratulated him for countering such "pure Jew propaganda."[40]

After the Stopes fiasco Gates married two more times. His second marriage was also quickly terminated. He fathered no children from any of these relationships. His failures have been taken by some as confirming Stopes's account of his physiological shortcomings. Moreover it is difficult not to see a sort of poetic justice at work here, inasmuch as an eugenicist, who declared himself a member of a "superior race," condemned interracial marriages for producing "mongrels," and pontificated on who should and who should not reproduce, proved himself to be incapable of siring offspring.[41] But was Gates, as Stopes claimed, impotent?

After his death in 1962, Gates's account of his humiliating first marriage was, as he had instructed, deposited in the British Museum. These papers make interesting reading. Stopes's followers had for thirty years lauded her as a saint, he grumbled, while unnamed "professional blackmailers and others" spread lies about him. He finally realized that he had been wrong to be silent. He recalled that they had met in Minneapolis and he proposed in St. Louis. Looking back on the whirlwind courtship he was now convinced that she had hurried the marriage so he would not learn more about her. "Had I known that she was a suffragette," Gates fumed, "I would never have proposed to her." More importantly, she claimed to be sexually ignorant, but Gates asserted that before they married in Montreal she had insisted that he go to a doctor and learn methods of contraception. The doctors only agreed to help when Gates promised to stop using the contraceptives once he obtained an academic position. Stopes herself, he claimed, employed a pessary. His argument was that it was the use of these contraceptives that "detracted from the joy of these experiences and doubtless acted as an impeding factor in my own sexual activity."

And even after the sacrifices he made, he stormed, she had the gall to have the marriage ended on the grounds that it had never been consummated. "She got annulment 1915 or 1916 by swearing I was impotent! On my solicitor's advice I was examined by Sir Alfred Fripp and given a certificate of perfect normality. This stopped the slander for a time but it was destroyed in the bombing of London, 1940." [42] Subsequently in 1947 he had himself tested by the Farris Institute for Parenthood which provided him with statement that his sperm were highly mobile. Mobile sperm do not, of course, prove potency.

Interestingly enough, though denying that he was impotent, Gates did admit that when he married he was still a virgin. "At our first sexual congress she had twitted me with having had no sexual experience. This was true. Although I had been greatly tempted many times, I had managed to lead a celibate life as a result of my strict religious upbringing combined with hard scientific work. I was probably clumsy at first, through lack of experience, but we were soon having intercourse frequently enough to satisfy a normal woman." [43] Gates's use of the term "normal" is telling. Moreover he complained that biographers of Stopes such as Keith Briant failed to note that she "was supersexed to a degree which was almost pathological."

So why did Gates concede the nonconsummation suit? He claimed he did not defend himself because it was the simplest way to end a disastrous marriage. This might appear a self-serving and rather weak argument, but if he had successfully fought the nullity suit, what would have been his reward? He would continue to be married to a woman he now hated. To obtain a divorce he would then have had to undertake the messy business of producing evidence that adultery had been committed by either him or Stopes. Gates, in accepting Stopes's nullity suit, clearly presumed that few people would ever hear of it. Little did he know that his lack of manhood would be cited by her and her disciples for decades to come as having launched the career of Britain's leading sex expert.

We will never know for certain what happened in the Stopes-Gates marriage. Yet there is no reason to be disappointed by the fact that their accounts differ so dramatically, with the combatants using such terms as "sex-ignorance," "normal," and "supersexed." If middle-class couples in the past had different opinions on the success of their sex lives, such information remained private. In the twentieth century such conflicts were to become central to the discussion of marital happiness. Moreover, prior to the twentieth century, doctors drew a sharp demarcation between impotent and nonimpotent men. If not completely impotent, the man had to judge his own sexual performance. The question was whether or not he was satisfied. No respectable woman could claim the right to judge. In the twentieth century, however, commentators began to blur the purportedly clear line separating the impotent and the nonimpotent. Impotence became all the more worrying as it ceased to be as clearly distinguished and isolated a phenomenon as it once had been.

In this redefining of male potency, Marie Stopes played a key role. She was representative of a generation of writers who argued that a successful sex life was the bedrock on which marital happiness was based. She noted that nineteenth-century sex manuals spoke primarily about restraint and not nearly enough about married couples' need for a regular, satisfying sex life. A number of historians have shown that many middle-class men and women in the late 1800s did believe that the wife should find as much happiness in the marital bed as the husband. Irregular practitioners like the phrenologist Orson S. Fowler maintained the old notion that a couple's climaxing together was required for conception to occur. Nevertheless most mainstream physicians assumed that the woman's passions were normally dormant and never as demanding as the man's. Many believed that only about 10 percent of women enjoyed sex, wrote one commentator in 1895, because of the feeling "that it indicates a lack of feminine virtue to feel a desire for sexual intercourse at all, and it is something to be proud of if you have never felt such impulses."[44]

Attempts in the early twentieth century to establish standards of what constituted normal and healthy marital relations took place in the context of an emerging awareness of new types of families that unembarrassingly pursued consumption and pleasure. Marriage counselors and birth controllers informed men and women that the first purpose of marriage was sexual happiness; children came second. The significance of sex in marriage was accordingly heightened to an unprecedented degree. Stopes's main argument was that a woman could and should experience the same pleasures as the man; accordingly, a happy marriage was one in which the husband continued to court and woo his wife. She condemned the state of affairs in which confused and ignorant young people entered wedlock. Some men had been brutalized by previous experiences with prostitutes while others were undersexed. She dedicated *Enduring Passion* to "married lovers." They had to adore each other, she insisted; no other relationship was as rich in interests and possibilities. Sexual compatibility provided their essential bond and it followed, Stopes declared, that the single bed was the enemy of marriage. She went on to explain in some detail how the man's duty, in the comforting confines of the marital double-bed, was to pleasure the woman so that she along with him obtained orgasm. She claimed that some had attacked her for letting women know what prostitutes knew, but her goal was simply to provide the man with a joyous companion. The recognition that women have sexual needs, she rejoiced, was "perhaps now at last, as a result of the recent frank attitude towards sex and its problems, openly recognized once more."[45]

At the moment, Stopes claimed, about 30 percent of professional and upper-class women were deprived, or in her words "starved" or "neurotic," because of their thoughtless spouses. Men had to be trained on when and how to arouse their partner. First, men needed to understand the female psyche and the fundamental female pulse that demanded at times abstinence and other times scheduled unions, perhaps several in one day. For Stopes full penetration was essential. "Far too many marriages depend on the external clitoris-orgasm alone for the woman. This would be rectified to a great extent were men more cultivated in self-control so as to secure the cervical-orgasm for their partners." She accordingly lauded the hardworking penis. Penetration she described as a "racial act" that "should only take place at special times and at rather infrequent intervals. Yet on account of the vital importance of this duty to the race, the penis, even from the hour of birth, is constructed as to be specialised to perform this duty."[46]

Deep penetration was essential because Stopes believed that it provided the woman with, in addition to semen, the "subtle absorptions from the complementary sex." Masturbation she necessarily condemned as harmful. "To play with sex and to indulge in premature and partial enjoyment is like eating small, bullet-sized green apples instead of waiting for the ripe sweet fruit." Stopes similarly castigated lesbianism as it tended "to unfit women for real union." It was only a form of play that could not satisfy. "*Hunger* for nourishment in sex union," she asserted, "is a true physiological hunger to be satisfied only by the supplying of the actual molecular substances lacked by her [the woman's] system." Stopes went so far as to claim that this need mitigated some female promiscuity. Self-control was impossible to those whose "sex-system cries out for chemical molecules."[47]

As bizarre as some of Stopes views were, she was not as original as she claimed. Her stress on the need for the exchange of "chemical molecules" was unusual, but Edward Carpenter had earlier suggested that sperm was absorbed by the tissues of the woman, and the cells of the female by the man. More importantly from the turn of the century onward women were increasingly presented in many English-language marriage manuals as the victims of clumsy spouses. Men were informed they had to sexually awaken their partners. Writers defended the woman's right to pleasure while continuing to assert that the man should take the initiative.[48]

American writers led the way in advancing this new conception of marital sexuality. The concern for the "synchronized orgasm" was voiced by George W. Savory in *Marriage: Its Science and Ethics* (1900), who believed that it would result in both happier marriages and superior offspring. W. F. Robie found that couples wanted to climax together if possible, and that a man was disappointed if his wife was not happy. In *The Sexual Life* (1907), Charles William Malchow paraded his American values in comparing intercourse to a well coached baseball game. "If the copulators intend to make the act count," he counseled, "the team must work together and be active in the nick of time." Another commentator likened sex to a track event: "Husbands and wives should be made to realize very forcibly that intercourse is a scientific procedure requiring training, not a haphazard act to be left to the direction of blind and wasteful nature." The goal was mutual orgasm, which took careful preparation and perhaps years of practice. C. B. S. Evans fell back on an even more curious metaphor in *Man and Woman in Marriage* (1932) when he asserted that it was the duty of the man to sexually satisfy his spouse. To disappoint her, he suggested, would be akin to promising a child a trip to the circus and then "at the very tent turn homewards."[49]

Such studies also assumed that their male readers needed a good deal of basic information on the female anatomy. If the female genitals were imagined to be boat-shaped, C. B. S. Evans helpfully suggested, "the clitoris lies where the flagpole would be on the bow of the boat." He strongly advised the husband to attend to it, meanwhile postponing his own climax by thinking of business or the movies. André Tridon suggested the man concentrate on the "recurring patterns of the woodwork of the bed, or possibly of the wall paper."[50]

Detailed instructions on how the male spouse could continue to be a lover were provided in a host of studies. Bernard Bernard in *Sex Conduct in Marriage* (1926) devoted a chapter to "The Husband's Function to Woo." Le Mon Clark in *Emotional Adjustment in Marriage* (1937) enjoined the man not to be a brute, but to satisfy his partner. Joseph Collins in *A Doctor Looks at Love and Life* (1926) argued that the husband had to avoid being selfish and learn about his wife's slower arousal. Helena Wright in *The Sex Factor in*

Marriage (1930) likewise asserted the man's need to "awaken" his wife. Only a minority of women were "spontaneously ardent," but most would respond to the spouse's "magic touch."[51]

Women who were not so pleasured began to be cited in texts such as Robert Latou Dickinson and Lura Beam's *A Thousand Marriages: A Medical Study of Sex Adjustment* (1932). "The several cases of male impotence are no more bitterly commented upon than the husband whose wife says he is potent but has 'no creative concept.' 'He just goes right to it.' She wants an artistic form, with the tempo of beginning, middle and end. When he says she is unresponsive, we nearly always find that she says he is 'too quick.'" One bride told Margaret Sanger that her disappointing first marital embrace had been like "a hurried meal over a lunch counter." The marriage experts presented women's desires, rhythms, need for foreplay, and dislike of routine as problems that men would have to confront if sexual harmony were to be achieved.[52]

Schedules on the timing and duration of intercourse were provided in *Hygiene of Marriage* (1923) by Isabel E. Hutton. She thought once a week was reasonable. Men took between one and two minutes to climax, reported M. J. Exner in *The Sexual Side of Marriage* (1932), whereas women took between ten and fifteen minutes. C. B. S. Evans reported that his sample of men said they lasted on average between five and fifteen minutes whereas the women—or at least those who did not fake their orgasms—asserted they needed up to thirty minutes. It was commonly reported that for many men premature ejaculation was a major problem. Exner for example asserted that it was especially rampant among the better educated and demanded a quick remedy. Male readers must have been shocked to discover that some experts went so far as to claim that any ejaculation that took place before the woman climaxed could be technically speaking classified as premature ejaculation, and it in turn was regarded as a form of impotence. Most interwar writers recognized the importance of clitoral stimulation, but like Stopes, regarded vaginal penetration as superior. Helena Wright held that a woman was not sexually mature until the pleasure of the vagina was as acute as that of the clitoris. A woman needed "full erection and deep penetration," stated Van de Velde, to provide the "full sensation and relief due to her."[53]

Despite all the references to romance, sex play, and the romantic wooing of one's partner, the marriage manuals' stress on techniques, schedules, and the employment of contraceptives inevitably created for some the sense of sex as work. Both sexes were faced with new pressures to perform. Wilhelm Stekel noted that women once denied their feelings. "No more is the frigid woman the model of virtue; she feels she is a poor sick soul! . . . Today the hypocrisy is much more on the side of passion: frigid women affect to be passionate, impotent men to be experienced." "Love is essential," enjoined Margaret Sanger. "Passion is essential. Virility is essential. Mastery of the instruments of expression is essential." Women who failed to be aroused might be condemned as frigid and men who did not match the new standards could find themselves labeled as impotent. Marie Stopes was particularly outspoken in attacking men who could not make the grade. She had a word or two to say about overly virile men—recommending cold baths and bromides—but was far more concerned with those she referred to as the "under-sexed."[54]

Stopes differed from most writers of marriage manuals in the amount of attention she devoted to undersexed men. She drew on her own experiences and, if she were to be believed, no one had ever discussed impotence until she arrived on the scene. Physicians, Stopes told a correspondent, had been of little help to her. "I had a family *doctor*, & when, after 3 years, I went to him & said 'Look here, I really don't believe I'm properly married, I wish you'd examine me or my husband or something, as it is beginning to worry me & I do want to know.' He *refused* even to look into the facts. So I wasted a whole year." Her point in making impotence a public issue was that it was a "self infliction" from which she hoped to save youths. "Men don't know & can't know (not even men medical practitioners) these things about other men unless I tell them, & their imaginations can't work correctly when the thing is put 'delicately.'"[55]

Stopes asserted that the completely impotent husband, though rare, did exist. There were marriages that were never consummated. Some deluded women mistakenly suspected their cool and distant husbands of infidelity. Other, more ignorant wives were not unhappy, thinking their blighted lives were normal. Doctors were of no use. Stopes gave the account of a woman married for five years. The family doctor told her husband that his lack of ardor was nothing to bother about and would probably "come right." The woman was left agitated and sleepless by his futile caresses. In discussing impotence most medical men reserved their sympathy for the man. "An impotent man," declared the American sex reformer William Robinson in *Sex Morality* (1919), "is a more pitiable man than a venereally infected one."[56] If culture had weighed concerns for the man, Stopes would tip the balance for the woman.

What were the modern causes of impotence? Stopes noted that shell shock, the stresses of motoring, and self-abuse could all contribute to the problem. The moralistic side of her argument was that youthful indiscretions, masturbation, and perhaps public school homosexuality might also play a role. V. S. Whitehead and C. A. Hoff agreed that most debility was due to indulgence, libertinism, and secret habits. The thoughtless man, according to Stopes, was doubly guilty: first of his own impotence, and secondly of thwarting the healthy woman's desire for a child. Employing the old notion of a spermatic economy, Margaret Sanger, the American birth controller, concurred, cautioning that a man who made "mistakes" in his youth would find in his thirties and forties that his "bank account of virility" was exhausted while the man who had practiced restraint could look forward to enjoying his "dividends."[57] Such views clashed with the progressive aspects of Freudian theory.

Stopes did strike a new note (perhaps thinking of her own situation) in raising the issue of the "under-sexed" man mismatched with a woman who had "an unusually strong and over-frequent desire." Both would inevitably suffer. She coined the term "semi-impotence" to describe the affliction of such a husband who wilted before the daunting prospect of his oversexed wife. The ranks of such undersexed males could only increase as once passive women began to make demands that their mates could not meet. Some Protestant churchmen agreed that impotence was the cause "of much domestic unhappiness and much unfaithfulness."[58]

Given her hostility to undersexed males, Stopes was surprisingly optimistic about their chances of being cured if they turned to her. Psychic impotence, she claimed, could be mastered in an hour by simply removing the patient's sense of guilt. She advised those suffering from premature ejaculation—which she found to be widely prevalent in the middle and upper classes—to avoid abstinence and to desensitize the penis with a lotion consisting of Listerine and alum. She opposed the use of aphrodisiacs and the rejuvenation operations offered by Eugen Steinach and Serge Voronoff, but had great faith in the ability of gland extracts to renew vitality. Though she believed that men, like women, went through a midlife "change" that might entail a decline in potency, she assured her readers that it was only a passing stage.[59]

Stopes drew on a stock of old notions about the causes and cures of impotence. For example, her portrayal of the undersexed exploited well-known stereotypes of the weakling. In *Vectia* she described the husband's "pale, dun-colored hair and face." Such an account mirrored earlier French texts in which "frigidité chez l'homme" was associated with the blond, grey-eyed, and beardless. Yet, if Stopes was in many ways curiously old fashioned and moralistic, she did tap into new preoccupations in raising the specter of "semi-impotence." Havelock Ellis, the English sexologist, agreed that many modern men suffered from "a relative defect of potency." "Erection more or less completely occurs and is followed, though too rapidly, by ejaculation."[60]

At the very time Stopes was seeking to end her marriage on the grounds of her husband's impotence, the American physician W. F. Robie was suggesting that such tragedies could be avoided. He noted that not infrequently one partner became sexually "incompetent." The solution, he suggested, was not divorce or adultery but the search for a way to provide physical comfort. As an example he cited a case in which a man had become impotent. "This husband, a religious but sensible man, remembered that he had been able at times to awaken desire in his wife by titillating her clitoris; so now, when her desire for intercourse became strong, he resorted to this maneuver, continuing the manipulation until she had an orgasm. He repeated this procedure as required during the period of his functional impotence. He was happy in thus being able to relieve her desire, she was gratified and contented and they have always been very happy together." In another case a woman who found intercourse repugnant nevertheless would masturbate her husband. "This couple," Robie reported, "have been absolutely faithful to each other and very happy." In *Hygiene of Marriage* Isabel E. Hutton also attempted to calm readers by assuring them that temporary impotence was not uncommon in the early days of a marriage, often as not precipitated by stress and excitement. The groom was advised to simply refrain for a week and return confidently to the task with help of his understanding wife. These writers were unusual in providing such composed accounts of marital problems.[61] Other commentators tended to describe difficulties in alarmist tones.

Following Stopes, impotence was increasingly noted in sex manuals as the greatest possible danger to marriage. "If fear of impregnation is woman's chief fear," argued James Oppenheim in *The Common Sense of Sex* (1926), "that of man is often the fear of impotence." Joseph Tennenbaum in *The Riddle of Sex* (1930) regarded woman as the real victims and noted some needed more than one orgasm to be relieved "of sexual tension." Women became more outspoken about their unhappiness. Katherine Bement Davis, in *Factors in the Sex Life of Twenty-two Hundred Women* (1929) reported, "Where the wife's desires are greater we find the higher percentage in the unhappy group." Dickinson and Beam in *A Thousand Marriages: A Medical Study of Sex Adjustment* (1932) gave as an example "Case 463. They are continuously unhappy after fifteen years. He is impotent. She says, 'He wants to hold on tight with one hand while he devils around with the other, and I am to await results, to be ready to welcome with open arms, to comfort and solace if expectations are to be realized. I'll be eternally damned first.'" In *A Research in Marriage* (1929), G. V. Hamilton found 15 percent of men in his sample had sexual difficulties that appeared to be linked to later age of first copulation. The American statistics were cited by Kenneth Walker in *Physiology of Sex* (1940).

He concluded that the fact that 41 percent of husbands had potency problems and 24 percent of wives regarded their husbands as defective was due to the neurosis of civilization.[62]

Most male performance problems, claimed the experts, were psychological in nature. A number of authors attributed men's difficulties to the repressive milieus in which they had been raised. Stopes had referred to the "psychic guilt" some men suffered. Walker claimed that 90 percent of the cases of male impotence he saw were psychological in nature, the result of puritanical and prudish upbringings. Van de Velde, the most successful of the interwar marriage manual writers, noted physical causes of impotence such as gonorrhea, diabetes, nephritis, tuberculosis, obesity, and overuse of drugs, drink, and tobacco; but he attributed most failures to psychic fears of sin, disease, discovery, and worries about one's virility. The temporary loss of erection was common. He saw the need to talk to both partners and employed psychotherapy as his "main remedial method." Among the genuine neurotics, Van de Velde included those with inferiority complexes, those fixated on another woman including a mother or sister, and those whose disgust revealed a homoerotic element.[63]

Van de Velde in addition attributed many males' inability to perform to practical considerations such as lack of privacy. "Since the war, these symptoms of erectile impotence have been very frequently observed in married men who have been obliged, owing to economic and housing shortage, to make their homes in furnished lodgings, or with their parents or parents-in-law as sub-tenants. It is easy to understand that these conditions destroy all the impulsive gaiety and spontaneity normal to the sexual function, and that a continuous undercurrent of embarrassment and anxiety, and expectation of spying or interruption, must be most harmful to masculine potency." He also echoed Gates's comment that contraceptive preparations turned off some men. "The often necessary but wholly utilitarian precautions of certain contraceptive measures—the preparation of douches and towels ready to hand, before contact begins, may dissipate all atmosphere of exaltation and romance, and completely 'cool off' men whose sexual temperament is not very robust and direct." George Ryley Scott reported the same phenomenon. "There are hundreds of men who find that the use of a condom destroys or weakens an erection; and there are others who find the smell of rubber, whether connected with male or female contraceptive appliances, is so repugnant that all desire for intercourse is destroyed. Anxiety in connexion with the possible bursting of a condom or failing to withdraw in time where *coitus interruptus* is practised, may easily cause the attempt at intercourse to be a failure." Male sexuality emerged from such discussions as appearing to be a far more fragile sprout than was customarily believed. Impotence was, asserted Bernard S. Talmey, "the anomaly which strikes the hardest blow to masculine vanity."[64] Whereas women told their friends about their ovariotomies, men always kept their sexual problems a secret.

In *Love Without Fear* (1941), Eustace Chesser summed up the gloomier findings of the spate of interwar marriage manuals. According to Chesser only one in twelve husbands knew the right sexual technique, most wives never knew "supreme joy," and 80 percent of marriages were "failures in the true sense," by which, of course, he meant the sexual sense of the term. It might have been anticipated that the increase in the reportage of impotence would have empowered women. Stopes certainly was intent on holding men primarily responsible for marital unhappiness. But the argument that bedroom disasters were the man's fault did not go unanswered. Some continued to deny a woman's right or ability to judge her mate. Indeed it was men's very fear that they were being tested, many argued, which led to honeymoon fiascoes. "Men have been known to 'disappear' on the eve of marriage," wrote one commentator, "because this fear has grown to tremendous proportions." Some went on to contend that if men were found lacking, it was the woman's fault. "The indifference of the wife who, as a rule, is about forty to fifty years of age and has either passed or is very near the climacterium, accounts for the husband's impotence in her company. Such men are able to perform the act only when the woman actively or at least cheerfully and willingly yields herself. The sullen, supine position of the frigid wife is not enough to hold a man's love forever." Indeed Talmey went on to claim that "the sour shallow, sexless shrew is surely an imposture as a wife. Her marriage is nothing else but a fraud." He asserted in 1912 that, though not as important as impotence, female sexual anesthesia was increasing, with probably 20 percent of women being frigid.[65]

In *Problems of Human Reproduction* (1926) Paul Popenoe attributed the majority of male problems to mental factors. "Most impotence is due to fear, disgust, aversion, excessive nervousness, or other abnormal psychic state [sic]." In fact, it was the woman who could rescue or destroy her partner. "The woman who is indifferent to coitus, still more the woman who is averse to or disgusted by coitus, is likely to produce impotence in her husband." And Popenoe went on to conclude "for this reason, a woman's testimony that her husband is impotent should never be accepted, in applications for divorce."[66]

The critics of the frigid woman rebutted the argument that the man should postpone or hold up his climax. G. Courtney Beale warned that it "means the imposing of a severe and probably injurious strain upon the nerves and emotions alike." Though he recognized that many married women never experienced orgasm, the Spanish scientist Gregorio Marañón insisted that men were biologically designed for quick love making. Evolution resulted in "abbreviating the reproductive act, diminishing its duration, and leaving the normal man free time to work for the progress of Humanity. In the cases of frogs, which have nothing better to do, coitus lasts for several weeks." Margaret Sanger's advice that the husband should, "like a skillful driver, at every moment hold himself under intelligent control" was refuted by a later contributor to the *Lancet:* "For a man to attempt restraint," he warned "is equivalent to trying to drive his car at full speed with the brakes on. Men, like motorcars, do not last long under such treatment."[67]

If some women were blamed for being too cold, others were blamed for being overly amorous. The English reactionary Antony Ludovici asserted that man had fallen to the station of the subordinate of woman due to the growth of maudlin attitudes. He attributed rising rates of male impotency to the growth of feminism. A common notion was that the woman, by being too bold and demanding, or by her reproaches, teasing, and sarcasm could destroy the romance of intercourse. Joseph Tennenbaum commiserated with the victims who were often "the object of cheap witticism." "Would their no less unfortunate wives know how much harm they do with their retaliating sarcasms, blundering reproaches and veiled threats, they would probably be more merciful to their husbands." A number of male commentators ungallantly took the position that a man's disgust could easily be caused by the woman's lack of hygiene. Van de Velde included as causes of impotence too much female resistance on wedding night and the abhorrence or resentment a man might feel for the immodest or indifferent woman. Her scorn and mockery could be fatal. Even in more placid households the monotony, hostility, and antipathy that marriages naturally produced resulted in a loss of passion. Van de Velde flippantly concluded by citing Napoleon's quip that the best way to become impotent was to remain faithful to one's wife.[68]

According to Joseph Dülberg, some male impotence was due to the "awkwardness of the female partner" in not knowing the appropriate positions. Still other wives were so insatiable that they caused "nervous disease" in the husband. Dülberg noted that one reason ladies were sent to the spas on the continent was so that men might be given "a chance to recover some of their lost virility." Before the onset of actual impotence, warned another alarmist, the exhausted husband would experience such tell-tale symptoms as "pressure in the lumbar region, nervous irritability, a feeling of pressure in the head, stupidity, restless sleep, ringing in the ears, spots before the eyes, shunning of light, a feeling of trembling and actual shaking, and a tendency to sweating." Van de Velde alerted husbands that their potency was not related to their overall strength and their wives were not as exhausted by the act. "I would warn husbands not to recklessly *habituate* their wives to a degree of sexual frequency and intensity which they (the husbands) may be quite unable to keep up for any length of time." [69] Women of southern Europe in particular could not moderate their desires, so there was all the more reason for the male to assert himself as teacher and guide.

Abraham Buschke and Friedrich Jacobson, whose *Sex Habits* appeared in an English translation in 1936, claimed that impotence was such a worry on the continent that "one authority (Værting) has gone so far as to declare, that, as a counterpart to the movement for 'motherhood protection,' there ought to be a movement for 'fatherhood' protection to safeguard husbands against premature impotence resulting from the sexual demands of their wives." Buschke and Jacobson warned that those who preached the need to pleasure the woman did not realize the costs. Such "false prophets who abound on all sides may, with their erroneous doctrines about the way to ensure the happiness of the married life, provide innumerable recruits for the great army of neurasthenics and greatly increase the number of persons affected with purely psychical impotence." [70] That German writers appear to have been especially sensitive to the new demands men had to face no doubt reflected the central European backlash against feminism that followed the war, but the fact that such works were translated demonstrates that many readers in the English-speaking world shared their concerns.

German sex reformer Max Hodann was one of the rare commentators to question the assumption that the stresses of the modern world led to an increasing rate of male sexual dysfunctions. "I am inclined to believe that these pessimistic conclusions are based on an oversight. The former taboo on sexual discussions, even between doctors and patients is disappearing, and many men now confide their difficulties and seek relief; whereas even a generation ago they would have concealed their sexual inadequacy as carefully as a secret crime, or put on a mask of sexual swagger and boasting, or simply accepted their fate as part of Life's Great Fiasco, without complaint or revolt." [71] How far had the discussion of impotence advanced in the interwar period? On the one hand, as Hodann observed, a revolution of sorts had occurred. Men had for years discussed female frigidity. Now men and women were publicly dissecting the topic of male sexual incompetence. Marie Stopes and Margaret Sanger might scold indifferent or immodest wives, but they primarily criticized clumsy husbands who failed to pleasure their sex-starved spouses. The appearance of the the eroticized wife in the marital sex advice literature led to the reporting of female disappointments and male performance anxieties. These data were in turn tabulated in subsequent sex surveys and marriage manuals. Healthy sex, the counselors increasingly argued, did not come naturally; its techniques had to be taught. Marie Stopes, claiming the authority of a self-proclaimed victim of male impotence, played a central role in advancing this new model of marital sexuality. She intuitively recognized that a woman's right to pleasure could be most dramatically defended if played off against the specter of male sexual incompetence. If Gates had not suffered from impotence, Stopes would have had to invent it. And perhaps she did.

On the other hand it is clear that in the marriage manuals and in the psychoanalytic texts the issue of male impotence was incorporated into the traditional notion that in sexual matters the man would normally continue to be the active partner and the woman his responsive mate. By dealing with the issues that caused his impotence, the experts claimed, men would achieve both a strengthening of their position in the family and an easing of gender tensions. In such works masturbation, effeminacy, and homosexuality continued to be condemned, though in more sophisticated ways. The message clearly was that if men became more potent and uninhibited, women were less likely to be restive. Samuel Schmalhausen, a champion of sex reform, summed up this view in noting that some English suffragettes had once campaigned for "Votes for Women and Chastity for Men." Now, he asserted, "the happy slogan for the newer generation of feminists, honoring love as a radiant passion, is: orgasms for women." [72]

Far from seeking a reversal of sex roles, the writers of marriage manuals and the popularizers of Freud denigrated the undersexed man for failing to play his part as initiator. And when one turns to the accounts that purposely defended men, one is struck to discover that, while they acknowledged the increased reportage of impotence, they to a large degree held women responsible for such incidents. In a dramatic demonstration of the tenacity of old ideas about the sexual division of labor, discussion of impotence did not, as expected, undermine assumptions of male power and self-confidence, but rather reinforced them. Yet those who made such attempts to reestablish a stabilized notion of the male body were, albeit unconsciously, providing the most telling evidence of the new concerns about its inherent instability. As much as they differed, the writers of the sex manuals and psychoanalytic texts also tended to share the belief that the causes of most forms of impotence were psychic in nature, be it at the conscious or unconscious level. Both groups were to be soon challenged by the appearance of a new school of medical scientists who argued that the glands rather than the mind dictated sexual behavior.

SEX GLANDS, REJUVENATION, AND EUGENICS BETWEEN THE WARS

In *The Conquest of Old Age* (1931) the German surgeon Peter Schmidt listed a few of the many amazing cases of sexual rejuvenation that resulted when men underwent the so-called Steinach operation, the cutting of the vas deferens. A seventy-one-year-old man was soon having erections and erotic dreams, a sixty-four-year-old journalist who had been impotent for eighteen months was returned to full health, and a fifty-seven-year-old retired doctor whose impotency had occasioned, he confessed, "some (physical) disharmony in the relations with the wife, who is a great many years younger," proudly reported vigorous erections. When he had a relapse in 1927, Schmidt injected him with testicular extracts to restore his sexual powers, and in 1929 ingrafted him with a testicle from a forty-year-old man. Schmidt went on to claim that such operations saved a forty-five-year old engineer from premature ejaculations, cured a twenty-seven-year-old man of epilepsy, and provided a fifty-year-old merchant with his first experience of penetrative intercourse. "The happy conviction that a powerful erection will persist long enough for the proper performance of the act," reported the patient, "relieves me from all worry I used to feel because the mechanism would not work properly."[1]

Schmidt was only one of a number of early twentieth-century doctors who turned to such radical new ways to restore manhood. They moved on from "organotherapy"—the transplantation of animal or human sexglands—to stimulation of the patient's own gonads by either radiation or the cutting of one of the vas deferens, and finally to the injection of hormones. Such undertakings represented both the old quest to overcome impotence and the first halting steps of the new science of endocrinology. The public was fascinated by what it learned of hormones, magical substances that in the tiniest of quantities could have life-altering effects. Their discovery overturned old understandings of the origins of sexual behavior and sexual characteristics, and revolutionized the way in which sexual dysfunctions could be treated. And for staid medical professionals uncomfortable with discussing sexual matters so often associated with quackery, they appeared to legitimize the scientific study of the male reproductive system.[2] Aside from having a placebo effect, none of these therapies could actually have been effective, but that is not terribly important. Far more interesting were the ways in which the cultural preoccupations of the age framed the discussions of the sex glands. The investigation of the internal secretions appeared to reconfigure understandings of the causes of impotence, yet doctors turned to them to shore up traditional notions of masculinity and femininity. The search for cures for male sexual dysfunctions was similarly implicated in contemporary eugenics concerns for "race improvement." Medical scientists who promised "rejuvenation" took it as a given that the reproduction of the "fit" should be encouraged while that of the "unfit" should be curbed.

Hormonal treatment of sexual dysfunctions naturally interested those doctors who felt that both psychoanalysis and surgery had proved to be of little value. Most general practitioners, if dismissive of Freud, did assume that impotence was primarily psychic in nature and that consequently they could do little more than offer supportive counseling. Nevertheless they prescribed hydrotherapy, electrotherapy, acupuncture, the insertion of bougies and sounds, massage, gymnastics, and hypnotic suggestion. "It is proper to use electricity, the vibrator, or any other means that will impress the patient with the thought that you are doing something, and that you have the ability to give him relief."[3] Rest, drugs, diets, baths and douches, and psychological treatment continued to be recommended in the belief that they could do little harm and might even do some good.

A few surgeons endorsed more heroic measures. In the late nineteenth century urologists thought venous occlusion was the key cause of erection and proceeded to affirm that by ligating the dorsal vein of the penis they could ensure erections. Their claims were soon rebutted. "The resection of the dorsal vein of the penis has been suggested some years ago," Victor Vecki noted in 1912, referring to the work of Chicago physician Dr. G. Frank Lydston. "Lydston reported that he was unable to secure as satisfactory results from this operation, as other more enthusiastic advocates. Still he claims 25 percent of the properly operated cases giving perfect satisfaction, in about half the remaining cases some improvement, failures for the rest. I have never seen the slightest effect of this operation, and agree fully with Lydston when he says that many of the sudden and complete cures are probably but cases of psychic impotence." Other doctors flatly declared that such operations either failed or led to painful erections lasting days if not months! Trying another tack, surgeons shortened the muscles of the penis. The so-called Lowsley operation also proved futile. Frank Hinman, a leading American urologist, conceded that surgeons' search for an organic cause of impotence was only helpful in an indirect fashion. "The suggestion that an organic cause has been found and can be treated may give the encouragement needed to effect a cure." That is, surgical intervention might act as a placebo. Some surgeons admitted to faking such operations to calm especially demanding patients.[4]

Doctors denounced the patent medicines that promised to fill "weak and nervous men" with "rampant vigour." In England Phosperine, Damaroids, Osogen, Neurovil, Law Palmetto, Dr. Lecoy's Invigoroids, Gordon's Vital Sexualine Restorative, and the Marston Treatment, were only a few of the "Lost Manhood Restorers and Nervous Debility Cures" that the British Medical Association sought to ban. The leading medical journals also denounced as frauds the proliferation of contraptions designers claimed could assure a sturdy erection. "No sufferers are so afflicted with credulity and gullibility as are the victims of sexual impotence," grumbled one progressive physician, "and the market is flooded with various appliances which are guaranteed to be sure cures. It goes without saying, that most of them are worthless frauds." He cited Bier's Erectruss as one of the worst. Having declared that "all forms of splints, rings, pumps and similar mechanical contrivances have proven such failures that I consider it a waste of space to give them any attention," another doctor went on to describe an "electric chair" that had a hole in it which allowed the genitals to hang down into a basin of water. "Suggestion was given that as the treatment progressed the organs would regain their old time power." The U.S. Postmaster General prosecuted for fraud the seller of a number of such devices, including C. Julius Saur who sold the Potentor, a rubber ring designed to squeeze the base of the penis to retard ejaculation, and Vim Manufacturing, which offered the Juvenator, a glass vacuum pump.[5]

Some physicians did recommend sex aids. "The penile splint, devised by Dr. Thad. W. Williams is really practicable and enables the introducing of the non-erected penis into the vagina under all circumstances," wrote Vecki. "Acting as a suggestive safety-valve it may be considered a legitimate therapeutic measure in neurasthenic and so-called psychic impotence." Dr. Joseph Loewenstein provided the fullest account of such "mechano-

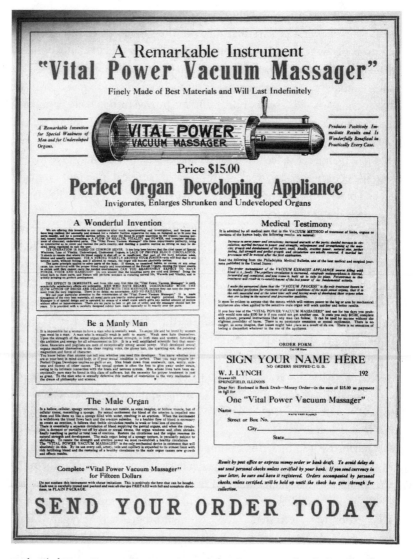

6. The Vital Power Vacuum Massager. A 1920s advertisement touting the benefits of a tubular device with a crank at the top that supposedly increased blood flow to the penis. By permission of the National Library of Medicine.

therapy." He noted that suction pumps such as those of Dr. Zabludowski provided only an illusionary erection that disappeared as soon as the penis was removed from pump. Equally flawed were the Erector-Sleigh, Gassensche Spirale, Gerson's Constriction Bandage, and Virility, a double cylinder connected to a bellows to produce a vacuum that, Loewenstein reported, "gives great bulk to the penis and makes it look grotesque." Loewenstein sang the praises of penis supports made of light metal. On the market already were the Sklerator and Virtutor, but he vaunted his own Coitus Training Apparatus, a sort of training wheels for the penis. Consisting of two rings for each end of the penis and rubber covered wires in between, the support was covered by a condom before penetration. Though he cautioned that care be taken that the support and the penis went in the same direction, Loewenstein promised that the partner of the "dexterous man" would not know he was using it. He called it a "training" apparatus because he believed that in many cases the erection of the flaccid penis would occur after entry, and once learnt could occur normally. Women were presumably entranced by neither the device nor the care needed to "extricate the apparatus." Lowenstein had the decency to admit that, "in most cases it will be inadvisable to forgo the co-operation of the partner."[6]

In displacing the need for invasive operations, years of psychoanalysis, or purchase of useless penile supports, the hormonal treatment of impotence was obviously attractive. The emergence of new therapies was the culmination of decades of scientific investigation of the process of reproduction. The spermatozoa had been first observed in the seventeenth century, but as far back as the Greeks it had been known that the testes were responsible both for a man's fertility and for his secondary sex characteristics. In the 1800s doctors began to ask if the gonads did more than simply produce gametes. That the testicles had both a reproductive and endocrine function was dramatically demonstrated in 1849 when A. A. Berthold produced male sexual behavior in castrated roosters by transplanting testicular tissue. In 1905 E. H. Starling coined the term "hormone" to refer to the chemical messengers produced by the various ductless glands that produced such effects.[7]

The first endocrinologists assumed that men and women produced antagonistic "male" and "female" hormones. Such a belief underpinned the work of Charles Edouard Brown-Séquard, a pioneering neurologist, famous for his early work on the adrenal glands. Brown-Séquard created a sensation in June 1889 by asserting that he had carried out testicular experiments on human subjects including himself. In his report to the Société de Biologie in Paris, the seventy-three-year-old scientist reminded his colleagues that castration, masturbation, and all other forms of seminal losses resulted in physical and mental debility. Semen obviously had to contain some special strengthening substance—a "dynamogenic power." To test this theory Brown-Séquard subcutaneously injected himself with a solution of water mixed with the blood of the testicular veins, semen, and juice from the crushed testicles of dogs and guinea pigs. Claiming that as a consequence his bodily strength had been miraculously restored, he strenuously denied that the results were due to autosuggestion. He discreetly referred to the restoration of his sexual powers, in claiming that after the injections the jet of his urine went 25 percent further. Despite the scientific community's skepticism, a number of enterprising medical men in Europe and North America followed up on Brown-Séquard's assertions in producing for "weak men" a variety of glandular extracts such as "spermine." Though many cures were claimed, such testicular material could have been of no value given that the male hormone was produced—not stored—in the testes and was not water soluble. It made no difference. Brown-Séquard had launched a craze for organotherapy.[8]

Human sex glands were soon being harvested. In 1913 Victor Lespinasse, a Northwestern University professor of genitourinary surgery, reported that he had planted slices of human testicle into the muscle of a man who had lost his testicles. Four days after the operation, Lespinasse claimed, the patient had strong erections and insisted on leaving hospital in order to gratify his desires. The first experiment in grafting an entire testicle was performed by Dr. Lydston on himself, on January 16, 1914. Expressing his disappointment that vulgar prejudices heretofore had prevented the exploitation of the sex glands of the dead, Lydston coolly reported how he transplanted into his own scrotum a suicide victim's testicle. The doctor admitted to one small mishap. "The awkward position necessary to the work and the distance of the field from the operator's eye were such that the tunica vaginalis inadvertently was cut." Otherwise Lydston was happy with the outcome of the operation and concluded that only a portion of testicular tissue might be needed to provide renewed vigor. He later cited the case of an impotent fifty-eight-year-old man who immediately after surgery had nocturnal erections and the return of "natural" sexual reactions. Though Lydston conceded that in such cases the psychic element could not be dismissed, he noted that two years later the patient was still happy.[9]

L. L. Stanley, resident physician of the California state prison in San Quentin, reported in 1922 that he had first implanted testicles from executed convicts and then moved on to inject into his subjects via a dental syringe solutions of goat, ram, boar, and deer testicles. Altogether he made 1000 injections into 656 men. Though he argued that more work had to be done to rescue the field from quacks, Stanley's own experiments smacked of the sensational. While stressing that his injections increased overall energy levels and so countered the effects of general asthenia such as acne, asthma, and senility, he also noted that they led, in some though not all cases, to improved erections. What he failed to explain was what interest a prison doctor would have in curing his inmates of sexual lassitude and impotence.

Such reports certainly won public attention. By 1923 an American sex reformer could claim, "We are justified in saying that testicle implantation is a useful procedure, giving, in most cases, good results in senility and in impotence, by increasing the general well-being and the libido." [10]

Stanley had been inspired by work of Serge Voronoff, an eminent Russian-born medical scientist working at the Collège de France. Voronoff began his career experimenting with skin and bone grafts. Led on by the notion that the aging process could be reversed by transplanting the testes of young animals into the old, Voronoff in 1919 scandalized many by transplanting the testes of chimpanzees into men. He asserted that "marked psychical and sexual excitation" typically resulted, followed by a resurgence of memory, energy and "genital functions." He supported his argument by peppering his books with before and after photographs of rams, lambs, boys, and men. In defending the respectability of cross-species glandular therapy, Voronoff asserted that the most important benefits were in physical and psychic invigoration rather than simple sexual rejuvenation. At the same time he argued that ardent lovers like Goethe were long lived. If a man's sex glands were decayed, so too were the "moral and physical energies" of manhood. The world's press naturally broadcast such sensational accounts of cross-species transplants, the *New York Times* reporting in 1921, for example, that students of Voronoff had invited interested physicians to the Majestic Hotel to watch a monkey gland transfer into the noted Western artist Irving R. Bacon. Thousands of such expensive operations were carried out on wealthy men including Maurice Maeterlinck, the Belgian poet and Nobel laureate. [11] Though Voronoff and his patients were convinced that his procedure worked, by the 1930s the scientific consensus was that the body would reject transplanted glands and only quacks could continue to advocate such procedures.

In the United States the most successful of such charlatans was John Brinkley, a product of the Eclectic Medical University of Kansas City where surgery (including circumcisions and clitorodectomies) were carried out for a variety of sexual complaints including masturbation, lust, frigidity, and enlarged prostates. Asserting that his experiences in a meat packing plant impressed him with the health of goats, Brinkley began in 1918 to graft their testicular tissue into male patients, claiming the operation would stop masturbation, alleviate schizophrenia, and most importantly of all, cure sexual dysfunctions. "Wives come to me," he reported, "and say 'Doctor, my husband is no good.'" Presenting himself as a heroic, small-town surgeon warding off persecuting professors, Jews, and easterners, Brinkley won over a rural clientele and made a fortune. By 1924 it was estimated that 750 doctors in America were charging hundreds of dollars for similar operations. [12]

Not until the 1940s did the American Medical Association succeed in using the laws against false advertising to silence Brinkley and his kind.

The operations of Voronoff and Brinkley easily lent themselves to spoofing. According to one wit a patient of Brinkley's dropped his prescription down the well and when asked if he had drunk any water from it replied, "No, we haven't even been able to get the pump handle down." In the film *Evergreen* (1934, dir. Victor Saville), a character jokes that a young singer looks so much like her famous mother that the audience might believe the latter took "monkey glands." In the 1920s Ethel Waters won laughter and applause in belting out the suggestive "You Can't Do What My Last Man Did."

> You know, you sure ain't loved me sufficiently,
> To make me forget my used-to-be, and he was seventy!
> He could love; oh, he loved me like a lover should,
> Always could, when he would, he was good,
> So, you've lost your nest, go east or west, or back to jail, you know
> where I got you from,
> [Slow Kid Thomas interjects] Well, you know I got two good feet and I got
>   two good hands!
> Yes, but as it is, you so weak I'll find out you still need some monkey glands!
> Now, you can't do what that last man did!

When running for governor of Louisiana in 1944, Jimmie Davis made similar allusions in singing "Gonna Get me Some Monkey Glands, Be Like I Usta Wuz." Such jokes were made worldwide. In France a satiric magazine suggested that since priests did not need their sex glands, Voronoff should use them. "God only knows what the effects of monkey glands are," wrote the Italian novelist Italo Svevo. "Perhaps a rejuvenated man on seeing a beautiful woman will be driven to climb the nearest tree."[13]

Others were more alarmed than amused by the notion of tampering with the body. Some believed that transplants produced sex monsters. Writers of fiction were particularly alive to such dangers. In novels male characters portrayed with missing limbs had often been coded as impotent. Now talk of swapping glands conjured up memories of Dr. Frankenstein. In Arthur Conan Doyle's "The Creeping Man" (1923), a professor of sixty-one (roughly Doyle's age) takes a testicular drug to rejuvenate himself before marrying a young woman, and turns into an ape. Sherlock Holmes spells out the moral. "When one tries to rise above Nature one is liable to fall below it. The highest type of man may revert to the animal if he leaves the straight road of destiny. . . . There is a danger there—a very real danger to humanity. Consider, Watson, that the material, the sensual, the worldly would all prolong their worthless lives. The spiritual would not avoid the call to something higher. It would be the survival of the least fit. What sort of a cesspool may not our poor world become?" In C. P. Snow's *New Lives for Old* (1933) a rejuvenation hormone proves a disaster since only the wealthy can afford it. It exacerbates class hatreds in allowing well-off seniors to pursue sexual adventures previously restricted to the young. In *Heart of a Dog* (1925) the anti-Stalinist Mikhail Bulgakov reversed the scenario, portraying a dog, accidentally humanized by being given a man's seminal vesicles, turned into a crass Communist hack.[14]

Unlike Voronoff, the Viennese physiologist Eugen Steinach, was not so much interested in offering therapeutic treatments as in understanding the process of sexual development. In the 1890s he undertook animal experiments, in particular the reimplantation of gonads, to trace the transformation of sex character. By implanting testicles into female animals and ovaries into male animals, he produced feminized males and masculinized females; that is he changed not their actual sex, but their sexual characteristics and behavior. Steinach deduced that in males the seminal vesicles contained two types of cells; germinal cells produced sperm, and Leydig or interstitial cells produced an active substance that entered the blood stream. He concluded that "the sexual life of every creature—whether in the male, female, hermaphrodite, or some other transitional, that is, intersexual, form—is determined by the hormone-producing sex glands, and by the quality, and quantity, of the hormone they furnish."[15] So far, so good, but Steinach went on to surmise that aging was a sort of castration resulting from the decay of the hormone-producing Leydig cells. He believed that if these cells could be rejuvenated, the aging process would be reversed. Vasectomies carried out on rats, Steinach reported, did just that by causing an atrophy of the testicle's seminal cells but a proliferation of the Leydig cells and subsequently greater sexual activity.

Since the 1890s doctors had performed vasectomies to either sterilize patients or to help (they hoped) shrink their enlarged prostates. Steinach now proposed the technique for rejuvenation and, in 1918, asked the surgeon Robert Lichtenstern to test the procedure on the first human subject. The beauty of Steinach's operation was that it was a unilateral ligation of the vas deferens—that is, cutting only one of the two vas deferens. The patient, though not sterilized, in effect received a hormonal boost from himself. To achieve the latter effect, Lydston and Stanley had employed the more unseemly methods of harvesting the human testicles of accident victims and the executed while Voronoff used the tissues of primates. Steinach declared his operation an astounding success. Believing his procedures could alleviate a host of ills ranging from impotence and premature ejaculation to tuberculosis and cancer, his most devoted followers likened the importance of rejuvenation to Darwin's theory of evolution.

Steinach's operation received world-wide attention. UFA, the leading German film production company, assisted in the making of a movie on his surgical procedure. Thousands of Steinach operations were carried out in Europe and North America. Unfortunately Mr. Alfred Wilson, a satisfied patient who paid £700 for the service and booked the Albert Hall in London for May 12, 1921 to speak on the subject "How I was Made Twenty Years Younger," dropped dead just before his presentation. Nevertheless Steinach was hailed by sex reformers such as Eden Paul and Norman Haire. The leading Spanish medical scientist Gregorio Marañón accepted many of Steinach's findings and carried out both testicular transplant and vasoligations. Perhaps the most extravagant claims for Steinach's methods were made in America. Even a cabbage, declared George Corners, could be "Steinached" if its reproductive function were checked. William J. Robinson stressed that the operation was cheap enough for "ordinary workingmen" to afford and concluded that, "in view of the fact, that the operation is harmless, practically painless, without danger, can be performed under local anesthesia and confines the patient to bed for only a very short period, it is worth trying in selected cases." [16]

In the United States Steinach's most vocal advocate was Harry Benjamin. In 1921 he spoke on the benefits of vasoligation to the Academy of Medicine. Though admitting that it would be more accurate to say that "reactivation" rather than "rejuvenation" of mental and physical vitality resulted from the procedure, Benjamin continued well on into the 1930s insisting that it worked. He argued that women could also be reactivated by applying heat to their ovaries by Roentgen and radium radiation, or by an electric current treatment known as diathermy, claiming to have successfully treated 300 male and 500 female patients. Rebutting the argument that such procedures only had a placebo effect, he cited the findings of Peter Schmidt who had performed Steinach operations on Chinese prisoners in Shanghai. Though they had no idea of the point of the surgery in 75 percent of cases, the prisoner patients experienced an improvement in their hearing, sight, blood pressure, erections, and potency. Sigmund Freud and W. B. Yeats were the most famous patients to undergo the procedure. Freud's operation on November 17, 1923 of both vas deferens was carried out in hopes it would alleviate his cancer of the jaw. He thought the operation had no effect. Yeats believed his sexual and creative powers were restored. His surgery, carried out by Norman Haire in 1934, won the poet the sobriquet of the "Gland Old Man." [17]

Though in hindsight their theories appear far fetched, Voronoff and Steinach were serious scientists, and accordingly sensitive to the notion that if they spoke too much about the sexual side of rejuvenation they would be regarded as quacks. Medical professionals shared the public's hostility toward doctors pandering to the requests of frisky oldsters. Julian Huxley, for example, was disgusted to find that his work on the use of the thyroid gland to accelerate growth in salamander-like creatures led to him being badgered by people looking for a sex stimulant. As one advocate of gland therapy noted, "Much of the hostility towards rejuvenation has been engendered through its association with sex. . . . The idea has been mooted abroad that those seeking rejuvenation are the immoral, the debauched, the libidinistic, the lecherous members of society; that the treatment prescribed appeals to men who have led dissolute lives, and are in search of a means whereby they can continue their careers of lust and excess." Benjamin accepted that in moralistic America the operation was a touchy issue. "Deep-seated puritanical complexes thus explain not only some of the antagonism against these methods, but also the silence by which this branch of medicine is so often treated." Researchers were accordingly ambivalent about publicizing the sex side of rejuvenation. Steinach always argued that his primary concern was not so much with the patient's potency, as with his more general well-being and vitality. The whole body was rejuvenated, not just one organ. And despite all his talk of "rejuvenation," he conceded that he sought only to make men more active and productive rather than actually younger. For Haire, the Steinach operation had some positive effects on sexual potency, but more importantly, it improved the patient's overall health and increased energy. Paul Kammerer studded his 1924 book on Steinach with obviously retouched before and after photographs in arguing that patients' metabolism, strength, skin, hair, and prostate functions all enjoyed a new vigor. He downplayed the operation's cure of impotency. "This symptom of returned manhood will hardly ever be beyond bounds and, in some cases, may be even scarcely discernible."[18] What Kammerer especially wished to stress was men's renewed enthusiasm for work.

Despite such protestations the public assumed that sex renewal was the chief goal of vasoligature and researchers obviously did believe that either the maintenance or reactivation of a man's usual sexual attributes remained a key way of measuring rejuvenation. After all, in his first experiments Steinach had taken the erections and coitus of rats as one obvious indicator. An enthusiast like Corners claimed that the sex life of patients was "marvelously intensified" by Steinach's operation. According to Kammerer, potency was "not only preserved, but often strengthened by vasoligation." Some opposed the operation for making men oversexed, but he assured his readers that "reawakened manhood up to now has always remained within the bounds of decency." Schmidt likewise asserted that it led to a "remarkable and constant" improvement in libido and potency. In the majority of his patients potency was regenerated, but not to the extent "to cause any trouble in the conduct of life." Striking a more practical note, Kenneth Walker reported the case of a naval officer whose fear of children had rendered him impotent. "Full potency was restored by the operation of vaso-ligature."[19]

Steinach also had his critics. Most of the opposition, said Haire, was founded on the histological controversy regarding the source of the testicular hormone, but it went beyond that. Columbia University professor Benjamin Harrow felt Steinach was on to something but asked why, since all kinds of glands had to interact, the change of only one organ should rejuvenate the whole body. In England, Kenneth Walker carried out some vasoligations and concluded that the results were capricious as the testis only provided one factor in the development of secondary sex characteristics. He also observed that the role played in rejuvenation by suggestion was hard to determine. This point was pursued by Morris Fishbein, editor of the *Journal of the American Medical Association*, who devoted a chapter in *The Medical Follies* (1925) to attacking rejuvenation claims. The success of Steinach and Voronoff's operations, he argued, was a mere placebo effect. Fishbein pointed out that before Steinach, vasectomies had been used for prostate problems but the elderly patients did not feel rejuvenated as a result because they did not expect to be.[20]

Steinach's theories, well received in the early 1920s, were derided in the 1930s. Because his operation was exploited by some, reported Walker, it came to be held in derision by the profession. Walker believed that "the treatment of sexual weakness by vaso-ligature rests on a more solid experimental basis," but it "has come to be regarded as a 'stunt' by the greater part of the profession, and a method of treatment that used properly might have taken its place in therapeutics has fallen into disrepute." More and more scientists reported that gland transplants and vasoligations either clearly did not work or were not proven to work. By 1939 a pamphlet observed that the term "rejuvenation" had "fallen into ill repute because of its use as a catch word to exploit certain pseudoscientific devices and 'cures.'"[21]

Nevertheless similar therapies dressed up in new trappings continued to surface. During the 1940s and the 1950s Professor Paul Niehans offered from his Swiss clinic what he referred to as "live cell therapy." Arguing, as had Steinach, that a loss of the secretions of the sex glands resulted in premature aging, Niehans injected patients with sheep, calf, pig, and human fetal cells. Diminished libido, degeneration, and a range of sex problems from small organs and acne to inferiority complexes and impotence could, he claimed, all be cured. Many members of Europe's social elite including Somerset Maugham, Charlie Chaplin, Winston Churchill, Nöel Coward, and Pope Pius XII availed themselves of his services.[22]

Though later endocrinologists tried to disassociate themselves from the earlier practitioners of organotherapy, in the 1920s Steinach was highly regarded in the scientific community and indeed nominated several times for the Nobel prize. In the decades he and Voronoff were garnering newspaper headlines, less well-known endocrinologists were working their way toward the identification and isolation of the male hormone. Frederick Banting and Charles Best's discovery of insulin in 1921 inspired hope that other diseases aside from diabetes could be conquered by hormonal treatment; yet experts admitted that though some endocrine therapies might work, they were still not fully understood. Urologists, once unable to deal with the commonest of ailments, placed particular hopes in the new science of endocrinology. A contributor to the *Lancet* noted in 1931 that the issue of impotence lay in the no-man's land between surgery and psychology.[23] Endocrinology promised to fill the gap.

Since male bodies contained only minute quantities of the sex hormone, subjecting it to analysis posed enormous challenges. Only in 1931 did German scientists finally succeeded in isolating and distilling a scant 50 milliliters of the male hormone from the 25,000 liters of urine contributed by the Berlin police barracks. Supported by the Organon Company of Amsterdam, Ernst Laqueur in 1935 worked out the molecular structure of the hormone named testosterone. The same year Adolph Butenandt (working for Schering-Kahlbaum) and Leopold Ruzicka (working for the Ciba Corporation) simultaneously reported they had developed the means of turning cholesterol into synthetic testosterone.[24] For their efforts they were to share the 1939 Nobel Prize for chemistry.

Now that one had testosterone, what was one to do with it? Many scientists in the 1930s still believed that it was too early to say that it could be used on humans. Nevertheless in 1937 James B. Hamilton reported using testosterone to provide sexual maturity to an underdeveloped twenty-seven-year-old man. In the United States assertions were soon being made that it helped circulatory problems, nervousness, and general sexual dysfunctions including impotence and reduced libido. The most extravagant claims were made by the popular writer Paul de Kruif who argued that sexual vigor was a sign of brain power but that most scientists were still uncomfortable discussing sex. He asserted that treated patients were cured of their midlife melancholy and "grew more strong-thinking and less sissified."[25]

Since testosterone could be administered by pills and injections there was no longer any need for the discredited gland transplants and vasoligations. Steinach dropped his operations and went on to employ synthetic hormones. Aware that impotence could be caused by psychic or physical factors, he called for the urine test of impotents to determine which patients suffered from psychic impotence and which had a hormone deficiency and required the male sex hormone. Others like Kenneth Walker and Harry Benjamin also moved on from vasoligations to administering hormone shots. What they had difficulty comprehending was that the so-called sex hormones were needed for a host of nonsexual physiological activities and that both women as well as men had the "male hormone." Moreover testosterone, though apparently effective in some cases of the male climacteric, proved to be of no use for impotence: it actually caused azoospermia (the decline in sperm production), and could exacerbate prostate cancer. With the synthetic production of hormones one had what one historian has called a case of "drugs looking for diseases."[26] Pharmaceutical companies had products to sell and now had to convince doctors and patients that they needed them.

Well before the identification of testosterone, commercial firms had been in advance of the scientific community in claiming that sexual dysfunctions could be remedied by hormone treatments. "The endocrine glands and their secretions, singly or in combination, are used most extensively, and great claims are made for their efficiency. I am using them in my practice every day, and I find them useful; particularly those preparations which can be used intermuscularly or subcutaneously," wrote William J. Robinson in 1923, but he went on to say that most advertised combinations were "perfectly worthless." Aphrodisiacs were now advertised as hormones. In Russia papers carried advertisements for Spermokrin. In Germany much of the work of Magnus Hirschfeld's Institute for Sexual Science was funded by the sales to the medical profession of a pharmaceutical called Testifortan; after 1929 it was sold to the general public as Titus Pearls. Whereas in Ernst Toller's play Hinkemann (1923) street vendors are seen selling Cantharoids and Damianiox, in Alfred Döblin's novel Alexanderplatz (1931) the hero is subjected to advertisements for Testifortan.[27]

In England in the 1920s the G. W. Carnick Company advertised Hormotone for menstrual and climacteric disorders, Viriligen for "lowered virility and sexual neurasthenia of functional origin," and an Orchic-Prostate

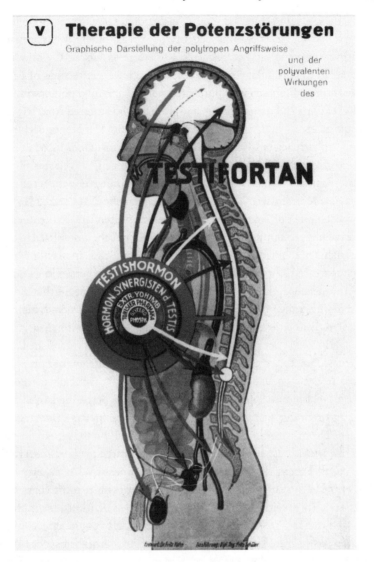

7. Advertisement for Testifortan, by permission of the Magnus-Hirschfeld-Gesellschaft. Beginning in 1927, Magnus Hirschfeld's Berlin Institute for Sexual Science sold to doctors a hormone pharmaceutical under the name of Testifortan. After 1929 it was sold to the general public in Germany and abroad as Titus Pearls.

Compound for sexual neurasthenia and enlarged prostates. The Harrower Laboratory produced Gonad Co, a formula mix of adrenal, thyroid, pituitary, plus "spermin" made from Leydig cells for "asexualism" and hypogonadism. The company lamented the idea that some debauchees would take advantage of such drugs. "Unfortunately, perhaps, there is quite a large class which includes the senile and roué, who do not deserve to recover their lost powers, for they have been misused, in whom organotherapy has been used with just the same kind of good results." More explicitly, the Middlesex Laboratory of Glandular Research claimed to have the records of 64,000 patients, including men who purchased normal and high potency pills for weak erections and neurasthenia, and women who suffered from frigidity, "sex quiescence," and "inability to reach orgasm." The laboratory's pamphlet for pharmacists advertising Middlesex Sex Hormones listed Emelgemal tablets for "loss of virility in middle and later life," Prejacrin for premature ejaculations, and Sterility Gland Tablets for barrenness. Its window display cards promised "The Fire of Life Replenished" and asked "Do You Wish to Renew Your Youth?" Once testosterone propionate was synthesized in the late 1930s, commercial firms were claiming it should be used in cases of eunuchism, hypogonadism, impotence, and prostatic hypertrophy.[28]

The fact that a network of doctors' offices and mothers' clinics existed that routinely examined women's reproductive organs meant that doctors could more readily prescribe hormones to women than to men. A historian has noted that by the 1920s, "the gynecological clinic functioned as a powerful institutional context that provided an available and established clientele with a broad range of diseases that could be treated with hormones." Thanks to estrogen, endocrinology and gynecology "practically merged" in the 1930s. Hormones began to be offered for late puberty, menstrual problems, and even the "unhappiness" occasioned by menopause. Doctors complained that in contrast, doing endocrine research on male sexuality was far more difficult. Changes in the testes that required medical observation were so infrequent that clinical observations were rare. As experimentation on male human subjects was usually not possible, researchers often based their conclusions on random cases. The conscientious, in any event, admitted that as the glands were interrelated, isolating the effects of any one was extremely difficult. In sexual matters the role of the psyche further complicated matters. Doctors attempting to gauge the success of hormones in treating men for sexual dysfunctions fell back on either observation of secondary characteristics, social indicators such as interest in the opposite sex, or the patient's own subjective account as in, it "feels better."[29] Such findings did not impress many. Little was still known about testosterone. It had worrying side effects and was very expensive to use, but the main reason why few men were prescribed hormones was simply due to the fact that they saw their physicians far less frequently than women did.

The medical scientists and commercial firms, in talking up the range of injections, pills, and surgical procedures that would provide sexual rejuvenation, no doubt created anxieties in some men and incited others to prove their manhood, but they did not simply force themselves on unwilling consumers. There was a demand for such products, fueled by changing cultural currents. As we saw in the previous chapter, the writers of the early twentieth-century sex and marriage manuals played up the man's role as lover and spouse and downplayed fatherhood. Similarly, the rejuvenators explicitly favored the recreational over the reproductive side of sex. Steinach's interest was in the virility rather than the fertility of his subjects.[30] Indeed in cases of vasoligations where both of the vas deferns were cut, increased potency was bought at the price of reproduction. That such trade-offs were taken for granted revealed the extent to which Western twentieth-century culture accepted the shift in male priorities. Hormones were thus a cause and effect of a reconfiguration of both masculinity and impotence. Whereas once it was the possession of a penis or the production of sperm or the fathering of children that made one a man, now it was having the right hormones.

Much of the explanation for the rejuvenation craze also stemmed from the twentieth-century attack on aging. One doctor tellingly noted that men were willing to accept that not all stomachs were the same but believed sexual performances should be. "If a man's natural capacity for sexual congress is only once a month," he protested, "it is hopeless to try and tune him up to three times a night." In the modern world sexual potency was taken as a key indicator of male well-being. This desire to be "normal" (which in fact was to approach the ideal) justified increased interventions in the body. Men of the 1920s were exhorted by the media to embrace a new model of masculinity represented by tanned, athletic youths. Like women, men were now supposed to have sex appeal.[31] At the same time it was still believed that the business life of the man was as important to him as the woman's sex life was to her. Given the social and political disruptions of the post–World War I years it is no surprise that some men sought out new means of rejuvenation. They found themselves under pressure to keep up with modern women and to counter the challenge of younger business rivals.

Of course, the need to demonstrate sexual vitality was not accepted by all. Most men no doubt continued to accept old age gracefully. They admitted that because they were aging their potency might decline, and spurned the new idea that it was their declining potency that made them old. Traditionally doctors had repeated the adage that moderation in all things was the best way to prolong life. "A certain abundance in the power of generation is favorable to longevity," asserted Christopher William Hufeland, but excesses and masturbation led to a drying out of the body. The argument that the old should direct their limited energies to living rather than to sex still made sense to some. "Many aging men," reported Norman Haire, "are glad to be rid of what has been at times a disturbing element in their life, glad to have reached an age at which they are no longer troubled by the lusts of the flesh, and yet are loath to lose their physical and mental efficiency."[32]

There were also doctors who expressed an unease with male patients who did not have erections yet still sought sexual release. "It often occurs that old men, no longer capable of performing the sexual act, will persist in coming to the physician for treatment, for the reason that they experience a sensation of sexual pleasure in having their prostate massaged. Especially is this true when the massage is continued to the point of forcing out the secretions (milking the prostate). Many of these old men secure all their sexual pleasure through these treatments." A sympathetic physician advised such gentle massage every five days or manipulation of the prostate to relieve congestion. Other doctors found old men's sexual desires distasteful. "To some hyperesthetic individuals, massage of the vesicles is so nearly a suggestion of the sexual act that I fear it is quite as likely to do harm as good."[33]

Was aging "natural?" In 1903 Elie Metchnikoff coined the term "gerontology," thereby launching the notion of aging as a medical problem that could be tinkered with. In arguing that many men were old before they needed to be, Steinach and Voronoff clearly represented a similar mindset. In the 1920s doctors increasingly referred to the "male climacteric," which they likened to the female menopause. A man's critical age had more diffuse symptoms than the woman's and occurred later; many doctors placed it in the man's fifties. One writer asserted that it could occur any time. Early starters ended early; sexual excesses led to senility. He warned that false hopes should not be raised in men over fifty; most could not be rejuvenated. Yet he went on to say that family life would be improved and marriages strengthened were a cure for such men's impotence found. "It will also diminish the ever-increasing number of cases of sexual neurasthenia ending in many instances in complete mental deficiency and even self-destruction. . . . These patients should not be dismissed with an exhortation to 'forget it,' a so-called aphrodisiac pill, which is valueless, or possibly the passage of a urethral sound or a cold rectal irrigation." Often the man was at the height of his professional power when his erections declined. If his libido was still strong, his interest in young girls, warned Marañón, might be a sign of inversion since youths were really androgynous. Or the older man in his increased emotionality, impatience, and conservatism might take on many of the unpleasant features of the older woman.[34]

Those investigating the aging process naturally interested themselves in the notion that the retention of sexual vigor could delay senescence. Having made his reputation with his classic study of adolescence, G. Stanley Hall produced a work on aging in which he provided a short overview of rejuvenation theory. "Sex glands," he wrote, "stimulate not merely amourousness but all kinds of cerebral and muscular energy, pouring into the blood a species of vital fluid, and give a sense of vigor and well-being and plenitude of life, which later vanish when their source begins to run dry in age." [35] Concluding that the only hope for postponement of death lay in the glands, Clarke noted that the leading thinkers of the age—like Steinach and Freud—agreed on the centrality of sex in the life of man.

The rise of the "midlife decline novels" such as those of Mann, Fitzgerald, and Hemingway in the 1920s and 1930s was one symptom of the cultural preoccupation with the aging male. A few writers directly tackled the issues of gland transplants and rejuvenation, often as not exploiting the "new wine in old bottles" theme by portraying old men seeking rejuvenation treatments to pursue young girls. Inspired by the Brown-Séquard affair, Jack London wrote "The Rejuvenation of Major Rathbone" (1899) in which an old man who drinks a youth serum becomes a lusty lout. His inappropriate behavior leads a scientist to see the need for an antidote, an "emasculator." In Germany and France several novels were devoted to rejuvenation. In the Shrove Monday's carnival parade in many parts of Germany performers had traditionally acted out the story of "The Old Wives' Mill" in which wives were remade; in twentieth-century novels it was the husbands who had to be rejuvenated. [36]

Perhaps the most entertaining exploration of rejuvenation occurred in the works of the Italian novelist Italo Svevo (Ettore Schmitz). In "An Old Man's Confessions" the narrator refers to himself as a "man who thought he must be decrepit, because he had given up women." In "Regeneration" (1927–28) the man who has been operated on believes he has changed, yet he tells his nephew he only wants women "who were young when I was young." As his maid reminds him of an old love he tries to seduce her as a way of testing the operation. "If you will cooperate in this noble, health-giving work you'll have your reward, I swear to you. First of all, you'll have it from me; and then in Heaven. . . . I'm sure all religions tell us to honour, help and protect old men. And I'm still an old man, even though I've become a young one too." Svevo raised the bothersome question whether rejuvenation—should it be possible—would liberate the elderly or add to their burdens. A similar point was made by a character in Aldous Huxley's *Brave New World* (1932): "Now—such is progress—the old men work, the old men copulate, the old men have no time, no leisure from pleasure, not a moment to sit down and think." But the American writer Gertrude Atherton—treated by Harry Benjamin with X-rays for her "mental sterility"—was convinced the rejuvenation process worked. In her best-selling novel *Black Oxen* (1923), which was subsequently made into a film, she portrayed a dazzlingly beautiful woman who looks thirty (though actually fifty-eight) seducing young men and revolutionizing Austrian politics. An old-fashioned doctor like Mary Scharlieb attacked such women for their "quasi-insane desire to prolong sexual life, or to bear children. It is extremely pathetic to find women well on to 50 years of age who are apparently as keen on sexual enjoyment as a bride might be."[37]

If the rejuvenators reflected their culture's concern for aging, they were even more marked by early twentieth-century preoccupations with improving the race. They spoke about returning potency, not to all men, but to otherwise "fit" men. In doing so they were echoing the widespread eugenic belief that reproduction was too important to be simply left to nature. Such sentiments were ultimately taken to their logical extremes by the Nazis. Though attempts to cure impotence might appear to be worlds apart from campaigns to eliminate social inferiors, the two undertakings did share some common obsessions.

Harry Benjamin claimed that "reactionaries" held back progress in hormonal research. Paul Kammerer asked his readers if they wanted to be "Slaves of the Past or Captains of the Future?" The sex researchers tended to see themselves as radicals. Though they at times recognized the need to disassociate sex and rejuvenation, they were self-consciously free of the shame that prevented others from investigating the reproductive process. Yet their views on sex and gender were far from revolutionary. Many maintained nineteenth-century notions of the spermatic economy. Brown-Séquard asserted that masturbation and sexual excesses result in impotency. Voronoff listed sexual excesses, protracted abstinence, and prolonged residence in warm climates as the causes of sexual debility. The old fear that a man was exhausted by the waste of his vital fluids resurfaced in the notion that vasectomy and ligature offered ways to retain energy. Sexual abstinence itself could be viewed as a sort of Steinach operation since in glands that were not used the generative tissue purportedly atrophied allowing self-insemination.[38]

Hormone research, in revealing how fluid the boundaries were between the sexes, might have destabilized notions of a clear male/female divide, yet the rejuvenators were clearly intent on maintaining—not eroding— traditional gender relations. Some were alarmed that women were becoming so aggressive that they were emasculating their mates. Lydston provided the most sensational reports, stating that he had treated a number of men who had had their penises amputated. "Cases of mutilation of the penis by jealous women are more frequent than generally is supposed." He produced photographs as proof. More commonly doctors argued that arrogant wives found it easy to boss about hormonally deficient husbands. Gregorio Marañón stated that a typical scenario was one in which a sexually timid, often sterile, hen-pecked husband was overmatched by a domineering wife. This suffragist type of woman was trying to oppose the laws of nature. Indeed Marañón asserted that if she had strong orgasms, it had to be because she had an enlarged clitoris and was therefore actually virile. Kenneth Walker also believed that the "emancipated" woman was often the cause of her partner's impotence. He argued that "the male must still play the dominant part, and if he has sunk to second place in the home he is unlikely to be successful in the sphere of love." Walker recalled that he had dealt with one virago who had "succeeded in producing impotence in two successive husbands, both of whom in the end escaped from her clutches through a nullity suit." [39]

The sort of gender expectations that doctors brought to their clinics, researchers brought to their labs. Steinach, for example, looked for ardor and aggressiveness in rats as signs of masculinity, and flirtatiousness as a sign of femininity. He took as a given that sex was reflected by behavior and character. Males were supposed to be strong and females gentle. Likewise when researchers turned to human subjects they read off a man's secondary sexual characteristics—voice, beard, muscles, and assertiveness—as indicators of his potency. Male and female hormones, Steinach assumed, were sharply antagonistic and he and his followers took any blurring of gender as a sign of trouble. Therapies were employed to reestablish boundaries and accordingly hormones were made part of gender politics. Steinach's procedures were aimed at returning to men and women their culturally appropriate virtues—for women good looks and for men sexual potency and strength. Likewise the larger goal of Voronoff's grafts was to "enhance 'normal' familial ties, social relations, and gender roles." Accordingly researchers boasted of their abilities to sexually reinvigorate elderly men while showing far less enthusiasm for the rejuvenation of older women. [40] Twentieth-century medical scientists thus gave new life to the nineteenth-century belief that women were not supposed to be as vigorous as men and once past childbearing had far less need to be sexually active.

Some argued that hormones, in addition to restoring the potency of individual men could indirectly restore the power of states. Linking the private and the public, doctors pointed out that the danger posed by impotence was that "the race cannot be propagated." It was no accident that the interest in rejuvenation research first crested in the 1920s. Given the huge population losses during World War I and the subsequent Spanish influenza epidemic, any undertaking that promised regeneration of the population would likely win a hearing. Rejuvenation became the rage in the same decade in which Fascists in Italy, Nazis in Germany, and Communists in the Soviet Union all asserted their intentions of creating new men and new societies. The notion of science making humans more efficient, virile, and productive was very much in the air. Lydston argued that "physiological efficiency" led to "social efficiency." As such he was voicing the common eugenic argument: for the Western world to flourish the fertility of the "unfit" would have to be curbed and that of the "fit" rewarded.[41]

Not surprisingly, in Germany the parallel was often drawn between the defeated nation and its exhausted male citizens. To restore them both Peter Schmidt went so far as to suggest that rejuvenation treatments, like vaccinations, be made obligatory. Yet links between eugenic thought and hormone research were also apparent elsewhere. In expressing his concern in 1924 that the "best stock" were not the best breeders, Frank R. Lillie sketched out the notion of establishing in Chicago an Institute for Racial Biology. In England, Francis Marshall lamented a marked drop in the fertility of the "servant-keeping class." Malthus's faith in nature restricting population growth had proven wrong: "The problem before the modern economist is not how to place a check on population generally, but rather how to secure that future generations shall be sufficiently recruited from that section of the population which is industrially capable, while at the same time to prevent indiscriminate propagation."[42] Such musings led Aldous Huxley to sketch out a vision in *Brave New World* of a future in which test tube babies would play a role in the engineering of different biological classes.

The rejuvenators' attempts to cure impotency can be fruitfully viewed as a form of "positive" eugenics. They unabashedly argued that their efforts were aimed at restoring the vigor and potency of fit, white business men and professionals. Benjamin, for example, wished that all the world's "aging intellectual, political and industrial leaders would be 'Steinached.'" In Germany, Kammerer seemed to suggest that the operation would ultimately open a "path to the Superman." The rejuvenators also supported "negative" eugenic policies aimed at limiting the fertility of the "unfit." Their prejudices were made clear enough. L. L. Stanley subjected to experimentation San Quentin inmates and Peter Schmidt operated on Chinese prisoners in Shanghai. G. Frank Lydston, a racist whose works including *Sexual Crimes Among the Southern Negroes* (c. 1893) and *That Bogey Man the Jew* (1921), expressed particular interest in Stanley's harvesting of the testicles of an executed Afro-American inmate because it demonstrated the possibility of "cross-racial" implantation.[43]

Seizing on the idea of using hormones to discipline the heretofore incorrigible, eugenists hailed the emergence of endocrinology. "The internal secretions . . . control human nature, and whoever controls them controls human nature." Charles Davenport argued at the Second International Congress of Eugenics that criminals had inherited bad glands, and therefore they were not to be hated, but treated. In the 1920s the *New York Times* carried a rash of such pronouncements. In 1921 the Pennsylvania Medical Society was told that truancy, dishonesty, and criminal tendencies were due to diet and thyroid problems. Pupils in the Chicago subnormal classes, the press reported, were to be fed a sheep gland diet. The Board of Education doctor expected to thereby put "new brains into the heads of subnormal children." The next year similar experiments were tried on prison inmates. The mystery writer Dorothy L. Sayers spoofed such undertakings when one of her characters claims unscientific attempts to deal with young criminals had failed: "Flogging and bread-and-water, you know, and Holy Communion, when what they really needed was a little bit of rabbit-gland or something to make them just good as gold." Now it was possible "to make everybody good by glands."[44]

If the goals of the rejuvenation researchers and eugenic theorists were similar, so too were their methods. Though Steinach's vasoligations were aimed at increasing the potency of the fit, they were ironically the same surgical operations that had been previously used to restrict the fertility of the unfit. They differed in that he usually severed only one vas deferens so the "fit" patient remained fertile. In 1899 Chicago surgeon A. J. Ochsner related that the operation restored a patient's flagging sexual powers, but his main point was that sterilizations should be used to prevent the births of habitual criminals, perverts, and paupers. At the Indiana Reformatory Dr. Sharp carried out this eugenic agenda, operating on some forty-two inmates. He too asserted that vasectomies both prevented procreation and improved health. The proponents of sterilization stressed that unlike castration, it did not unsex the patient and was not to be viewed as a sort of punishment. Paul Popenoe, America's most vocal defender of sterilization in the interwar years, asserted that of the sixty-five "normal" men he had interviewed who had had a vasectomy for birth control purposes, nine actually felt more potent.[45]

The obvious intent of the eugenicists in supporting sterilization was, of course, not to improve the health or sex life of the institutionalized. The goal was to prevent them from reproducing and so burdening the state. In England the program was aggressively defended by Robert R. Rentoul who in 1903 proposed the sterilization of the country's 100,000 asylums inmates, 50,000 tramps, and 60,000 prostitutes. The latter two groups had, Rentoul argued, by their choice of profession demonstrated their mental defectiveness. In the United States, Lydston was only one of many medical men to call for the sterilization of the tubercular, the insane, the epileptic, criminals, imbeciles, and perverts.[46] The argument that social deviancy was at heart a biological problem that doctors were best qualified to deal with met ready acceptance in the more progressive parts of the world. By the mid 1930s compulsory sterilizations programs were established in thirty American states, two Canadian provinces, and the Scandinavian countries, well before Nazi Germany began its campaign.

Eugenic proponents frequently succeeded in having "perverts" included as potential subjects of either castration or sterilization. A number of the medical scientists interested in rejuvenation techniques saw gland transplants and hormonal injections as "curing" rather than punishing their patients. Hence the limerick:

> Ah, Vienna, the fortress of Freud!
> Whose surgeons are always employed;
> Where boys with soft hands,
> Are provided with glands,
> And two-fisted girls are de-boyed.[47]

Alarmed by what he believed was a surge in the number of homosexuals, Lydston recommended testicular grafts as a cure. "Defective and aberrant psychic or physical sex development and differentiation—inversions and perversions—are definite indications for sex gland implantation." In 1923 Corners suggested that transplants be carried out to deal with "inborn sex inversion," followed up by psychoanalysis to remove psychological complexes. Voronoff claimed he had successes in four of the seven cases in which gland transplants were employed to remedy sexual inversion. Steinach asserted that homosexuality was due to a hormonal deficiency. After the urologist Robert Lichtenstern did a testicular graft for an accident victim, Steinach asked him to provide a homosexual with the testicle of a "healthy man." Homosexuals were obviously not healthy. Steinach asserted that the testicles of five of his homosexual patients in fact had cells resembling those found in ovaries. Though Marañón believed Steinach's observations could not be right, he still felt his colleague was on the right track. Marañón advised two homosexuals to undergo the Voronoff treatment. In one of the cases it appeared to work though Marañón concluded that suggestion played a role.[48]

Strikingly enough, a number of homosexual doctors enthusiastically supported offering hormonal therapy to those who wished to be "cured" of their sexual orientation. Norman Haire, for example, praised the attempt made by Robert Lichtenstern in 1916 to cure a homosexual by providing him with normal testicle. As Haire told it, within a short time the patient destroyed the will in which he had left all his money to a male friend, developed secondary sex characteristics, flirted with his nurse, and finally married.[49]

Magnus Hirschfeld, Europe's leading campaigner for the rights of homosexuals, supported such experiments. Since he previously claimed that true males and females were only ideals and the vast majority of individuals found themselves somewhere on the continuum in between, his new stance appeared somewhat contradictory. He took this position because those hostile to homosexuals commonly argued that they simply had made the choice of being perverts. Hirschfeld countered that scientists had established that homosexuality had a physiological basis, it was neither a vice nor a disease but a "developmental error." He asserted that the interstitial cells of homosexuals were distinctly different from those of heterosexuals and elaborated a theory that their testicular secretions led to development of a more "feminine" type of brain. He naturally took great interest in Steinach's work. So, on the one hand Hirschfeld used hypnotism to heighten the desire of heterosexual men suffering from impotence, and on the other he sent a handful of patients who wanted to overcome their bisexuality or homosexuality to surgeons like Richard Mühsam. The failure in one case he attributed to the fact that though the patient received a "normal" testicle it had to share a scrotum with its homosexual counterpart. Arguing that homosexuals had no choice in deciding their sexual orientation made tactical sense for a man seeking an end to the law that declared them criminals, but in going on to argue that homosexuals were physically different from normal males, Hirschfeld implied that they were in some way sick and so could possibly be cured. Walker more cautiously noted in 1930 that some doctors thought homosexuality was "the result of disturbances of the endocrine function of the sex gland, or some other organ of internal secretion," yet he maintained that "the surgical treatment of homosexuality cannot be considered a practical measure until much more is known, not only of the cause of homosexuality but also of tissue grafting in general." Nevertheless decades later Paul Niehans continued to give cellular injections to counter "homosexual and lesbian tendencies."[50]

Although only a few gland grafts were carried out on homosexuals in the interwar period, they provided a dangerous precedent for the Nazis who set out to eliminate homosexuality by the most barbaric of means. An example of this genealogy was represented by Knud Sand, a Danish professor of forensic medicine, who like Steinach began by experimenting on animals to demonstrate how hormones influenced sexual development, and proceeded to support the notion of curing homosexuality by testicular transplants. He played an influential role in the passage of the 1929 Danish law that allowed for the castration of sex offenders and the sterilization of the feeble-minded. During the World War II his colleague Carl Vaernet experimented on homosexuals rounded up by the SS.[51]

Is it fair to regard the rejuvenators as harbingers of the Nazis? On the one hand Paul Kammerer happily declared in 1924 that the "sterilization of inferiors," a form of negative eugenics, was now being balanced by a "productive eugenics," the "race-hygienical" exploitation of the ductless glands. Voronoff was inspired by Alexis Carrel, the 1912 Nobel Prize winner, for his work on animal transplants and who in *Man the Unknown* (1935) called for a "biological aristocracy." "Eugenics is indispensable for the perpetuation of the strong. A great race must propagate its best elements."[52] John Brinkley, the American goat-gland doctor, decorated his swimming pool with swastikas and paraded his anti-Semitism. Adolf Butenandt, who received the 1939 Nobel Prize for his work on testosterone, remained in Germany right through war, insisting that true science could never be tainted by politics. Only in the 1990s was it discovered that he had done research on the blood samples of Auschwitz inmates. Yet the leading rejuvenators were exactly the sorts of the people the Nazis reviled. They were sex reformers. Harry Benjamin, Eugen Steinach, and Norman Haire all participated in the 1926 International Congress for Sex Research organized in Berlin by Albert Moll. Benjamin and Haire also attended the conferences of Magnus Hirschfeld's World League for Sexual Reform. Haire and Hirschfeld were homosexuals. Furthermore, Haire, Hirschfeld, Benjamin, and Steinach were all Jews. Steinach had to flee Austria for Switzerland. Hirschfeld, whose Institute for Sexual Science was destroyed by the Nazis, died in exile in 1935. Both eugenics and rejuvenation theories had such broad appeals that they attracted support across the political spectrum. If a sex radical and leftist like Hirschfeld thought something good might come from hormonally treating homosexuals, it speaks to the faith so many had in the early twentieth century that medical science could solve every sexual conundrum.

Though curing the impotence of the otherwise healthy and limiting the reproduction of the "inferior" might appear to have little in common, they were regarded by some in the decades between the world wars as two sides of the same coin. Rejuvenation, eugenics, and endocrinology were each in their own ways symptoms of the twentieth-century desire to improve the body.[53] Though their adherents might not all have believed that human behavior could be standardized, they were convinced that sexual behavior could be measured against scientifically established norms. In the postwar years, Alfred Kinsey set out to demolish just such theories and in doing so provided yet another reappraisal of impotence's cultural significance.

THE "IMPOTENCE BOOM"
From Kinsey to Masters and Johnson

Under the caption "The Impotence Boom (Has it hit you yet?)," *Esquire* carried on its October 1972 cover a photo of an apparently nude Burt Reynolds casting a worried look at his loins. Philip Nobile's inside story played off claims by alarmists such as Dr. George L. Ginsberg that in recent years there had been a marked rise in impotence, against the reassurances of Dr. Albert Ellis that only reports of such dysfunctions had risen. The general tenor of the story was that worrisome changes explained why impotence was now a topic that novelists, magazine writers, and moviemakers avidly exploited. Men were on the defensive. Nobile titled his story "What Is the New Impotence, and Who's Got It?" The "old impotence" was attributed to tired, older men bored with their middle-aged partners; the "new impotence" was experienced by younger men increasingly daunted by the demands of sexually liberated women. Nobile cited a Harvard undergrad who stated that in dating the question now was *not* "Will she or won't she?" but "Could *he* or couldn't *he*."[1]

Like any journalist, Nobile concentrated on the sensational, but he touched on a number of key issues in the shifting of gender relationships and the resulting recasting of impotence that took place in the decades between World War II and the 1980s. In these years the media portrayed incapacitated males as casualties of the war, of the social pressures of the consumerist, conformist culture of the 1950s, and finally of the sexual revolution and the feminist movement of the 1960s and 1970s. These were the decades in which preeminent sex surveyor Alfred Kinsey and the therapists Masters and Johnson became household names. In rewriting the sexual script, they popularized notions of new models of the sexual body, and in their very different ways advocated a shift in treatment of male dysfunctions away from psychotherapy and toward sex therapy. Such sex experts presented themselves as freeing the anxious from the burdens of old taboos and restraints. They defended or legitimated a number of common sexual practices previously regarded as sapping male sexual vigor. They provided accounts that should have reassured the anxious. But the "sexual revolution" they helped sponsor had its inherent tensions and contradictions. The experts justified the increased attention they paid to a man's sexual practices on the gravity of his "performance anxieties." Yet the very fact that a sex therapy profession emerged and increasing numbers of "patients" allowed themselves to be subjected to the most intrusive forms of help imaginable suggests that in a so-called age of liberation, the pressure to meet sexual norms increased rather than decreased.

In 1950s America discussions of male sexuality were colored by the notion that individual men, like the nation as a whole, were vulnerable to attack. Films and novels tapped into such insecurities, representing virility as a means by which to beat back the perversions of communism and homosexuality. Employing a transparently sexualized rhetoric, politicians accused opponents of being "soft" and prided themselves on being "hard" on subversives. They warned the citizenry that in the outside world lurked communism and other forces of evil that might "penetrate" and overwhelm democratic societies. At home sexual pessimists bemoaned the growth of suburbanization, white-collar work, and youth culture to which prosperity had given rise. They pointed to declining fertility and rising divorce rates as symptoms of the erosion of family values. These problems were in turn traced back by a new generation of experts to the notion that men, women, and young people were failing to fulfill their prescribed age and gender roles. The war-time economy had lured countless women into doing "men's jobs." A host of sex counselors in the 1950s accordingly sought to correct the war's corrosive impact on notions of masculinity and femininity by exaggerating "traditional" gender divisions.[2] Believing that New Deal welfare legislation, military regimentation, and stultifying office work had all undercut masculine forcefulness, they looked to sex surveys for evidence to back up their assertions.

In his 1948 best seller, *Sexual Behavior in the Human Male* Alfred Kinsey set out before the public an exhaustive account of American men's private practices. Kinsey boasted of drawing on tens of thousands of interviews to report on the variety of sexual acts ordinary white Americans actually engaged in. When Kinsey asked men about their sexual "outlets," he found that over the course of their lives "true heterosexual intercourse" occupied only fourth place; masturbation, wet dreams, and heterosexual petting preceded it. Masturbation, Kinsey pointed out, was ubiquitous and, though psychiatrists were still reluctant to admit it, harmless. So too was the homosexual sex play that 60 percent of his subjects recalled having as boys. Once males began their sex lives they never stopped. Countering the old notion of a "seminal economy" that held that one had a limited reserve of sexual energy that should not be squandered, Kinsey declared that sexual activity was a sign of health.[3]

Though he said relatively little about impotence, Kinsey's key argument that abstinence impaired performance—"use it or lose it"—was later on taken up by a host of popularizers. There was no need to worry about excesses. "The ready assumption which is made in some of the medical literature that impotence is the product of sexual excess is not justified by such data as are now available."[4] In fact Kinsey argued just the opposite. The age at which one began to be sexually active was the main predictor of sexual longevity; those who started early, ended late. Equating inhibitions with ill health, Kinsey surmised that the sexually apathetic were most likely poorly educated and religiously devout.

And despite what the rejuvenators had claimed, Kinsey found no evidence of a sudden male climacteric. The sexual activity of the male peaked in his teens and then began a slow life-long decline; male rates of intercourse crested in a man's twenties and then they too fell. Most men did not experience a sudden decline of sexual vigor in their fifties. At age sixty, 5 percent were sexually inactive; at seventy, 30 percent. Kinsey concluded impotence was actually quite rare and doctors specializing in the subject had inflated its importance. Kinsey found erectile impotence in less than 1 percent of men under age thirty-five; one-quarter were impotent at seventy, and over one-half by seventy-five.[5] Yet even in old age impotence was often attributable more to psychological than physiological causes.

Kinsey's 1953 report *Sexual Behavior in the Human Female* created another sensation. Perhaps the most important finding of this study, based on nearly 8,000 subjects, was Kinsey's rediscovery of the importance of the clitoris for female pleasure. He was consequently led on to defend clitoral stimulation against the psychoanalysts who insisted that women needed training in "vaginal response." Yet in marital intercourse, the wife's desires seemed to be of secondary importance to Kinsey. Since three-quarter of the males he interviewed took two minutes to climax, he assumed that their haste could not be deemed "abnormal." He noted that chimps only took ten to twenty seconds. In any event, many women never climaxed during intercourse and it was therefore all the more unreasonable to expect men to prolong it. Indeed Kinsey believed that doctors had been mistaken in labeling premature ejaculation a type of impotence. "It would be difficult to find another situation in which an individual who was quick and intense in his responses was labeled anything but superior, and that in most instances is exactly what the rapidly ejaculating male is, however inconvenient and unfortunate his qualities may be from the standpoint of the wife in the relationship." Kinsey suggested couples work out their "sexual adjustments in marriage" and he included chapters dealing with the physiological, psychological and hormonal factors in sexual response and orgasm. He was not terribly interested in therapies. Priding himself on simply cataloging what men did, he was disdainful of the psychoanalysts and marriage counselors who tried to cure or change them.[6]

Kinsey's findings should have dampened down fears of loss of male virility yet, each subsequent decade saw some publication gloomily allege that a surge in male impotence was occurring. In the 1960s one study showed impotence jumping from about 7 percent for men age fifty, to 25 percent for those sixty-five, to 55 percent age seventy-five. In the mid 1970s, impotence was described as an "epidemic," affecting a third of men. Medical doctors had little new to offer. They continued to believe that most cases were psychological in origin though some were linked to disease. The treatments available in the late 1960s still included local measures (including circumcision, Lowsley's operation, urethral diathermy, and employment of splints); hormonal therapies (the use of testosterone derivatives, thyroid compounds, and the Steinach operation); chemotherapeutic therapies (including doses of yohimbine, strychnine, apomorphine, amphetamine); and finally the psychological therapies (psychotherapy, counseling, hypnosis and relaxation, and behavior therapy).[7]

If in theory there were numerous medical treatments available, in practice few doctors knew much about them. Before the 1960s physicians received almost no formal training on sexual matters. Most knew little more than their patients. Donald W. Hastings, the head of psychiatry at the University of Minnesota, recalled in 1963 that when he was in medical school in the 1930s only one hour was spent on the study of contraception and that as a young intern he was embarrassed to be put in charge of a ward of prostitutes who knew far more about sex than the medical students who attended them. Little had changed in thirty years. Urologists in the 1960s dealt with surgical matters, not with the decline of the libido. In any event the vast majority of men did not seek sexual advice from their doctors. Dysfunctions were self diagnosed and purchases made of quack remedies to increase vigor. The latter included in the late 1950s "Stagg Bullets for Men,"

"Passionala," royal jelly, and pega palo, a Caribbean weed that purportedly enhanced virility.[8]

Medical doctors largely conceded the discussion of impotence to psychoanalysts and marriage counselors, and a vulgarized Freudianism permeated much of their commentary. Though Kinsey believed psychoanalysis was just another means for instilling guilt, the science peaked in popularity in the 1950s. Leaders in the profession such as Edmund Bergler and Helene Deutsch attributed impotence to castration fears, homosexual tendencies, mother fixations, and infantilism. A man's overattachment to his mother led to feelings of guilt and fear of castration. Such fears were reactivated by any woman "identified" as the mother. His inhibitions and impotence ensued as a protection against a symbolically incestuous relationship. In the first instance such interpretations attributed much of the blame for men's dysfunctions to their mothers. Drawing heavily on Freud, Philip Wylie in *Generation of Vipers* (1955) attacked what he termed "momism." Legions of destructive, idle, middle-aged women, he asserted, had destroyed their sons, leaving them "limp and querulous." Psychiatrist Edward A. Strecker held such "apron-stringing" moms responsible for the hundreds of thousands of men rejected or discharged by the army. Establishing "momarchies" by usurping the rightful role of the father in the family, such "moms in pants" doomed their boys to immaturity if not homosexuality.[9]

For the psychoanalyst a potency disturbance could not be understood without understanding the underlying neurosis. In a typically elaborate example of such psychoanalytic sleuthing Bergler traced back a young man's marital impotence to his having seen the film *The Human Beast*, a dramatization of Emile Zola's novel.

> In it [the film] the protagonist shrinks from having intercourse because he fears that in his sexual frenzy he might strangle the heroine. The young man could not forget that central scene, applied the situation to himself and feared that he, too, would commit such a crime. He became completely impotent, and felt close to a "nervous breakdown." ... His fear pertained to castration threats, meted out by the father in his fantasy, and Father is undoubtedly an external person. In short, he played the role of the aggressive transgressor of educational commands, who is threatened by an outside danger of retaliation. In his enforced "abstinence" (after a few fiascoes, he did not touch his wife), he secondarily avoided the "bad boy" situation. More, he preventively executed the sentence of castration upon himself, since an unusable organ is unconsciously synonymous with a castrated organ. This, in turn, immediately brought him into the orbit of "negative Oedipus" which in itself was

but a duplication on a "higher" developmental level of the passivity he had experienced on the pre-Oedipal level.[10]

Such inventive reasoning was all the more impressive given that psycho-analysts noted that neurotics, presenting other problems as a façade, rarely mentioned sexual difficulties in their first therapy sessions. But Freudians could detect impotence—even if the patient could not—because they saw it manifested in a variety of behaviors. Bergler argued that neurotics felt that every sex act was a test of their potency. "The wolf is (contradictory as it may sound) *an impotent man who conceals that bitter fact from himself and others by constantly exchanging women.* Were he to stay for any length of time with *one* woman, he, the great seducer, would be proven impotent. In an unconscious preventive action, therefore, he does not allow the situation to arise." Bergler repeated the argument in *Counterfeit-Sex* (1958). Psychoanalytic-psychiatric studies revealed that "nine-tenths of all infidelity in women is based on frigidity, and nine-tenths of the 'running from one woman to another' in men is reducible to open or hidden impotence." Bergler likewise pronounced that promiscuous women were actually frigid. Many mistresses were lesbians who really wanted a wife. "Paradoxical as it may sound, Lesbians are not woman-lovers but woman-haters and, in the deepest layer, gluttons for punishment administered by a woman. All Lesbian relationships, therefore, are suffused with hatred and suffering." Such outbursts explain why Kinsey regarded Freud's followers as simply carrying on the moralizing tradition of priests and philosophers.[11]

In looking for the cause of impotence, Freudians placed much of the guilt first on the man's mother and secondly on his wife. In a study of un-consummated marriages, the English psychoanalyst Michael Balint stated that treating frigid women often cured men's impotence. Balint noted how powerful such women often were. Those who sought artificial insemination were actually demonstrating a desire to have their own penis and thus to devalue men. Most of the women in the study suffered from tightness, or vaginismus, and had unconsciously chosen timid husbands. These women, according to Balint, had to learn to be passive and less independent. Simply instructing the woman to permit her husband to be more manly often solved the problem. "There is no question that if the woman allows her husband to be aggressive, and even enjoys it, it might give more to him than any psychiatric treatment. We agree that to treat impotent men is a very long and difficult task, whereas here in a few weeks we can make them potent by treating their wives—heaven knows how."[12] In fact he did know how—by restoring the appropriate gender roles.

Bergler also accused the frigid wife of claiming her husband was impotent as an alibi for her own shortcomings. A colleague stated that "not infrequently a husband's potency reflects a wife's frigidity. If she is cold, indifferent, or averse to intercourse, he is likely to be overwhelmed by feelings of futility and frustration which may lead to impotence." Of course frigidity, according to many Freudians, was true even of women who had the wrong (that is, the clitoral) sort of orgasm. The man's failings were thus displaced onto a woman declared to be nonorgasmic or repressed. Books with such titles as *How to Hold Your Husband: A Frank Psychoanalysis for Happy Marriage* that purported to inform their readers on how to overcome female frigidity, were often in fact indirectly addressing the problem of male impotence.[13]

If many Freudians instructed women on the importance of being dutiful wives, they also warned men that any lack of interest in the opposite sex could be taken as a sign of latent homosexuality. Charles W. Socarides provided a classic Freudian explanation of how impotence and homosexuality were linked.

> One's happy experiences at the breast exert a favorable influence in promoting genitality. Only when there is undue oral stimulation and frustration does the organism undergo an intense fixation to the oral phase and produce an undue degree of fear because of the rejection of its oral hunger. The object relationship of the genital phase becomes filled with a pattern acquired at the oral zone including the unconscious fantasies and feelings of desire and fear. In many men this may be interpreted as a fear of being devoured by the vagina. This is probably the most important factor responsible for psychosexual impotence in men.[14]

According to Bergler homosexuals were, unconsciously, "simply frightened fugitives from women, fleeing in their panic to 'another continent.'" Their mother had been too strong and their father too weak. In treating homosexuals, therapists looked for the patient who had such a dad: "A father who is sexually inhibited, impotent, fearful of women, bisexual and/or homosexual." Those who embraced the notion of the "flight to homosexuality" held that since virility in the modern world increasingly had to be proven by woman's sexual response, weak men retreated into less demanding same-sex relationships. Socarides coined the term "variational homosexuality" to refer to those who because of their impotence or near-impotence, sought out homosexual experiences.[15]

Some therapists held that impotence led to homosexuality, others postulated that the homosexual was impotent. "Homosexuality is a form of impotency, although at times it may not evidence itself anatomically or completely," asserted John Cavanagh. He went on to state that as a psychiatrist he had to "insist that the homosexual is psychologically impotent in heterosexual relations." There was a positive aversion to the act itself. Furthermore, "the homosexual lacks the capacity for that unselfish love which is necessary for marriage." While asserting that there was no necessary relationship between impotence and sexual deviation, psychiatrist George Henry described a case in which homosexuality and impotence were closely linked. "Egbert's latent homosexuality was associated with impotence. He was troubled by panicky feelings about losing his health and his mind, by impulses to punch pregnant women in the stomach, and by obsessive thoughts such as: 'I'm not of any value; nobody wants me. I'm a failure.'" Even progressives in favor of decriminalization of homosexuality like Eustace Chesser asserted that homosexuality was related to self-love, failure of sublimation, and arrested development. The liberal English sex expert Joan Malleson described homosexuals as neurotics who like bisexuals needed psychotherapy to draw them to "normal paths." Like Bergler, such experts tended to regard homosexuality as a "curable disease." The transition from homosexuality to a "sustained premarital relationship" with a woman would, however, noted Lawrence Hatterer, be marked by sexual complications. "Premature ejaculation, transient impotence, low frequency of intercourse, and an inability to abandon himself or to achieve mutual orgasm are just a few possible difficulties that may arise at this time in the patient's new sexual adaptation."[16]

Doctors "rediscovered" the problem of homosexuality in the postwar years. In 1952 the American Psychiatric Association developed the *Diagnostic and Statistical Manual of Mental Disorders* (DSM-1) that declared homosexuality a sociopathic personality disorder. Fears of homosexuality also underlay the postwar panic over sexual psychopaths. Between 1947 and 1955 twenty-one American states passed laws targeting deviants, the purported purpose being to better protect women and children. In the 1960s doctors continued to suggest that impotent inverts were prone to commit sex crimes. "Many sexual offenses occur because the individual is seeking the stimulus necessary to overcome his impotence. The individual who has lost his potency frequently becomes obsessed with the idea that if he could receive a certain type of stimulus he could then perform a sex act quite satisfactorily. He may have enjoyed such stimulation or (more likely) has enjoyed it in fantasy. This stimulus may vary from some simple form of stimulation such as pornographic pictures at one end of the scale to sadistic murder at the other." Patricia Sexton stated that the typical murderer was a "nice guy" like Sirhan or Oswald (the killers of the Kennedys) who were quiet "feminized males" whose normal impulses were so warped they had to prove their virility by killing. Such accounts of "sick" perverts deflected attention from the fact that the vast majority of assaults on women and children were carried out by heterosexual male friends or family members.[17] In the decades in which men were egged on to be more virile and manly, few arguments were more unsettling than the suggestion that impotence could lead to homosexuality, which in turn could lead to sadistic sex crimes.

Psychologists and psychiatrists dealt with impotence as a problem affecting the individual. Marriage counselors treated it as a problem affecting a couple. Sexual dysfunctions were spoken of far more openly in the 1950s, especially by the professionals who assumed the task of ensuring that unhappy couples not even envisage separation. Their premise was that the higher expectations of marriage in the twentieth century largely explained the upturn in divorce rates. Marriage counseling had begun in the 1930s. In the United States the Marriage Council won the support of eugenicists and progressives because of the fear of the impact that the depression had on families. A dangerous combination of economic and sexual disappointments could, they believed, topple many fragile marriages. Quaker Emily Mudd founded the American Association of Marriage Counselors. Similar religious preoccupations colored the views of the National Marriage Guidance Council in Great Britain, which beginning in 1938 produced such texts as *How to Treat a Young Wife*. The gist of their message was captured by E. F. Griffith's declaration that sexual incompatibility was the root of most marriage problems. David Mace, Britain's chief advocate of marriage guidance, described marital disharmony as a "disease."[18]

Marie Stopes had led the campaign in the interwar years for the eroticization of marriage by portraying unhappy marriages as resulting from clumsy husbands and sexually restrained wives. Marriage counselors similarly hoped that by improving sex, it would be restricted to the marriage bed. Women had to find marital sex pleasurable, and Emily Mudd accordingly provided advice on how the husband should "court" his wife. To counter husbands from straying, wives were enjoined to make themselves more responsive and attractive. Reports on marriages in the years following World War II suggested little had changed. In England data drawn from Family Planning clinics in the 1940s revealed that 50 percent of women were still not sexually satisfied. Few men knew much about the importance of clitoral stimulation. In 1950 a doctor who noted that potency was usually defined as the ability to initiate, sustain, and conclude sexual intercourse "to the satisfaction of the male" went on to state that "if we include the words 'and the female,' some 50 percent of potent males might be classified as impotent." Professionals thus came round to the notion that in cases of impotence, there were not one but two sufferers. Who complained of impotence? Doctors reported that wives were more likely than their husbands to talk of the latter's lack of interest in sex. When Hannah and Abraham Stone published an article on female frigidity they were surprised to receive letters from women insisting it was their husbands who had deficiencies.[19]

The problem grew as the population aged. In 1965 one in every eight people in the United States was over the age of sixty. Progressive doctors stressed the need to recognize the normality of sex for the elderly, though some counselors thought it shocking. Alex Comfort found as had Kinsey that early starters were late finishers. "What we are seeing in cross-sectional studies, therefore, is a mixture of high and low sexually active individuals, in which those whose sexual 'set' is low for physical or attitudinal reasons drop out early—often using age as a justification for laying down what has for them been an anxious business. So much for the obsession with loss of sexual function which has so heavily influenced gerontology—senile asexuality is a sociogenic disorder." But Kinsey had also revealed a gender gap in sexual desire. Men's sexual activity peaked early and their libido declined well before women's. A 1961 study found that the mean age of ceasing regular coitus was 68 for married men and 58 for the unmarried. The decline in marital coitus was usually due to the husband's lack of desire, not the wife's. In fact the woman's enjoyment of sex often increased after menopause, in part due to her no longer being worried about getting pregnant.[20]

Despite such findings, the writers of marriage manuals continued to attribute to the man the instrumental role, while portraying the woman as less active if not sexually dormant. It is true that from the 1950s on, the acceptable sex acts discussed in such manuals expanded. Mutual orgasm was no longer insisted upon as always being the ultimate goal. Yet given the premise that the man was to be in charge and the woman was to respond, the issue of impotence posed an obvious problem. The cautious began by noting that one had to be careful in using the term "impotence" since illness, worry, or even a wife's sarcasm could be expected to inhibit most men. Occasional erectile dysfunction, declared Joan Malleson, was quite common, likening it to a sportsman "who has 'bowled a wide' or 'served a double'"; only when such failures were habitual was it true impotence. The counselor needed to see what sort of sexual dysfunction the man had and how it related to what was happening in the marriage. Perhaps the problem could not be "cured," but it could at least be exposed.[21]

Others were more intrusive. Edwin W. Hirsch asserted that civilization, prudery, bad education, and fears of masturbation produced sexual cripples.

Psychic impotence could be cured only by force of will. "Nature does not reward cowards and mental slackers." Some still clung to the discredited notion of a spermatic economy. Premarital experiments often led to poor marriages, asserted one expert, but the healthy man could go on into his sixties if he had "exercised his sexual powers in a legitimate way." The promiscuous would have their just desserts. "The man who has had many mistresses and has lived in a way that was sexually exciting to the extreme, is going to find that he is not sufficiently stimulated by the same woman, his wife, day after day, and he therefore tends to become impotent at a much earlier age than if he had been more saving of his sexual powers."[22] The more current writers followed Kinsey's line that those who were sexually active soonest lasted longest.

Therapists reported the complex interactions that resulted in impotence. One sketched out the picture of the typical noncommunicative couple where the libido of each partner had waned. Each night the man could be found with the "evening paper, highball in hand, relaxing after a rigorous day of encounters with the business world. After dinner there come the television wrestling matches. . . . Smarting under this kind of treatment and tired herself at the end of the day, understandably the wife may be more than a little difficult to arouse sexually." Impotence or frigidity could, psychiatrists also surmised, be related to fantasies of extramarital relationships. When frustration through impotence or frigidity was combined with a sense of guilt, the result could be emotional disorder to the point of mental illness.[23]

Like the psychoanalysts, the marriage counselors placed much of the blame for impotence on women. The point was well made in the title of Maxine Davis's work *The Sexual Responsibility of Woman* (1957). Davis coyly stated that as the spouses were climbing the same mountain, the man should not walk too fast. The wife's job was to "adapt herself to her husband," depending on whether he was inhibited or randy. The young groom was often as jittery as the bride and she had to reassure him: "Don't be upset, sweetheart. The doctor and all the books say this can happen, especially to a really sensitive person like you. It's because we're both wound up. Everything is going to be all right." Calming words would do the trick. "The average healthy young fellow will respond like a new tennis ball to his bride's trust and belief in him as a potent male." Men were not to be held responsible for all fiascoes. Some women, said Hirsch, were "tardy" or straight-laced but, "a wise and encouraging wife can convert a so-called impotent husband into a sexually potent spouse." Another expert argued that the wife needed to help if the husband were "to escape from his sexual imprisonment." A colleague noted that the wife could obviously not deny that she was at fault when her vaginismus or "flinching" made penetration difficult. Nor should she believe that she should have an orgasm every time like the man. Too many women read too much and overvalued the physical. And for the woman to criticize her spouse was an absolute betrayal. "The moment a woman acts as though her husband is not capable or is actually losing his potency, she is bringing into play a devastating destructive factor."[24]

Men suffering from impotence were presented in much of the literature as being victims of changing social norms. An American text gave the case of husband who, priding himself on being the sole economic support of his wife, lost his potency when she began to earn her own income. "The ability to perform the sexual act has been a criterion for man's evaluation of himself from time immemorial," observed a marriage expert. "Virility used to be conceived as a unilateral expression of male sexuality, but is regarded today in terms of the ability to evoke a full sexual response on the part of the female. . . . The urgency of the problem of impotence may arise also from the psychological need to buttress masculinity in one area safe from female competition, and it may also be that sexual prowess represents an alternative to economic success in validating manhood. Any deficiencies in this realm, therefore, are much more ego-threatening to men than to women. Sexual adequacy affects the relationship of men not only to women, but also to other men."[25] A number of doctors likewise attributed the increased reportage of vaginismus, not to physiological difficulties but to women's financial independence.

More common was the assertion that because now marriage was supposed to assure the sexual happiness of both partners, males felt under increased pressure. It was suggested that people worried too much about their capacities. Feeling more responsible led men to exaggerate their failures. Potency was in effect a "fear of fear" problem. Men simply had to become more skilled lovers. More conservative commentators flat out advised men to ignore the wife's reaction. J. F. Tuthill, who worked for the London and Birmingham Marriage Guidance Councils, claimed that trying to prolong the sex act simply increased a husband's anxiety. In the first half of the twentieth century, some sex experts had set the simultaneous orgasm as the goal toward which every couple had to strive. From the 1950s on those writing about marriage increasingly warned that such efforts should not be exaggerated, that most women preferred "romance," and that over strenuous attempts could have the unanticipated effect of incapacitating the male.[26]

Such cautions were to be expected given that the "sexual revolution" of the 1960s was widely perceived as increasing the pressure on men to perform. As measured in rates of pre- and extramarital sex, women changed more than men in this decade. Studies appeared showing that young women were making unprecedented sexual demands. Wives changed as well. Robert Bell advanced figures showing that two-thirds of wives in the 1920s wanted less sex, whereas only one-sixth in 1940 and one-thirteenth in 1964. Numerous reports were published of men being disconcerted by female overtures. Pressure built as it became more common for women to have had premarital sexual experiences. Women had always been blamed for intimidating men, but in the 1960s a particular type of woman—the feminist—was singled out for attack. In a 1964 article denouncing sexologists, the psychoanalyst Leslie H. Farber asserted that when the woman did not know about the orgasm she did not miss it; it was not "isolated from the totality of her pleasures." Now experts had "enshrined" the orgasm as her right. By the 1970s a conservative doctor like B. Lyman Stewart, was asserting the "passive male" was rendered impotent by a "paternalistic or socialistic form of government" and by the fear of the sorts of aggressive women who supported the Women's Liberation Movement. He pointed to the fact that younger men and non-Caucasians were now showing up in doctors' offices as a sure indicator of a rise in male difficulties. Since more aggressive women had appeared, Stewart saw as the only answer the need for even more powerful men. Some liberal commentators were bemused by such calls to arms, interpreting them as an inability to imagine egalitarian relationships. "We are in a situation where the bluff of male potency has been called by the militant sisterhoods of America and Britain, or so it would seem from the anger they provoke," wrote Karl Miller. "The penis has sustained its comeuppance, or rather putdown." Others argued that the increased popularity of oral sex was an indicator of men worrying about their ability to penetrate.[27]

That symbol of 1960s sexual modernity—the contraceptive pill—played a central role in the emergence of the "new impotence." From the nineteenth century onward it had been reported that the need to employ contraceptives sapped the ardor of some men. In the 1950s and 1960s birth control continued to be cited as a cause of impotence due to men's dislike of the condom and the anxieties associated with coitus interruptus. The fact that the main methods of contraception were the man's responsibility compounded the problem. Finding that many men claimed they could not perform if forced to wear a condom, the birth control advocate Margaret Sanger saw the need to distance sex from contraception. Her goading of medical scientists and philanthropists finally resulted in the appearance of the birth control pill in 1960. With the coming of the oral contraceptive the sex act was finally divorced from both reproduction and the messy methods to avoid it. Most men were delighted that the pill relieved them of the responsibility for contraception and made women more sexually available. Yet, some were not sure. David Reisman worried that the pill allowed women to become "critical consumers of male performance." There were even men who lamented the fact that with the pill they were ignorant of a woman's intent. Given the chances of getting pregnant in a pre-pill age, a woman would have consented to sex only if she were serious about the relationship. Now she was free—like a man—to shop around. Almost immediately the cry was raised that easier contraception caused even more impotence. Dr. Herbert A. Otto claimed that "the pill and the IUD contribute to a male perception of women as sexually demanding and possibly insatiable, since the fear of pregnancy which has acted as a deterrent to her sexual appetites has been removed." In reality, the evidence suggests that the separation of intercourse and protection by oral contraceptive largely allowed gender norms to go unchanged. The very fact that women took the pill well before having sex meant that they could continue to play the passive role.[28]

It was hardly a coincidence that in the 1970s reports of a "new impotence" followed not only the widespread use of the pill and the emergence of second-wave feminism, but the discovery of the multiorgasmic female. The latter phenomenon was widely publicized by William H. Masters and Virginia E. Johnson, the most important of the sex therapists who in the 1960s presented themselves as replacing marriage counselors and psychoanalysts as the best qualified experts on sexual dysfunctions. Their best-selling *Human Sexual Response* (1966) claimed to provide the first scientific explanation of the mechanics of intercourse. Masters, who began his observation of orgasms in 1954 at George Washington University in St. Louis, in effect created the new field of sex therapy. In the late 1950s he married Virginia Johnson and they became a husband and wife team. At first they mainly saw men worried by impotence or premature ejaculation; in the 1960s their patients were primarily women seeking orgasm. Much has been written about their work on women but little about their work on men.[29]

Whereas marriage counseling had been all about communication and emotional adjustment, sex therapy was mainly about technique. It presented itself as more scientific, basing its recommendations upon the actual observation and measurement of sex acts. When Masters and Johnson's research was initially reported, the public felt an unease upon hearing that sex was being subjected to laboratory experimentation and—with miniature cameras inside plastic penises—observation. They skillfully defused such worries by presenting themselves as white coated medical scientists rather than as sex radicals. In referring to "erectile dysfunction" and "female sexual arousal disorder" rather than to "impotence" or "frigidity" they distanced themselves from the Freudians. More importantly, they presented themselves as a therapy team dealing with the "marriage problems" of both husband and wife, justifying their intrusiveness as serving the higher goal of marital harmony. They did not set out to cure individuals; the "marital unit" was the "the patient" and the interaction of the couple accordingly crucial.

While Kinsey had argued that sexual performance varied according to social class, Masters and Johnson began with the basic premise that sexual intercourse was simply a physiological process. They believed that men in particular were hard wired to be orgasmic. Based on their fifteen years of lab experiments and eleven years of clinical trials they claimed that existing types of therapy lacked physiological insights. In asserting that the clitoris was a woman's main source of pleasure and that her sexual capacities exceeded those of the man, Masters and Johnson made their name, yet they simply demonstrated much that was already known. Their declarations both increased men's sexual concerns and offered reassurances. Some men were no doubt daunted by the therapists' claims of having discovered the multiorgasmic woman. It was also humbling for some to hear that women could have more orgasms without men than with them.

Masters and Johnson dealt with both nonorgasmic women and impotent men. Their simple message was that, armed with new, scientific knowledge, overcoming marital problems was relatively easy. All that was required was a two week training session costing $2,500. They found that over the long term, negative thinking—depression, anger, fear, and boredom—were the main causes of the male's sexual decline. Like Kinsey they reported the key factor was "consistency of active sexual expression" from middle age on. Nevertheless they claimed that those over fifty could still be "trained" out of "secondarily acquired impotence." A man's virility could be "reconstituted" or "restimulated." In the short term, monotony, preoccupation with one's job, fatigue, overindulgence in food or drink, and physical infirmities, all played roles, but they singled out the heavy burden of male responsibility in intercourse as the leading cause of the performance anxieties that led to erectile dysfunctions.[30]

Stopes and Sanger had given their correspondents some general instructions on how to improve their sex lives. Masters and Johnson provided intrusive coaching aimed at behavior modification. They shifted the focus from Kinsey's concern for the quantity of sex to the quality of the orgasm. By teaching techniques of orgasmotherapy, starting with an education in masturbation, they claimed it was possible to ignore cultural conditioning and circumvent the psychoanalytic preoccupation with the psyche that might demand years of treatment. They reassured their patients that penis size was not important. Men needed only to relax, knowing that sexual intercourse was simply "a natural physical function."

If established patterns blocked healthy, natural reactions, the individual needed reconditioning. "Negative conditioning"—due to bad memories, fears, and hostilities—were the chief causes of anxiety. A "repressive upbringing," a dominant mother, or notions of sin might all play a role. Embracing a behaviorist psychological model, the therapists believed an impotent man would inevitably respond to stimulus-response. The purpose of subjecting him to training or "sensate focus sessions" was to remove his unhealthy responses and develop his pleasure-giving abilities. These might include self-stimulation. Nineteenth-century doctors said masturbation caused impotence; Masters and Johnson claimed that in providing an "education" that overcame "performance fears," masturbation could help cure it.[31]

In some ways Masters and Johnson raised the sexual bar for men. Whereas Kinsey refused to view premature ejaculation as a problem, they went so far as to assert that a man who failed to bring a woman to orgasm at least half of the time had to be counted as suffering from the condition and well on the road to having the secondary form of impotence. They regarded premature ejaculation as a conditioned response resulting from petting and coitus interruptus. Neither the traditional attempts at distraction—the reciting of baseball statistics and so on—nor the use of sedatives and calming ointments worked. Instead the therapists explained how the wife in the female dominant position, should employ the "squeeze technique," allowing the husband "to become acquainted with the sensation of intravaginal containment in a nondemanding, therefore nonthreatening, environment." Better than other therapies like hypnotism, drugs, tranquilizers, barbituates, and the creams and jellies used to reduce sensitivity, Masters and Johnson claimed the "squeeze technique" resulted in the curing of 182 of 186 cases.[32]

Masters and Johnson defined "secondary impotence" as failure in 25 percent or more attempts at penetration. Here the goal of training was to remove the man's fears and teach the couple to communicate. The wife was instructed to mount the man so he would not be distracted by the "hunt" for the vagina. She was instructed to "tease" and warned that "a demanding pattern of female pelvic thrusting is indeed threatening to any man with erective insecurity." With just such simple training over a two week period they claimed to achieve an unbelievable success rate of 75 percent. They even claimed to have cured nineteen out of thirty-two cases of "primary impotence," which they attributed to psychosocial causes, homosexual preference, and prostitute traumas. As a colleague reported, they prided themselves on doing more than restoring a man's potency. "They add that the husband's ability to perform effectively and securely in the sexual sphere has also profoundly affected his ability to play the male with confidence in other spheres of his life, and has revolutionized the marriage relationship."[33]

In some cases unmarried men brought "replacement partners" to the training sessions and in others Masters and Johnson provided "partner surrogates" for married men. Their justification was that such women were needed to service the "anxious, tension-filled male."[34] Such a form of therapy was hardly new. For centuries doctors had advised men to experiment with prostitutes. Given Masters and Johnson's pose as objective scientists it was curious that they did not spell out why they did not also provide women with surrogate lovers. The employment of strangers certainly ran counter to the therapists' stress on the importance of a married couple's communication.

Masters and Johnson's emphasis on the purely physical aspects of sex, their seeking to reverse symptoms rather than to improve relationships, appears stultifying in hindsight. At the time critics pointed out that their suspiciously high success rates resulted from preselecting candidates. Nevertheless they laid the basis for a whole new profession of caregivers, each of whom gave the impotence problem a particular spin. Albert Ellis claimed to have preceded Masters and Johnson in developing RET (rational-emotive therapy). His view was that patients with rigid views of themselves and others created their own sexual problems like impotence. Having "awfulized" their situations or resorted to "must-urbation," they needed homework to break the spell. Helen Singer Kaplan agreed that it was "surprisingly easy" to cure the 50 percent of the male population that experienced occasional impotence or what she preferred to call erectile dysfunction. Since anxiety was the key problem, she enjoined men to abandon an "over concern for partner" and "be selfish." Such therapists called on the woman either to avoid touching the man's genitals altogether or to provocatively fondle him in the back seats of cars, at films, concerts and plays, or under a blanket at the beach. A whiff of the 1960s was carried in the suggestion made in an English text that music—"Indian evening ragas, African drumming, reggae, madrigals"—could distract and so ease a man's anxieties.[35]

One came away from a reading of the works of such therapists with the sense that intercourse was now regarded as a highly organized event for which one had to train and carefully prepare. The popular sex manuals that followed in the 1970s set out problems and provided strategies, scripts, exercises, and illustrations. Calling for programmed spontaneity, they promised that the goal of the orgasm could be achieved if sexuality was approached in a conscious, calculated, technical fashion. Masters and Johnson did note the risk of making sex work, yet fell back on the use of economic and industrial metaphors, referring, for example, to a man who "simply cannot 'get the job done.'"[36] They instructed the man both to relax and to get on with his "job" of pleasuring his partner. Given that the sex therapists popularized the notion that women could have multiple orgasms, the task appeared all the more daunting.

The sex therapists did help educate the public. They highlighted the ability of individuals to learn how to please their partners. They popularized the notion that Freud had been mistaken in denying the importance clitoral stimulation. Such insights were diminished, however, by those who presented the body as being little more than an assemblage of buttons that had to be pushed to produce an orgasm. Thus Hirsch attacked the "anticlitorine propaganda" of the psychoanalysts and instructed the husband to vigorously attack the "torpid" or "frozen" clitoris no matter what the wife said. Reclaiming the clitoris, like the increased public acceptance of oral sex, should presumably have made penetrative sex less important. The therapists and writers of sex manuals continued to assume, however, that penetration was the ultimate goal. They did not disabuse men of their preoccupation with genital sex. On the one hand it was in the professional interests of sex therapists to exaggerate the rates of impotence and their significance. Indeed some writers asserted that male sexual dysfunctions were the cause of a range of social problems including alcoholism, divorce, drug use, suicide, and homosexuality.[37] On the other hand it was also in their interest to reassure the anxious that if the right lessons were followed, cures were assured.

Though the sex therapists' manuals daringly discussed a range of once tabooed sexual practices, a dreary faith in behaviorialism pervaded much of their work. They set out to condition men to respond appropriately to women. In the most extreme cases, some went so far as to advocate the use of punishments. "The technique employed to reduce the patient's aversion to the female genitals," reported Helen Kaplan, "was a modification of the 'stop-shock' technique described by Feldman and MacCulloch, which is reported to be highly and rapidly effective in reversing the sexual orientation of secondary homosexuals. Briefly, the technique consists of pairing pictures of the female genitals with relief from an electric shock." It would be hard to imagine a more striking example of compulsory heterosexuality. A similar sense of desperation was evident in therapists' injunctions that penetration, no matter how achieved, was good. An American doctor gave instructions on the ways in which to "shoehorn" a limp penis into a moist vagina. An English team of therapists explained how after oral sex and masturbation had provided the man with the rudiments of an erection, the woman could employ the "stuffing method" to get him inside her. Another expert described how she should use the two-handed method, "exactly like the action used in milking a cow."[38] Though such stratagems might have given the partners some sense of accomplishment, they seemed unlikely to provide much delight.

Did the sexual revolution, as so many claimed, result in a rise in impotence? There is no way of telling. As skeptics pointed out, if more men played baseball, more would inevitably report difficulties in hitting the ball. So too, with the more relaxed mores brought on by the 1960s more intercourse was taking place and more people were willing to confess to their disappointments or difficulties. There were thus more reports of impotence, though it was possible that the actual rate was declining. Sexual norms were certainly maintained despite the rhetoric about "revolution." If women became more sexually active than they had been in the past, men were still supposed to be dominant. The feminist researcher Shere Hite accepted that due to such pressures, over 10 percent of men regularly had potency problems, but she went on to point out that their concerns for their erection stemmed more from their competition with other men than in the desire to pleasure women. If the latter had been their chief concern they would have been far more prepared to engage in oral sex. Homosexual men—in contrast to straight men—had a less limited repertoire.[39] Yet the very visibility of the growing gay movement might also have increased the fears of impotence of those heterosexual men who took as a given women's penetrability and men's impenetrability. The homophobic implication was that a man who could not penetrate would be penetrated.

The 1960s also witnessed a resurgence in the old preoccupation that white males had with the threat of black sexuality. A number of black writers produce classic accounts of the function served by such panics. In *The Fire Next Time* (1962) James Baldwin argued that white men believed their masculinity depended on denying it to others, but that due to their insecurities they projected their own fears and longings on to blacks. The psychiatrist Frantz Fanon reported that in their racial fantasies some of his patients saw the black man as simply a penis. Such delusions helped explain why lynchings had been so frequently accompanied by castrations. Pointing out that particularly in America white men were "torn by repressed dreams of sexual virility" and "fantasies of masculine inadequacy," the psychologist

Calvin C. Hernton agreed that whites had constructed out of their own guilt an image of the black macho male. But if such writers had as one of their goals the dampening down of white sexual anxieties, Eldrige Cleaver took the opposite tack in *Soul on Ice* (1968). Playing on the worse fears of white males, he boasted that freedom for a black man was symbolized by having a white woman. Indeed white men were so enervated, claimed Cleaver, that they even paid to have their wives provided with "black rod."[40]

A relatively small proportion of the population read the books of either the sex therapists' or their critics. Turning to the works of social commentators, fiction writers, and moviemakers provide us with a fuller sense of how the public discussion of male sexual dysfunctions played itself out in popular culture. One response to the purported changes brought about by the sexual revolution was a spate of writings that presented men as victims. Books appeared with titles like *The Male Dilemma: How to Survive the Sexual Revolution*. Similarly headlined articles appeared in the new pornographic magazines such as *Penthouse* and *Mayfair,* which never tired of attacking feminists for emasculating men. In academia anthropologist Lionel Tiger in his classic *Men in Groups* (1969) claimed that if men could not get away from women they lost their maleness. They needed their pubs or huts or haunts. As proof that North American male academics in college towns had lost their "constructive maleness" because their work and family interests were intertwined, Tiger cited Kinsey's figures that showed them having the lowest rate of sexual intercourse of any occupational group. Choosing to title his book *Sexual Suicide* (1973), George Gilder made it even clearer as to what he thought of a world in which women were more sexually aggressive. To end biological differences would be suicide. If men were not in control they could not perform. "Fear of impotence," he stressed, "is a paramount fact of male sexuality." Feminists failed to see "that for men the desire for sex is not simply a quest for pleasure. It is an indispensable test of identity." If the culture did not reaffirm men then they had all the more need for sex. They needed to be aggressive to be secure. "The man who is expected to have a rigid penis at all times," protested the Australian feminist Germaine Greer, "is not any freer than the woman whose vagina is supposed to explode with the first thrust of such a penis." Gilder responded: "Aggressiveness on the part of the woman can jeopardize the whole process if it destroys the man's rhythm of control and enhances his insecurities. If the conditions are right, he may succeed anyway. But the likelihood of impotence is increased. The key contingent variable in sex is the male erection, and it emerges from an internal psychochemistry of trust and confidence that is usually undermined by female activity. Germaine Greer's attempt to suggest that greater female aggressiveness will overcome male impotence reveals the complete failure to understand males that is omnipresent in her book."[41]

Such issues were pursued by novelists who from 1960 on increasingly included in their cast of characters a man who was sexually intimidated. "The point of suspense in the modern novel is no longer focused on whether she will or she won't," a British marriage expert noted, "but on whether he can or he can't."[42] This was an exaggeration, but the impotence theme did receive unprecedented literary attention. And whereas male writers in the past had monopolized the discussion, now liberated female authors joined in. Disappointment in male sexual abilities were most famously and explicitly expressed by the narrator in Erica Jong's *Fear of Flying* (1973).

> I kept sucking away, but as soon as he got hard, he'd get soft again.... "I can fuck with the best of them when I feel like it," he said defiantly.
>
> "Of course, you can."
>
> I had been a feminist all my life . . . but the big problem was how to make your feminism jibe with your unappeasable hunger for male bodies. It wasn't easy. Besides, the older you got, the clearer it became that men were basically terrified of women. Some secretly, some openly. What could be more poignant than a liberated woman eye to eye with a limp prick? . . . No wonder men hated women. No wonder they invented the myth of female inadequacy.[43]

Male writers defended themselves as best they could. Kingsley Amis tried to laugh the issue away in a number of comic novels. In *Difficulties with Girls* (1981) a man complains to a friend that his wife's reading has led her to have unreasonable expectations:

> "It's these books and articles she's always reading that tell her about her right to things like physical fulfillment. I happened to take home a copy of Anthea Schmutzige's Trigger My Bomb which we published last spring and I don't think it's been out of Barbara's sight since. Of course it's all fantasy really but she takes it literally. It puts me in an impossible position. And I mean impossible."
>
> "Well, it would put . . . King Kong in a *delicate* position," faltered Patrick.
> "Women shouldn't be encouraged to take the initiative in my experience."
> "Absolutely asking for trouble."

Amis, who owned a copy of Patricia and Richard Gillan's *Sex Therapy Today* (1976), consulted sex therapists himself in the 1970s. His novel *Jake's Thing*

(1978) provides his take on the experience. The first joke in the novel sets its misogynistic tone. The narrator (an historian) is asked by his first therapist:

> "How much does your wife weigh?"
>
> "What? No, I beg your pardon, I heard what you said. How much . . . I don't quite know. But you're right. I mean she weighs a lot."

Jake is ordered into a "nongenital sensate-focusing session" with his wife and instructed to log his erections. Eventually he decides that he actually is potent, but just does not like women. Amis appeared to embrace this old self-exculpating line that men's impotence was due to women's failure to arouse them.[44]

Some of the world's most eminent authors chimed in, voicing the concern that women's demands were emasculating men. When in Alberto Moravia's *Two: A Phallic Comedy* (1971) a woman is astride the hero, he describes feeling as though he has lost his genitals, in much the same way as did sixteenth-century men who believed themselves cursed.

> I now had the impression. . . . it was Mafalda who was the male, if for no other reason than that it was she who moved, she who was, in her way, penetrating. I was indeed aware, at each of these powerful movements of her pelvis, of a violent pressure and, as it were an advance which alas, on "his" side, corresponded symmetrically to a yielding and equally noticeable retreat. To such a degree that I suddenly had the strange, disturbing sensation that I was no longer a man but a woman and that, in the place where once "he" had been, with all his cumbersome presence, there was now an emptiness, an absence, positively a cavity.[45]

Possibly the most explicit fiction that focused on male sexual dysfunction was Romain Gary's *Your Ticket Is No Longer Valid* (1977). The middle-aged Gary, who was married at the time to the young American actress Jean Seberg, presents his male characters wondering if women's vaginas are getting larger and then realizing that their penises are getting smaller. His men are so given to avoiding vaginal intercourse that one jokes that when asked to show the doctor his sex organ he sticks out his tongue. Men now depend on the kindness and pity of women. Believing that death would be preferable to humiliation, the narrator plans his own murder.[46] Gary no doubt intended to use his hero's impotence as a metaphor for the decline of the capitalist West, but most readers simply saw it as a lament for the loss of male power.

In Philip Roth's *Portnoy's Complaint* (1967), the best known of the sex novels of the 1960s, the mother-fixated hero flops on visiting his "homeland." "*I couldn't get it up in the state of Israel!*" And potency is so important for the main character in Roth's *The Counterlife* (1987) that he dies seeking to restore it. The drugs that thirty-nine-year-old Henry Zuckerman takes for his heart condition have rendered him impotent. "Impotence, Zuckerman had been thinking, has cut him off from the simplest form of distance from his predictable life . . . as long as he was potent there was some give in his life between what was routine and what is taboo. But without the potency he feels condemned to an ironclad life wherein all issues are settled."[47] He risks bypass surgery so he can continue his affair with his mistress. Ironically his wife believes that he had the deadly operation for her. Though it is unlikely that such novels reflected the actual thinking of many men, in conjuring up a "last stand" mentality in which death was seen as preferable to impotence they did capture the rhetoric of a time when some felt under siege.

Dramatists also found the impotence issue irresistible. In reviewing Edward Albee's *Who's Afraid of Virginia Woolf* (1962), Kenneth Tynan observed that the award-winning play dwelt on impotence, "a long established Broadway theme that has lately hardened (or softened) into an obsession. No serious play is complete without it." He backed up his argument by citing as other examples Tennessee Williams's *Cat on a Hot Tin Roof* (1955) and *Sweet Bird of Youth* (1959), Paddy Chayevsky's *Middle of the Night* (1956), and Lillian Hellman's *Toys in the Attic* (1960). The general public was exposed to such themes through films. Beginning in the 1950s, moviemakers recognized that there was an audience ready to regard impotent males as tragic casualties of their society. Impotence was blamed on the war. The theme of the disabled veteran had been exploited after 1918, but such fears were even keener following World War II. *The Men* (1950, dir. Fred Zinnemann) presented spinal cord injuries threatening not simply the veteran's mobility, but more importantly his manhood. "I'm not a man any longer," laments the character played by Marlon Brando. "I can't make a woman happy." His girlfriend's parents—wanting grandchildren—oppose their marriage. The hero's economic dependency on the government and his fiancée is presented as less a threat to his masculinity than his sexual incapacity.[48] Though Alfred Kinsey had just publicized the wide range of nonpenetrative sex acts in which Americans engaged, the film discreetly implies that the hero is doomed to a life of sexual frustration.

More commonly filmmakers depicted social pressures as incapacitating the anxious husbands and sickly breadwinners of a conformist society. Alfred Hitchcock exploited popular notions of Freudianism in presenting a series of frigid heroines and impotent males.[49] Imaginative film critics have regarded the hero of *Rear Window* (1954) as what in psychoanalytic terms would be described as a castrated/impotent voyeur. The never-married central character of *Vertigo* (1958) is similarly unable to master females. In *Frenzy* (1972) Hitchcock explicitly chronicles the career of a psychopathic murderer who can only overcome his impotence by strangling women.

Impotence was blamed on affluence. Numerous Hollywood movies re-hashed the old story of the upper class lacking the sexual vigor of the lower. Condemned as obscene by the Legion of Decency, *Baby Doll* (1956) was Elia Kazan's take on two of Tennessee William's one act plays. It has its virgin child bride, its blustering, drunken older husband who tells his doctor "I haven't been myself lately," and its seductive stranger bemused by the "un-occupied nursery," all characters reminiscent of early modern bawdy tales. In Douglas Sirk's *Written on the Wind* (1957), the rich Texas playboy has a "weakness" that makes his ever having children unlikely, leaving his wife and sister to lust after his manly, lower-class boyhood friend.

Predictably, impotence was blamed on women. Despite its title *The In-credible Shrinking Man* (1957, dir. Jack Arnold) made no direct references to the central character's sexual abilities (his fate was due to accidental expo-sure to radiation), but in depicting the once dominating man of the house reduced to the size of a mouse, the film exploited existing gender anxieties. Albee provided a thorough dissection of the battle of the sexes in the black comedy *Who's Afraid of Virginia Woolf?* (1966, dir. Mike Nichols). George, a professor of history, and his wife Martha are childless, and have a night of vicious game-playing with a new faculty couple. Martha, who pursues men, refers to one as a "flop," another of her "impotent lunkheads." She has already emasculated George. When Martha says some would give their right arm to marry the college president's daughter, he dryly replies: "Alas, Martha, in reality it works out that the sacrifice is usually of a somewhat more private portion of the anatomy." Misogynistic musings peaked in *Car-nal Knowledge* (1972, dir. Mike Nichols). The character played by Jack Nich-olson complains that as a result of the sexual revolution "the women today are better hung than the men." [50] This dedicated womanizer ultimately finds himself having difficulty in performing except with prostitutes and makes his hatred of women clear. "When you think of what he's got to dip into, any guy with a conscience has a right to turn soft. Am I right, Louise?"

A few films also picked up on the linking in popular culture of impo-tence and homosexuality. In Tennessee Williams's play *A Streetcar Named Desire* Blanche's husband commits suicide after she catches him with older man. In the 1951 film version Elia Kazan responded to the censor by having Blanche discover her husband is "weak," that is, impotent. [51] In Williams's *Cat on a Hot Tin Roof* (1958, dir. Richard Brooks), the suicide of Brick's close college friend is presented as having plunged him into alcoholism and marital impotence. It says something of changing sexual mores of the first few postwar decades that while films could not sympathetically portray homosexuality, they could broach the topic of male impotence.

A key reason why moviemakers were allowed to allude to impotence was that it could be a source of humor.[52] In *Some Like It Hot* (1959, dir. Billy Wilder)—still widely regarded as the funniest American film ever made—Joe (Tony Curtis) fakes impotence in order to seduce Sugar (Marilyn Monroe).

SUGAR: You should see a doctor—a good doctor.

JOE: I have. I spent six months in Vienna with Professor Freud, flat on my back. (He lies on the sofa.) Then, there were the Mayo Brothers, injections, hypnosis, mineral baths. If I wasn't such a coward, I'd kill myself.

SUGAR: Don't say that! (She rushes over to him.) There must be some girl some place that could . . .

JOE: If I ever found the girl that could, I'd marry her just like that.

SUGAR: Would you do me a favor?

JOE: Certainly, what is it?

SUGAR: I may not be Dr. Freud or a Mayo brother, or one of those French upstairs girls, but could I take another crack at it?

JOE: All right, if you insist.

SUGAR: Anything this time?

JOE: I'm afraid not. Terribly sorry.

In the midst of the sexual revolution Curtis reprised the role in *Sex and the Single Girl* (1964, dir. Richard Quine), playing a sleazy magazine reporter who is preparing a story about a woman sexologist who has written the book *Sex and the Single Girl*. He makes several trips to her office incognito, pretending to have a problem with impotence. In a remarkable number of books and movies men were shown to be playing roles—the naïve pretending to be sophisticated, the potent impotent—which implies that the radical notion that gender was something performed, that masculinity was a sort of masquerade, had begun to percolate through society.[53]

The most popular way in which filmmakers treated impotence was in including it in accounts of clumsy young men fumbling their way towards sexual maturity, a common trope that reflected the self-conscious candor of the 1960s. In the Czech Academy Award winner *Closely Watched Trains* (1966, dir. Jiri Menzel), Milos recalls a girl crawling into his bed at her uncle's in Prague: "And I caressed her, too, and I was man enough until it came to the point of being a man, but then all at once I wilted, and it was all up with everything, Masha tried pinching me, but I'd gone quite dead, as though I was paralyzed in all my extremities." His embarrassment is all the greater because the uncle, a photographer, has an advertisement promising "FINISHED IN FIVE MINUTES" and Milos has to confess, "I was finished even before I began." It almost became de rigueur in coming-of-age films to present the naïve male and his understanding partner. In *Never on Sunday* (1960, dir. Jules Dassin), the incompetent young man is taken under the wing of the caring prostitute, while in *Bonnie and Clyde* (1967, dir. Arthur Penn), Bonnie fails at first to rouse Clyde who protests, "Ain't nuthin' wrong with me . . . I don't like boys."[54] In *Midnight Cowboy* (1969, dir. John Schlesinger) the young would-be stud flops the first time ("Ain't never happened to me before"), while in *The Last Picture Show* (1971, dir. Peter Bogdanovitch) 1950s Texas youths are sexually humiliated ("I don't know what happened"). Movie directors were reluctant to deal with the more complicated and sensitive issue of marital impotence. Even *The Family Way* (1966, dir. Roy Boulting), a British comedy portraying a young husband whose inability to consummate his marriage is caused by having to live with the in-laws, was regarded as scandalous by some when released in the United States in 1967.

Strikingly enough, when filmmakers portrayed the lives of disabled Vietnam veterans they provided the most audacious accounts of men dealing with sexual dysfunctions. The best known was *Born on the Fourth of July* (1989, dir. Oliver Stone) based on Tom Kovic's 1975 book of the same name. It begins with the narrator's wounding entailing his loss of dignity and sexuality. "It is over with. Gone. And it is gone for America. I have given it for democracy. It is okay now. It is all right. Yes it is all right. I have given my dead swinging dick for America. I have given my numb young dick for democracy. It is gone and numb. Lost somewhere out there by the river where the artillery is screaming in. Oh God, oh God I want it back!"[55] By exploiting Mexican prostitutes the narrator does reestablish a sex life of sorts and in engaging in antiwar protests ultimately restores his sense of self-worth. An earlier film, *Coming Home* (1978, dir. Hal Ashby), infused with both feminist and antiwar sentiments, presented a paraplegic having recourse to oral sex in his affair with a married woman. Unlike her virile husband, the "impotent" lover brings her to orgasm. In *The Big Chill* (1983, dir. Lawrence Kasdan), a group of 1960s college activists reunite for a weekend. Nick counters a woman's come-on with the question, "Did I ever tell you what happened to me in Vietnam?" and informs a friend that "the equipment doesn't work at all." The young woman who decides to live with him says it is not important. Such films, in enlarging the definition of manliness, gave some credence to the idea that the 1960s did see some relaxing of sexual attitudes.

The films, plays, and novels that broached the issue of impotence rarely pursued it at length and generally preferred to give it a comic rather than a serious treatment. Though some indirectly referenced the works of the sex surveyors and therapists, they shied away from discussing recourse to medical or psychological treatments. Most treated male sexual dysfunctions as just an embarrassing passing phase. Nevertheless right through the 1960s and 1970s novelists and filmmakers familiarized the public with the notion of impotence being one of the life's hurdles that at some time all men might face. Usually the story ended with potency restored, but the very fact that it was questioned undermined to some degree the notion of a monolithic masculinity. Although those who tracked changes in heterosexual norms from 1960s on quite rightly focused most of their attention on important shifts in women's beliefs and behaviors, they had to acknowledge that as female sexual scripts changed, so too did male.

Yet the specter of impotence still loomed large. A researcher who went through *Psychological Abstracts* for the years 1940 to 1983 was surprised to discover that although the number of articles on frigidity had dropped to zero by 1979, those on impotence had rocketed up, with over thirty articles on the subject appearing in the year 1979 alone. "Frigidity" was considered too loaded a term and had been replaced with "female orgasmic dysfunction," but therapists, while admitting that the term "impotence" was difficult to define and obviously carried all kinds of negative cultural baggage, still felt free to use it. The sexual revolution and the rise of the sex therapy profession had had the unintended consequence of inflating rather than diminishing the cultural fixation on the erection. The more investigations experts made of sexuality, the greater was their ability to fuel the concerns of pathology, though the notions of "normal" that were inculcated were cultural rather than medical constructs. Sex manuals enjoined the impressionable to indulge in self-diagnosis and to demand services not just to cure their problems but to improve and enhance their sex lives. This reflected the fact that in the modern world sexual competency was based on meeting "cultural standards" and sex accordingly was not simply a biological need but, as an British observer noted, a way "in which we meet our needs for social acceptance and approval."[56] As the spate of articles on the "new impotence" revealed, in the 1960s and 1970s the culture led many men to believe they might fail the test.

Though some observers lamented that sex increasingly seemed to have a "compulsive quality" that threatened to rob it of meaning, the enterprising recognized the possibility of exploiting the potentially huge market that the sex therapists had only begun to tap. If scientists could produce a simple pill that would cure impotence and thereby dispense with the psychoanalysts' years of investigations and the sex therapists' intrusive conditionings, a fortune could be made.

VIAGRA
Hard Science or Hard Sell?

On March 27, 1998, Viagra became the first oral medication to be approved by the United States Food and Drug Administration to treat erectile dysfunction. A flood of books and articles, which shows no sign of abating, has subsequently been devoted to analyzing the pill's impact. Among the more insightful is Meika Loe's *The Rise of Viagra: How the Little Blue Pill Changed Sex in America* (2004). Her title encapsulates the popular argument. But what does it mean to say sex is changed? Is Viagra a wonder drug? A magic bullet? The rejuvenating potion doctors sought for centuries? Supporters of the medicalization of sexuality certainly claim as much. Many have suggested that just as the contraceptive pill in the 1960s made possible a new age of relaxed sexual mores, Viagra is having an equally revolutionary impact in the first decade of the twenty-first century. Dr. Irwin Goldstein, a leading researcher in male sexuality, asserts that Viagra has begun a "second sexual revolution." The diamond shaped pill, agrees sex therapist Bernie Zilbergeld, has changed the way we think about sex, yet contradictorily he concedes that it has not changed men. That the fans of Viagra should tout its powers is to be expected. More surprising is the enormous impact attributed to the pill by its critics. Though feminist sociologist Meika Loe provides a trenchant analysis of Pfizer's marketing ploys, she also argues that the Viagra phenomenon "has changed our understanding of sex in America and, increasingly, is changing it around the world as well. . . . Normal sex now means sex on demand, sex for everyone, and sex for life." [1]

The historian has to be skeptical of such extravagant claims. As we have seen, each age has reconfigured the notion of male sexual failure. Foucault reminds us that sexuality is always controlled, what changes is the nature of the control. An analysis of Viagra's success is the central subject of this concluding chapter of our study, but the arrival of the little blue pill certainly did not end male sexual anxieties. Indeed there is a good deal of evidence that it actually heightened them. Specific social and cultural conditions were responsible for the appearance and profitability of a new generation of sexual pharmaceuticals in the 1990s. These conditions have to be understood. Some critics of Viagra have been so preoccupied by the ways in which it has purportedly overturned our views of aging or gender that they have slighted the more important point that Viagra was itself a product of the interactions of science, medicine, the media, and popular culture. We know a lot about the "supply" and little of the "demand" side of the story. The appearance of Viagra and the other erectile drugs of the late 1990s was clearly the culmination of developments that began decades earlier. To appreciate the Viagra phenomenon we need to trace the emergence of the new pharmacological agents that arose in the 1990s but then situate them in the context of changing cultural attitudes toward masculinity, medicine, and the enhancement technologies.

"For the first time in American history," writes Meika Loe, "biotechnology is being used to 'fix' or enhance heterosexual male confidence and power, and thus avert 'masculinity in crisis.'" Yet, as we have seen, for centuries men had turned to doctors for pills and potions to restore their potency. Indeed in the 1980s medical professionals were still recommending vacuum devices and herbs like yohimbine that had been around since the Victorians. There were also new remedies on offer including implants, injections, and bypass surgery of the penile arteries. The operation to reconnect the arteries (pursued by researchers such as Irwin Goldstein) was complex and risky. Success rates were low and the chief interest of such surgical intervention was that it first raised the question of whether American insurers would recognize and cover attempts to restore potency as a legitimate medical expense.[2]

An even more dramatic form of intervention was undertaken when surgeons from the 1970s on implanted silicon rods in the penis of impotent men. In the 1980s American Medical Systems offered three models, the Malleable 600 Penile Prosthesis consisting of two silicon rubber rods that could either be bent for comfort or straightened for penetration, the Dynaflex Penile Prosthesis with two fluid filled cylinders that when squeezed inflated the penis; and the 700 Ultrex Inflatable Penile Prosthesis complete with reservoir and pump hidden in the scrotum. These devices produced a formidably rigid member reminiscent of the body parts of the robot played by Arnold Schwarzenegger in the popular film *The Terminator* (1984). Advertisements had wives reporting they found their spouses bearing such contraptions "were more relaxed and confident." Such devices, claimed one doctor, "allow sex to be completely spontaneous." Likening arousal to turning on a switch or pumping up a flat tire, such enthusiasts apparently equated "mechanical" with "spontaneous." Late night TV comedians made the purchasers of such devices the butt of countless jokes. Serious critics such as Thomas Szasz, the libertarian psychiatrist, declared that the so-called satisfied patients were only deceiving themselves and their partners. He cruelly referred to such implanting (which could cost from $3,500 to $9,000 per operation) as "dildoization." Szasz, who had a good grasp on the history of medicine, also pertinently noted that doctors were again following a fad. They once had castrated those who were not supposed to perform sexually; now they implanted sexual prostheses to allow the impotent to perform. Such inflatable penile implants were not initially examined by the Food and Drug Administration and were plagued by failures and infections. Nevertheless it was estimated that within a decade 250,000 to 300,000 had been inserted.[3]

In the same decade surgeons were implanting prostheses, medical scientists stumbled across a number of vasodilating substances that caused an immediate erection when injected into the penis. The first report appeared in a 1982 article in the *Lancet* written by the Parisian researcher Ronald Virag. He had accidentally injected the muscle relaxant papaverine into a patient's penis and an erection resulted. Noting that the mechanism of erection was still not fully understood, Virag then moved on to trials, which showed good results. He speculated that the muscle relaxant had some sort of inhibiting effect. His British colleague Giles Brindley who experimented on himself with a similar muscle relaxant, created a furor at the 1983 meeting of the American Urology Association in Las Vegas when he presented his own chemically induced erection for public inspection.[4] It is impossible to read of Brindley's exhibition and not be reminded of Brown-Séquard's performance a century earlier. Virag and Brindley demonstrated to urologists how an erection could be instantly created; at the very least, the method allowed doctors to observe penal vascular flow so as to better understand the process of erection. It had long been known that blood flowing into the spongy corpora cavernosa of the penis created an erection. What kept the blood trapped there? Some had earlier thought that some microscopic valve played a role, but now it was observed that the muscle relaxant in allowing the corpora to absorb blood, increased it in size and so squeezed shut the veins that would otherwise have taken the blood away.

Injections served a useful diagnostic function; they had obvious drawbacks as a form of therapy. They were initially very expensive with shots of papaverine costing $1,200 to $2,400 a year. Some considered it a plus that injections instantly created an involuntary erection whatever one's state of mind. Doctors referred to a rapid reaction as a sign of one's being "spontaneous."[5] Critics—even those who were not particularly romantic—protested that the splitting of physical arousal from emotional desire was unseemly. Moreover injections could work too well, creating a painful erection that could last for hours and might require emergency medical intervention. Their most obvious drawback was that they entailed what for most men was a nightmare scenario, the plunging of a needle into their penis.

Despite these obvious problems, Virag and Brindley's work sparked a rush by the pharmaceutical companies. Envisaging the enormous financial potential of drugs like prostaglandin E-1 and papaverine, companies recruited teams of doctors and scientists as paid consultants. In 1995 the Upjohn Company received FDA approval for the first injected prescription drug for impotence; alprostadil was sold under the brand name Caverject and cost $20 to $25 a shot. The same year Vivus brought out the MUSE delivery system, which consisted of a tiny plunger that placed a chemical pellet into the urethral opening. The injected drugs almost immediately replaced penile implants, but good information was not available on the successes and failures of either. We do know that only a minority of the men who tried vasodilating substances had the courage to carry on with them. Nevertheless *Business Week* reported in 1995 that American men were spending $600 to $700 million annually on attempts to assure their virility.[6] In short, the medicalization and commercialization of male sexuality had occurred before Viagra appeared on the scene.

These developments represented a major cultural shift. In the post–World War II era, medical doctors had admitted they could do little for men suffering from impotence, and most were therefore willing to accept the common belief that the vast majority of cases could be attributed to psychological disturbances. Impotence was duly listed in the American Psychiatric Association's *Diagnostic and Statistical Manual of Mental Disorders* (1952) as psychologically based. Master and Johnson began their work with that premise. Psychoanalysts and sex therapists accordingly dominated the discussion of sexual problems through the 1970s. Sex counseling was moreover associated with the "sexual revolution" of the 1960s and the campaign for women's "sexual rights." As noted in the previous chapter, Masters and Johnson were best known for their stress on the importance of clitoral stimulation and the discovery of the multiorgasmic woman. Sex therapists did deal with impotence, but many regarded their message, which stressed improving technique and communication, as female-oriented in both its methods and goals.

The 1980s saw the emergence of a new paradigm, a swing toward the medicalization of male sexuality. One example of doctors' growing interest in impotence was the increased attention paid the subject in urology textbooks. The third edition of *Campbell's Urology* (1970) had only one page on impotence but four on masturbation; by the fifth edition (1986), the discussion of masturbation had been dropped and there were now thirty pages on impotence; the sixth edition (1992) devoted fifty pages to impotence; and the seventh (1998) had one hundred and eighteen pages on what were now listed as Erectile Dysfunctions. Another example of the medicalization of male sexuality was the establishment in 1982 of the International Society for Impotence Research, dominated by urologists. They sought to convince the public of the physiological causes of impotence, particularly the role of vascular obstructions. Advancing what critics regarded as a reductionist medical model, urologists began with the premise of penetrative and orgasmic imperatives and blamed breakdowns in normal sexual cycles on abnormal blood flows. As some cynics pointed out, with highly sensitive diagnostic tests there were few problems that doctors could not trace back to an organic defect.[7]

The message that impotence was a mechanical and therefore fixable problem was obviously what many men wanted to hear. In 1982 Bruce Mac-Kenzie, taking a urological tack, wrote *It's Not All in Your Head* and created Impotents Anonymous. Boasting of having invented a vacuum pump to deal with his own erectile problems, Gedding Osbon, a tire salesman from Georgia offered his help to fellow sufferers. Grassroots organizations such as the Impotence Institute of America, the Impotence Information Center, and the Osbon Foundation called on doctors for help.[8]

The press popularized the view that doctors were in the process of triumphing over an age-old problem. A 1988 *Time* article repeating the refrain "It's Not 'All in Your Head'" asserted that up to ten million men in the United States suffered from chronic impotence. Most problems were once thought to be psychologically based yet it was now known that 75 percent had physical causes. Doctors had for years linked sexual dysfunctions to such diseases as diabetes and warned of the dangers of excessive drinking, smoking, and bicycle riding. Now they associated impotence with vascular problems, the rise in the number of prostate operations, and the increased use of certain prescription drugs. Interestingly enough women's magazines took the lead in informing the public that doctors recognized that what was regarded as a psychological problem, could have physical causes and was treatable.[9] The popular press followed this trend in educating the public on the availability of drug-injection therapies, vascular-reconstruction surgery, and implants.

The argument that urologists were better qualified than anyone else to treat impotence did not go uncontested. Thomas Szasz attacked the notion that "impotence" and "premature ejaculation" should be viewed as medical diseases. He insisted that it made more sense to regard them as "the solutions of certain life tasks" that an individual had adopted. If he wished, he could learn new ones. A defender of sex therapy and a shrewd critic of the medicalization of sexuality, Leonore Tiefer agreed that sex was like dancing; to improve one had to practice. One did not ask a doctor for help. Her point was that sex therapy aimed at changing unhappy relationships; urology did not. Like other critics she complained that the medical model was strictly functional. It focused simply on the body and in effect reified the erection. John Bancroft of the Kinsey Institute tried to strike a balance in pointing to cases of impotence where the psychological and physiological issues were intertwined, an example being that of the diabetic who thought his illness would impede his performance and as a result it did. In dealing with sexual dysfunctions doctors had to be aware that both the patient's mind and body needed to be treated.[10]

Urologists, however, overcame such carping; by the end of the 1980s the media largely parroted their line that in 90 percent of cases the causes of impotence were physiological rather than psychological in nature. In shifting the focus from the psychological to the organic, urologists elbowed aside sex therapists. Why did doctors enjoy such success? Though all the treatments urology offered for male sexual dysfunctions had obvious shortcomings, the specialty, like almost every other, enjoyed increased status due to the enormous strides made by medicine in the late twentieth century. The public believed in medical intervention. Less apparent were the economic forces that helped push the medical agenda. Urologists turned to male sexual dysfunctions in search of more patients. It obviously served their purposes to medicalize the issue of impotence and exaggerate its extent. Urologists in turn were spurred on by pharmaceutical corporations that had a financial interest in advancing such views.[11] Health management organizations (HMOs) reimbursed patients for their medical costs, though they refused to do the same for the clients of sex therapists. With the medical profession, the pharmaceutical corporations, and the HMOs in favor, it is no wonder that a medical approach to male sexual dysfunctions won out.

It was still the case, however, that the vast majority of men did not turn to the medical profession to discuss their sexual problems. Doctors in the early 1990s complained that male patients were notoriously uncooperative. A 1985 survey revealed that in only 0.2 percent of visits to the doctor did men discuss their sexual concerns. Effective vasodilating substances were available but only a minority who tried injections carried on. The urologists' main lament was that older men simply accepted their impotence.[12] Doctors had long assumed that it was their duty to seek to stop patients from indulging in life-threatening behaviors like smoking or drinking. In the last decade of the twentieth century some began to regard it as their right to criticize patients for failing to improve their sex lives. With the arrival of Viagra doctors had a pill whose benefits only the most benighted could refuse.

Just as Marie Stopes claimed that her own unhappy experiences forced her into writing about sexuality, so the Pfizer Corporation asserted that, though not looking for a sex drug, it was compelled by events to discover one. The official story at least was that Pfizer scientists had hopes that a drug called sildenafil citrate would, by increasing blood flow to the heart, act as remedy for angina. Work on sildenafil began in the late 1980s and testing on human subjects started in 1990. The drug failed to do what it was supposed to do, but in 1991 an unexpected side effect was noted. Test subjects reported they had erections and the story was told of patients refusing to give their pills back or even trying to steal more. In other words, happy male patients pushed Pfizer into carrying out further research on sildenafil as a possible remedy for impotence. The story may well be true. At the same time the retelling of the tale was obviously a shrewd way of a corporation initially justifying work in what many still regard as a potentially down market product. In that same light Pfizer astutely recognized the need to replace the word "impotence" with the term "erectile dysfunction." By so doing it told its potential clients that they suffered simply from a vascular problem, not from any character flaw. The new nomenclature also spoke to the corporation's concern to appear soberly scientific and quite distinct from shady sellers of love potions and aphrodisiacs.[13]

Tests on sildenafil citrate revealed its link to nitric oxide. Nitroglycerin had been taken for heart problems for over a century but only in the 1980s was it discovered that it worked by releasing nitric oxide gas. In 1986 scientists reported the role of nitric oxide as a messenger in relaxing smooth muscles, in telling blood vessels to dilate and so lower blood pressure. Scientists also found that in the penis nitric oxide transmitted sexual arousal messages coming from the brain.[14] It sparked the production of cyclic guanosine monophosphate (cyclic GMP) that relaxed the smooth muscle so allowing the engorgement of the corpora cavernosa of the penis with blood. But if the blood was not prevented from flowing out a full erection would not be achieved. Sildenafil worked by suppressing the enzyme phosphodiesterase type 5 (PDE5). PDE5's normal role was to break down cyclic GMP, which initially started the muscular and vascular processes that created an erection. Sildenafil citrate did not create an erection; it sustained it by inhibiting the process that would otherwise allow an outflow of blood and resulting flaccidity. The drug accordingly might assist the man whose $PDE5$ overwhelmed his cyclic GMP; if they were in balance, as in most healthy men, the drug would serve no purpose. Pfizer quickly saw the potential of its product and marshaled a large research staff and millions of dollars in funds to bring it to market. In the small number of trials it carried out the drug reportedly helped 50 to 80 percent of subjects. Strikingly enough, almost one quarter of the men on placebos also got erections.

Pfizer had a product and the next step was to sell it. The drug was to be sold under the brand name Viagra. Even before the pill was produced the Pfizer advertising department had thought that "Viagra," in conjuring up "vigor" and "Niagara," would work well as a marketing tool. It was not named, as some thought, in honor of the researcher Ronald Virag. The little blue pill enjoyed extraordinary success. Viagra produced more or less the same results as had the injections but by a method men found acceptable. (In this regard the drug could be compared to the contraceptive pill, which was hardly more effective than the diaphragm but far more likely to be employed.) Some suspected that it was largely to protect itself from law suits that Pfizer stressed that sildenafil citrate was only a "natural" enhancer, and not an aphrodisiac. John Bancroft believed that Pfizer would not admit that Viagra had libido stirring qualities for fear that a rapist might subsequently claim the drug had caused his crime and so render the company liable. The corporation's law department was certainly aware of the dangers of being drawn into law suits in which abuse of or addiction to Pfizer's product was claimed. A "Viagra defense," based on the physiological and psychological effects of Viagra, was first advanced in 1999 by an Israeli man asserting the drug led him to commit a rape. In the United States a women accused of murder argued she acted in self defense against a man aroused by Viagra.[15] Both defenses failed.

Viagra immediately became the fastest selling pharmaceutical in history. Pfizer's stock went up 150 percent in 1998. Its sale of Viagra topped one billion dollars in 1999 and it enjoyed a profit margin of 90 percent. Was Pfizer's success due, as it claimed, to its reaching a large, preexisting "untapped market" or to its creation of a new market? Obviously it was a bit of both. One can only speculate about how many men were impatiently awaiting the arrival of such a drug. What we do know is that Pfizer launched a sophisticated campaign to convince millions that they needed its product. The publicity began years before Viagra was even released. Magazine stories prepared the public for the arrival of a wonder drug. In 1996 *Time* reported

Pfizer was working on sildenafil and *Newsweek* in the following year projected huge sales for erection drugs.[16] "The Potency Pill" was the cover story for *Time* for May 4, 1998. In that year an avalanche of articles were devoted to the topic. Viagra had arrived, making a private experience a public—and ultimately health-insured—concern.

Afraid of being associated with the sellers of sleazy love potions and sex toys, Pfizer initially was careful to strike an earnest tone. By continually stressing that it was dealing with a serious "medical condition," it sought to make its undertaking respectable. Yet the Viagra message was complicated. Though it was a product of years of highly technical research and required a man to carefully plan to take an expensive pill at least an hour before intercourse, Pfizer asserted that he would now be able to act "naturally." The drug would not inflame his passions, but simply allow him to "respond" to stimulus. On the one hand the drug manufacturers assured their customer that he should feel no shame inasmuch as he was only dealing with what was portrayed as a simple plumbing problem, yet on the other hand it was implied that a pill could magically transform his life, identity, and relationships.

Who needed the pill? Previous surveys suggested that when strictly defined as the inability to get an erection perhaps ten percent of men suffered at times from impotence. But in 1993 Dr. Irwin Goldstein, a central player in the 1993 Massachusetts Male Aging Study, equated self-reported unsatisfactory sexual experiences to erectile dysfunctions, and suggested that half of men over forty had experienced impotence of some sort. By conflating all categories that hindered "satisfactory sexual performance," the notion that perhaps ten million American men had potency problems was overnight inflated to a figure of thirty million. A frequently cited article in the *Journal of the American Medical Association* in 1999 asserted that 43 percent of women and 31 percent of men had a "sexual dysfunction," which accordingly posed "an important public health concern." A subsequent issue noted that the journal had "inadvertently" failed to disclose that the research of two of three authors had been financially supported by Pfizer. All the public remembered was that a third of American men had potency problems.[17]

Or did they? When does a difficulty become a dysfunction? Skeptics observed that it was perfectly normal to be sexually dysfunctional if tired, stressed, or poor. Such issues did not figure in the calculations of the pharmaceutical companies, indeed it was in their interest to assume that every case of impotence was physiologically based. With drug companies playing such a central role in research, it followed that often loose definitions of sexual dysfunctions were advantageous for marketing. Ambiguities in subjective reports were exploited in tabulating cases of what were vaguely

referred to as "mild erectile dysfunctions." Inflated numbers of men suffering from impotence—due partly to ongoing differences in definitions—
were to remain commonplace in the medical literature. Alarmist reports led
to the notion of America being swept by an "epidemic" of impotence that
had to be combated.[18] By such disease-mongering the pharmaceutical corporations presented a common problem as a worrying illness.

For whom was Viagra meant? With most medical complaints a doctor
would examine a patient, determine the cause of his distress, and prescribe
the appropriate remedy. In the pharmaceutical age the cause of impotence
held little interest for most doctors; they were more impressed by the fact
that a pill could make it go away. This was a case in which, as the authors
of a sociological study note, "the functional effect of the drug, not the disorder, defines the bodily condition." The only way the doctor could tell if a
patient "needed" Viagra was if he later reported that it had improved or enhanced his sexual performance. Doctors in effect conceded that they were
usually treating a "condition" rather than a disease. Sex researchers worried
that the popular view was now that a pill could solve any problem. Conservative congressmen, who had always been hostile to sex research, exploited
the new surge in biological reductionism by calling for cuts in the funding
of sex studies.[19]

Pfizer first targeted a respectable base of the middle-aged and elderly
married. As a sign of its caution it made a point of seeking the tacit support of a variety of churches and even contacted the Vatican. It chose as the
first public face of Viagra seventy-five year old Bob Dole, Republican presi-
dential candidate, Vietnam veteran, and prostate cancer survivor. Its focus
on the segment of the demographic that obviously did experience declining potency did not last long. With sales reaching a plateau by 2000, Pfizer
shifted the focus of its advertisements from older men to baby boomers. In
broadening the categories of suitable candidates to target a larger customer
base, the corporation's advertisements increasingly portrayed younger,
macho men. "We're talking about guys in their late 30s to 40s at the peak
of their professional careers," observed an admiring marketing strategist.
"They're burning themselves out with long hours at work. Their sexual lives
are suffering. Now to have a quick answer in a pill. It's no surprise Pfizer
is going after them."[20] In the television coverage of the 2002 World Series,
Viagra ads figured prominently. A well-known ball player declaring, "I hit,
I catch, I take Viagra" challenged viewers to "Step up to the plate." And by
2005 Pfizer was also edging away from the stress on respectability, running
ads depicting a trim, forty-something man with a devil's horns leering at
lingerie displays.

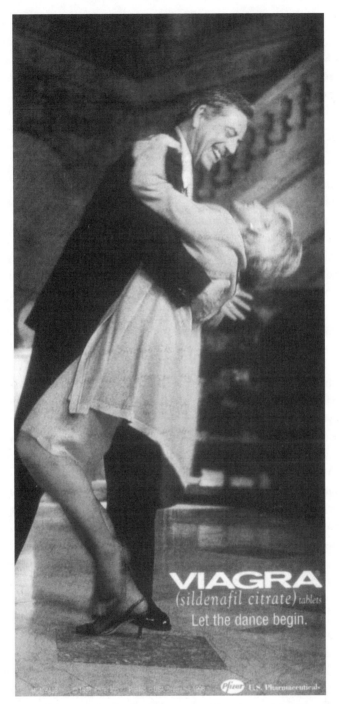

8. "Viagra: Let the dance begin." An example of one of the first advertisements for Viagra distributed in 1998, by permission of Pfizer Inc.

Though the placing of advertisements at baseball games and NASCAR events and offering free "six packs" of pills made it clear that Pfizer was pursuing a younger customer, it always denied it. Yet almost as soon as Viagra had arrived, young men were taking it. The changing public portrayal of young men's sexual concerns was captured in film. In the original version of *Alfie* (1966, dir. Lewis Gilbert), which enjoyed iconic status for its representation of the 1960s womanizer, the Michael Caine character's main worry is that his girlfriends will get pregnant. In the remake of *Alfie* (2004, dir. Charles Shyer) made almost forty years later, contraceptives are readily available and the hero (played by Jude Law) is only panicked by a bout of impotence. If the ravages of age could be defeated by pills, why not use them after a twenty-four hour rave? Films such as *Trainspotting* (1996, dir. Danny Boyle), *Permanent Midnight* (1998, dir. David Veloz), and *Human Traffic* (1999, dir. Justin Kerrigan) portrayed narcotics sexually incapacitating young men. Accordingly, the *Village Voice* reported in 1999 that Viagra now rivaled ecstasy in the singles scene. Partiers used it as "date insurance," bodybuilders to ward off the effects of steroids, and ravers to add to their drug cocktails. In 2003 Pfizer stated that only 10 percent of prescriptions for Viagra were written for men under thirty-nine, but clearly a much larger percentage obtained it by other means. Eighty percent of prescriptions for the drug were written by general practitioners who asked few questions. Some doctors offered telephone examinations; others made it available on the internet. Many young men exploited such networks to try a variety of erectile enhancers, doing their own "Pepsi Challenge." The effects of such drugs on young, party types were not known, since that population was never tested. [21]

Why was the marketing of Viagra so successful? Obviously, the drug company representatives would reply, because the pill worked. The hundred deaths linked to its use in its first year on the market they attributed to the victims' preexisting medical conditions. Pfizer did admit that healthy men might experience some minor side effects including flushed face, headaches, and blueish vision, but insisted that their product was highly efficacious. In the two double-blind studies Pfizer funded, Viagra was reported as having a 69 percent success rate as against a 22 percent score for the placebo. Though some suspected that the figures might have been inflated, pharmaceuticals appeared to have accomplished what surgery, psychoanalysis, and sex therapy had failed to deliver. Indeed Viagra was said to be effective even in unlikely cases. Psychiatrists noted that depression commonly caused impotence and the impotence in turn deepened one's depression. Viagra could break this vicious circle. [22] The drug also enticed more men into visiting their doctors' offices where they showed an increased willingness to discuss sexual matters. This was of some value given the difficulty of getting men to have prostate exams. For good or ill, Viagra's arrival had made the once taboo topic of impotence a subject of water cooler and dinner table conversation.

Those critical of pharmacological cures for impotence at times gave the impression that drugs like Viagra served no positive purpose. They noted that a sexual dysfunction could be a symptom of a serious complaint and if pills were automatically prescribed, there was the danger that problems such as those caused by illness, stress, and obesity could be missed. Their more important point was that to claim a pill to cure impotence "worked" was a far from simple assertion. Determining effectiveness was difficult. Many of the reports on the efficacy of the pill were suspect, coming as they did from researchers whose financial support was provided by the pharmaceutical corporations. In the modern scientific world in which corporations carried out their own research or funded much of that done in private or university laboratories, it was increasingly difficult to find a disinterested expert. Even taking at face value the studies that were carried out, it was often hard to determine what definition of dysfunction had been employed. Moreover the success or failure of a sex drug was usually based on self reporting and accordingly judged subjectively. The most obvious indicator of the unreliability of such accounts was that wives consistently reported lower success rates than their husbands. The high level of success achieved by men who simply took a placebo was an another indication of the powerful role the psyche played in sexual matters. On the other hand men who had high hopes that Viagra would work for them and found that it did not felt the drug actually exacerbated their distress.[23]

Investigators who interviewed couples found that of those who reported that Viagra "worked," there were some who felt that it had not so much restored a man's ability to function as it had created a new situation. Some men became addicted to it as a sort of sexual crutch and it led others into extramarital relationships as a way of testing their virility. Women often were not all that happy, feeling that their spouses' use of Viagra pressured them toward intercourse and away from cuddling and intimacy. Couples did not fully accept the medical model that made sex seem clinical and planned. They reported they preferred the "real thing." But perhaps the best indicator of the limited effectiveness of Viagra is that only half of the men who tried it renewed their prescriptions.[24]

Nevertheless Pfizer soon had competitors. The year 2003 saw the arrival of Cialis, made by Eli Lilly and Company and Icos, and Levitra, manufactured by Bayer AG and GlaxoSmithKline. Cialis boasted of being effective over a thirty-six hour time period and thus allowing "spontaneity." Its side effects could include dangerous four-hour long erections. In 2002 Pfizer spent $300 million in advertising, and sales of Viagra increased 13 percent to $1.7 billion. Only an 8 percent growth in the market occurred in 2004, though the big three pharmaceutical corporations devoted $373 million to direct to consumer advertising and a similar amount on marketing to professionals. In 2005 the number of new prescriptions actually fell.[25]

The pharmaceutical companies were already looking for new markets to exploit. Given that more men complained of premature ejaculation than impotence, a pill for that problem appeared to have enormous potential. In fact some doctors claimed that Viagra indirectly helped since it enabled some men to have a second erection. Johnson and Johnson is reported to have a drug called dapoxetine that works like a sedative and is tailored to postpone ejaculation. But what is "premature ejaculation"? One survey reports men who regard themselves as "normal" take seven minutes to climax, the precipitous, two. A *Wall Street Journal* article suggests that the drug companies are raising the bar of "normal" to swell the number of potential purchasers up to 15 to 30 percent of all males.[26] The company says the pill will only be meant for those with serious problems; critics foresee that inevitably the "normal" and would-be sexual athletes will seek it out. In other words many of the issues raised by Viagra—declaring a common condition a "medical problem" and "curing" it with a pharmaceutical—are posed once more.

Moving on from its success with Viagra, Pfizer has interested itself in the creation of a new category of illness, "female sexual dysfunction." A dozen other companies are also involved in popularizing the notion that such a medical condition exists. Armed with survey data reporting that a third of women lack desire and a quarter have difficulty achieving orgasm, the pharmaceutical industry is supporting the research of teams of urologists who presume that such unhappiness is due to problems with blood flow. Already testosterone-based pills, blood vessel dilators, and brain stimulators are being sold to women panicked by the worry that they are not normal. The companies' goal is to produce for women a pill whose profits will dwarf those of Viagra.[27] The fact that the most insightful discussions of Viagra today have been produced by feminist scholars is due not just to their concern for gender but to their realization that women are the pharmaceutical companies' next target. Relying in large part on the insights of these writers, this chapter now turns to an analysis of the shifting sexual and social terrain that was the site of Viagra's success.

In attempting to locate the discussion of impotence in its cultural context one has to resist the temptation to divide time neatly up into either liberal or conservative epochs. In the minds of many the 1960s and 1970s were progressive decades that saw the birth of the "sexual revolution," whereas the 1980s witnessed a backlash. They point to the rise of the Christian Right and its attacks on day care, affirmative action, and sex education, the recruitment of feminists into the antipornography crusade, the emergence of the men's movement, and the growing viciousness of antiabortion zealots that culminated in bombing women's clinics and killing doctors. Yet the general public's views were in the same years becoming more liberal. For example, levels of support for abortion and a tolerance of homosexuality generally rose. A more sexually pluralistic age was emerging in which the classic man and woman in the street found themselves discussing, if not approving, everything from test tube babies, transsexuals, "safe sex," pornography and "lip stick lesbians."[28]

A good argument can be made, however, that if it had not been for the political swing to the right, the success of drugs like Viagra would have been attenuated. The affluent 1960s and early 1970s were followed by a down turn in the economy, which resulted in the 1980s in the election of the conservative governments of Ronald Reagan and Margaret Thatcher. They explicitly set out to serve the socioeconomic interests of the major corporations by freeing them as much as possible from government regulations while assisting their research and marketing strategies. Viagra emerged in a neoliberal economic climate in which universities and science labs were linked to big business and research was geared to market needs.

Leonore Tiefer has described the FDA approval of Viagra as capping the long campaign of urologists and pharmaceutical corporations to medicalize male sexuality.[29] The pharmaceutical industry emerged as the most profitable in the United States. The huge profits that could be made in lifestyle drugs naturally led companies to focus their research efforts on products that were the most lucrative rather than on those that were the most needed. Perversely enough, that meant supplying expensive drugs such as Viagra and Prozac to healthy people in America and Europe rather than producing cures for the hundreds of millions of desperately ill and poor in the developing nations.

Pandering further to the industry, in 1997 the United States government allowed pharmaceutical corporations to engage in direct-to-consumer advertising. "For the first time in history," claims one account, "patients were asking their doctors for particular pharmaceutical products they saw marketed."[30] This situation was in fact not really new, but rather a return to the nineteenth-century world in which doctors were badgered by patients for the medicines they had read about in the newspapers. It is true, however, that the relaxing of FDA rules and the greater access to television gave the pharmaceutical industry an unprecedented ability to flog a range of lifestyle drugs.

Even in the Western world paying for the pills that the public was told it needed posed challenges. In the United Kingdom the government was so worried that the National Health Service would be bankrupted by the demands for Viagra that it rationed what it deemed a "recreational drug" to those who demonstrated medical need. The fact that insurers in the United States would reimburse patients for their purchase of Viagra guaranteed its success. America insurance providers quickly offered coverage for the pill after clients threatened law suits. Yet only 15 percent of insurance plans covered the oral contraceptive pill that had been on the market for forty years; companies knew women would pay to avoid unplanned pregnancies. Such egregious disparities led state legislators eventually to push for "contraceptive equity laws."[31]

The conservatives who pushed for open markets also defended what were called "family values." What that actually meant was not all that clear, and Viagra's success was largely due to its straddling the issue. The pill appeared at a time when commentators were bewailing high rates of divorce and remarriage. Viagra could be used by the masturbator, the homosexual, and the womanizer, but Pfizer implied that its product would protect marriage and was particularly meant for communicative, monogamous, married middle-aged couples. Even the churches rallied to the notion that good sex would maintain family stability, though no actual empirical data were advanced to prove the argument. The advertisements for Viagra and its competitors always showed happy couples slow dancing, holding hands, and laughing. Curiously enough, though the product supposedly only affected blood flow, the story line was always about romance. Children did not appear in such advertisements. We now lived in a culture in which—thanks to the contraceptive pill, abortion, and reproductive technologies—it was taken as a given that sex and reproduction were split. In the last decades of the twentieth century in vitro fertilization, donor insemination, and adoption had undercut any remaining reproductive necessity for male potency. Men were egged on to take Viagra, not in order to sire children, but to match a certain standard of masculinity.[32]

The story that the drug companies did not tell, but which became a staple of comics' routines, was that sex pills could destroy marriages by leading randy men to wander. Both scenarios exaggerated the significance of sex in marriage. In the mid 1990s a new United States national sex survey reported that despite claims of the sexualization of society, it found modest rates of partnered sex. Most respondents reported having sex a few times a month; only 8 percent four or more times a week. Sexual inactivity jumped once a man turned sixty. That only 75 percent of men and 29 percent of women said they always had an orgasm from vaginal intercourse was not regarded as posing a danger to marriage.[33]

Viagra was explicitly billed as propping up the traditional heterosexual marriage in which the husband took the sexual initiative. A number of scholars have suggested that at a time when white, middle-class men felt that they were being squeezed out of the labor market by downsizing and had lost power to feminists, homosexuals and African-Americans, such an appeal would strike a cord. Countering the liberalism of the 1960s, a backlash of sorts did take place in the 1980s and 1990s represented by a resurgence of biological explanations of gender difference. A "Men's Movement" emerged in the United States to counter feminism, with reform of the divorce and child custody laws the central preoccupation of the more militant men's groups. The Million Man March of 1995 saw an army of African-American men converge on Washington, D.C. to pledge to be better fathers and husbands. Two years later almost as many white male "Promise Keepers" assembled on the Washington Mall. Even *Playboy* and *Esquire* joined the fray, asserting that men had had enough of the emasculating sensitivity induced by bleeding heart liberals. There were, however, powerful counter currents. The growing popularity of common law relationships in which partners sought to be open about such issues as the domestic division of labor and sexual reciprocity provided evidence of a search by some men for more equitable relationships. The media particularly attributed the appearance of the "New Man"—sensitive, antisexist, confused, cosmopolitan—to the influence of gays and feminists.[34]

Did Viagra represent part of a backlash against advances made by women? Did the pill counter equality? Those who argue that it did have no shortage of evidence. Often cited as the most flagrant example was the way in which Viagra was rushed onto the American market. And in Japan, though the government had postponed for thirty-four years the approval of the contraceptive pill, it took only six months to OK Viagra. It has also been pointed out that the makers of Viagra, Levitra, and Cialis all exploited traditional notions of what it meant to be a man. Sociologists have noted that the advertisements for such products transmit "cultural scripts which serve as enforcers of normatively gendered expressions of sex and sexuality."[35] Should this occasion surprise? Commercial publicity campaigns are not aimed at changing society. On close examination, discussions precipitated by the appearance of the erectile drugs reveal that the views our culture has of sex, aging, and medical intervention are often more conflicted than they might first appear.

The first lesson to be drawn from such discussions is the extent to which physical performance was, at the start of the third millennium, still central to notions of masculinity. The defenders of the sex drugs propounded the old message that sex made the man. One did not say "he is a headache," but one did say "he is impotent" implying that a particular condition denoted the whole man. Viagra's implicit promise was that in dealing with a blood flow issue it would restore to a man all his masculine prerogatives. The old message that was so dear to nineteenth-century quacks was repeated by twenty-first-century scientists: a man's identity depended on his being able to have an erection. For example a doctor attached to the Harvard University medical school actually reported that a sign of the return of one particular patient's potency was that the man started to get decent haircuts.[36]

The great appeal of Viagra and its ilk was that it reduced the problem of impotency to a simple plumbing problem. Men preferred the medical model since it spared them shame. Urologists absolved men of failure by asserting that, if anything were wrong, it was with their penis, not with them. Critics complained that this led in a curious fashion to men being separated from their penises. In presenting the man as suffering from a medical problem doctors finessed the question of whether or not impotence was related to the relationship in which a man was involved. His condition ceased to have a history and he was spared the need to discuss it. Men were, of course, notorious for not wanting to broach such subjects. A New Zealand male psychologist reported that when injections were first made available sex counselors found that some men were so desperate to avoid discussing their sexuality that they actually preferred sticking a needle into their penis to talking to their partners.[37]

In their publicity material Viagra and the other erectile pharmaceuticals shored up an existing model of masculinity in which heterosexual male desire was taken as a given. The pill manufacturers followed urologists who constructed and diagnosed erectile dysfunction according to a normative hydraulic model. Narrowing the definition of male arousal, they implied that sex necessarily meant penetration. It followed that the harder the penis the better the sex and doctors set about measuring the "quality" of the erection. But here again, urologists and pharmaceutical companies did not invent these ideas. Men already used machine metaphors for the penis—hard-on, tool, pecker—making clear that they still bought into the myth of men always having to manifest control and hardness. Viagra was esteemed because it allowed performance, not necessarily pleasure. Indeed phrases such as "blow jobs" or "hand jobs" suggested that some men regarded sex as work or perhaps part of a commercial exchange.[38]

Feminists complained that urologists were only interested in genital intercourse and that they ignored the relational and cultural aspects of sexuality. Should one be disappointed that they were so mesmerized by the erection? Perhaps one should. Therapists pointed out that in fact an erection did not always indicate desire; men had them when asleep, when on bouncy buses, when frightened. Yet a flaccid penis could give pleasure and result in orgasm. Moreover lovemaking was changing in the late twentieth century. Nongenital pleasures—particularly those of oral sex—were increasing in popularity. The new focus on safe sex was also helping to shift attention away from penetration, which was not as linked to heterosexuality as it once was. One can argue that if erectile dysfunctions were a problem so too was the doctors' fixation on the erection, effectively reinforcing the old notion that men's sexual problems were always physical and the woman's always psychological.[39]

A second finding drawn from the discussions of Viagra is that many men appeared to feel under increased pressure to prove themselves. The tensions appeared to be mainly due to men attempting to sustain outdated ideals of masculinity that stressed power and control, when the social world in which they lived had dramatically changed. Viagra was seen by men, claim some researchers, as a "masculinity pill" that would fix the broken male machine.[40] Of course for centuries, every quack seller of restoratives had made more or less the same claim. Similarly, masculinity had been declared in crisis in almost every decade of the twentieth century. That said, it is true that in the 1990s men faced new challenges.

Given that a portion of Viagra advertisements were from the start directed at African-American consumers made it clear that the pharmaceutical corporations recognized that the pressure to perform was not restricted to whites. In the 1970s the fact that some non-Caucasians sought medical help for erectile dysfunctions had surprised doctors. They unconsciously accepted the racialization of masculine sexuality and its clichéd terms of the greater sexual potency and larger penis size of black men. Impotence was understood culturally as a white man's problem. By the 1990s such crude stereotyping was to a degree attenuated, but this evolution in turn posed challenges. How did blacks and Latinos, whom the culture had for centuries oversexualized, deal with the possibility of being "undersexualized?" That they had good reasons for being even more preoccupied than whites in restoring their potency was argued by Dr. Terry Mason, an

African-American urologist: "To the extent that the Black man is so deci-
mated in every other area of society, it's devastating for him to come home
and not be able to sexually satisfy his mate." Other doctors pointed out that
the situation was exacerbated inasmuch as black men—who might have internalized the notion that one had to be a stud to be a "real man"—were in
fact more susceptible than whites to diabetes and the cardiovascular problems that could lead to loss of erections.[41]

And white and black men's relations with women were changing. Were
increased concerns about impotence due to women's increased sexual demands? The idea that the contraceptive pill had unleashed female passions
was still strong. Some women did take umbrage at their partner's impotence,
regarding it as a personal insult. Interestingly enough, Viagra was initially
hailed as helping women's sex lives and the question was quickly posed if it
would also be used by women. Even *Ms* magazine lauded Viagra, arguing
that women had often been blamed by men for their impotence but now it
was proven to be an organic problem.[42] The romantic nature of so many of
the advertisements for the erectile drugs was no doubt due to the manufac-
tures' calculating that wives would often be the ones who would talk their
spouses into getting a prescription.

Misogynists took the view, however, that the new drugs could be used by
men against women. Ignoring the power issue, such men presented males
as having been victimized by the sexual revolution. They now crowed that
Viagra allowed them to turn the tables on women. "The penis is back," proclaimed an editorial in *Playboy.* "The sixties put the clitoris stage center.
The penis had been symbolic of male oppression. After 30 years of clitoral
tyranny, millions of hours of cunnilingus and battery assisted orgasm, Viagra offered a return to phallic-centered sex, the great god Cock." There was
more to this reaction than mere rhetoric. With the enormous profits offered
by attending to male sexual dysfunctions, the pharmaceutical corporations
placed on the back burner female-oriented research projects on contraception, abortion, and sexually transmitted diseases.[43] Even American medical
schools were affected. According to a 1999 survey of Medical Students for
Choice and general medical students, more course time was devoted to the
biochemistry of Viagra than to methods of contraception and abortion.

The Viagra discussions revealed that for some men the contemporary
sexual world was becoming more rather than less complicated. Men took
pills to improve their marriages, but then lied about it to their partners.
With rising divorce rates they worried about satisfying younger wives. In
a world that accepted "recreational sex," they reportedly found the dating
scene too rushed. Thirty-something men took Viagra to assuage date anxi-

ety, one doctor likening it to having snow tires in the trunk. (Automobile metaphors abounded in such discussions, some doctors suggesting that Viagra could "jump start" the sluggish.) And if the real dating world did not put enough pressure on men, more was added by the media's increasingly graphic portrayal of sex. Viagra was known to be used by male porn stars, leading Meika Loe to ask: "Is the porn star's pressure to perform that much different from that of the everyday American male?" Presumably it is, if he has to perform more than a few times a week. Yet there is some truth in Susan Faludi's argument that in the 1990s porn sexual standards entered the mainstream. Pornographers—like radical feminists—sustained the view that men necessarily sought to dominate women.[44]

Faced with such pressures, the argument goes, men turned to Viagra. What were rarely mentioned were their partners' views. Given that sex experts had for decades reported that women preferred clitoral stimulation to penetration, why was there this unprecedented male fixation on the erection? Who were the erections for? When Ann Landers carried out a poll of her women readers she found out that half were not interested in extending their sex life. They saw the dangers posed by effective erectile pills including coerced sex, adultery, and divorce. Women did not value penetrative sex to the extent men did, but knew that a man faced with erection problems tended to avoid engaging in other forms of affection.[45]

In the 1990s a feminist joke asked "Why do women fake orgasm?" and answered "Because men fake foreplay." In the masculinist version the question was "Why do women fake orgasm?" and the answer, "Because they think men care." Just as men had sex to pleasure themselves first and foremost, they had erections for the same reasons. Men candidly concede that there was a good deal of truth in such assertions, whereas the pharmaceutical corporations refused to acknowledge the narcissistic—some would say masturbatory—nature of their products.

The Viagra discussions brought special attention to bear on the sexual behavior of two male subgroups—the elderly and gays. As noted in earlier chapters, the attack on aging can be traced back at least as far as the works of Brown-Séquard in the 1890s. For much of the twentieth century, however, most men assumed that a loss of sexual vigor was a natural aspect of getting old. In the early 1980s when Clyde Martin asked subjects if they would take a safe drug to recover their youthful sexual vigor, most said they would not and looked forward to bowing out gracefully. Such stoicism came under increasing criticism. The marriage and sex counselors pushed the "use or lose it" ethos that implied the man who did not consciously attempt to prolong his sex life was a defeatist. With the medicalization of sexuality and the popularization by the urologists of a mechanistic notion of impotence, sexually inactive older men began to be described as suffering from a dysfunction. Doctors who failed to ask their male patients about their sexual health were chided. Researchers reported that men in their forties had erection problems associated with drinking, diabetes, and hypertension. The Massachusetts Male Health Study asserted that 52 percent of men between forty and seventy had some degree of impotence. But was this a medical problem? Given that declines in the flow of blood and in the velocity of the nerves due to aging were "the most predictive factor" of erectile difficulties the more obvious conclusion would be that a natural slackening of sexual vigor was to be expected. Certainly most older couples took that view, responding to a man's loss of erection by adopting various coping strategies including new positions. And some, of course, welcomed the end of their sex life.[46]

The pharmaceutical companies in contrast played up the notion that erectile dysfunctions were not natural, but problems that could be cured by a pill. Some older men's impotence did have an organic basis. As the number of prostate operations—rendered safer by newer techniques—increased from the 1980s onward, so did the number of men who experienced resulting erectile problems. Pfizer shrewdly selected Bob Dole, a prostate cancer survivor as its first spokesperson. In reality, Viagra had a low success rate with this sort of patient and the corporations really had their eyes on the affluent market made up of the growing number of healthy if aging baby boomers. It was estimated that by 2030 one in four Americans would be over sixty-five. The turn of the century has as a result witnessed an unprecedented commercial targeting of the "sex ageless consumer." Whereas it was once said that a healthy life would prolong one's sex life, the pharmaceutical corporations turned the formula around to argue that an active sex life improved one's health. The popular media contributed to this pressure on the aging by hailing personalities like Tony Randall and Saul Bellow who proved themselves by remaining sexually active late in life. Though the notion of men in their seventies siring "Viagra babies" led to a certain amount of disquiet, Western culture continued to find acceptable old men bedding young women, but not the opposite. What did cause concern was a rise in HIV among seniors, which investigators attributed to Viagra inasmuch as it allowed to become sexually active a generation that had not been educated about sexually transmitted diseases.[47]

When doctors first suggested that there was a male climacteric, few men embraced the notion because it seemed to imply that they would experience something akin to the unpleasant symptoms of menopause. Masters and Johnson speculated that only about 5 percent of men over sixty experienced such a dramatic life change. By the end of the century doctors were reporting far higher percentages because there were more older men and far more aggressive drug companies who could profit from such a diagnosis. Just when the risks of women taking hormone replacement therapies were being discovered, doctors sought to get men to take them. In February 2005, the North American Congress on the Aging Male held a forum for doctors and corporate representatives who were intent on convincing older men that they should subject themselves to testosterone treatments and other rejuvenating medications. Viagra, speaker after speaker noted, had opened the door to the notion that a decline of functions was not a "natural" part of male aging.[48]

Turning to gay men's use of Viagra, one finds that their experiences encapsulated many of the pill's contradictory influences. To win the support of the churches and middle-class America, Pfizer touted the ability of its product to rejuvenate marriage. Gay men were never portrayed in its advertising. Safe sex activists in fact pointed out the hypocrisy of Bob Dole's endorsing a cure for erectile dysfunction yet not protesting the television networks' embargo on condom advertising. But at the same time conservatives expressed their alarm that in its printed material Pfizer always referred to the man and his "partner" (rather than his wife) benefiting from Viagra. The continued use of the gender neutral term was presumably done so that a larger market could be accessed. The word "partner" was vague enough to cover both girlfriends and boyfriends, so that straight and gays, the married and single, the monogamous and philanderers were all implicitly targeted. Gay men certainly purchased the pill. Indeed a 2003 article in the *Advocate* cited a survey of HIV negative men that found 15 to 20 percent had used Viagra. It suggested that gays were more likely than straights to have taken the pill as the former were more open to experimentation. A later study found that in one men's health center two-thirds of the clients who used Viagra were heterosexual, and one-third gay or bisexual and their average age was thirty-two.[49] It was the rash of collapses in 1998 of gay men who had used Viagra along with amyl nitrate "poppers" that forced Pfizer to include warnings against combining its product with other medications that could dangerously lower blood pressure.

Gays' use of Viagra demonstrated that they too felt the pressure to conform to a specific standard of masculinity. Perhaps even more so than their straight counterparts, they bought into the idealization of youthful, virile male bodies. They also had their own specific reasons for using an erectile drug. Men who indulged in anal sex needed a firmer penis. Some young men experimenting for the first time in a same-sex relationship wanted a drug that would bolster self-confidence. Use among gays shows that Viagra appealed not just to the aging, but also to the young. As mentioned above, those who attended circuit parties often used recreational drugs like ecstasy and cocaine that could cause impotence and needed a pick me up. Unfortunately the combination of lowered inhibitions and a sexual stimulant increased the likelihood of high risk behavior. A 2005 issue of the *American Journal of Medicine* cited fourteen studies showing high risk behavior associated with Viagra. Its lead author, the director of sexually transmitted disease prevention and control services at the San Francisco Department of Health, noted that unlike contraceptives, Viagra was the only sexual health product associated with increased risk of STDs.[50] Pfizer warded off the notion that public health warnings be attached to Viagra prescriptions, insisting it was the behavior not the pill that was dangerous.

Gay men's experience with Viagra was not all that different from that of straights. Both groups shared a common belief in manliness being demonstrated by virile performance. Viagra worked for some and not for others. Some felt that it spoilt sex in making it unnatural. Feeling that they knew more about the penis than other men, gays were suspicious of an overly firm erection.[51] Echoing the complaints of some wives, one gay man described himself as feeling "pill fucked." In the main, erectile drugs maintained for gays as for straights certain normative notions of masculinity. The argument can be made, however, that a sexual minority that used such drugs in search of its own subversive pleasures turned these pharmaceuticals—despite the intent of their producers—to transformative purposes.

No account of the Viagra story would be complete if it were not compared to the other enhancement technologies that appeared in the last decades of the twentieth century. Though Viagra was approved by the FDA to deal with a medical dysfunction, all the evidence suggests that it was increasingly used to enhance pleasure or performance. As such it reflected the desires of a culture that sought to be "better than well." In part such an ambition reflected a peculiarly American impulse toward self improvement as well as the more general Western secular notion that to be ill somehow represented a moral failing.[52] Such compulsions were exacerbated in a service-oriented economy in which health and appearance were ever more important. But what if one was fat, bald, or impotent? Medical professionals and pharmaceutical representatives offered the reassurance that quick fixes were available for many of the medical conditions whose significance they themselves had conjured up. In addition, they popularized a biological language with which consumers could carry out their own pessimistic self-diagnoses.

Nostrums had been peddled for centuries but, assured by the media that it was living in age of miracle cures, the late twentieth-century public was led to assume that medical technology could deal with almost any physiological or psychological deficiency.[53] If one did not have a perfect body, recourse could be had in a shot of Botox, or a surgical procedure such as liposuction, breast augmentation, or limb-lengthening. If moodiness was a problem, a range of mind altering, psychoactive drugs including Ritalin, Prozac, and Paxil could be prescribed. The best-selling new drugs that came onto the market about the same as Viagra were Propecia (for baldness), Lipitor (to reduce cholesterol), and Evista (for osteoporosis). In a drug-addicted world where pills were taken for everything from ADD to PMS, it was hardly surprising that erectile dysfunctions should be similarly treated. What so many of these lifestyle drugs had in common was that they purported to deal with a medical condition, when in many cases the patient had a more profound problem of self-image and social confidence. This was made clear in the drug advertisements promising not just to cure but to provide happiness. And happiness, in turn, was assured by the drug to make people feel "themselves" (as Prozac boasted) or "normal" (as Viagra claimed). Thanks to market-driven cultural imperatives late twentieth-century, America was a nation in which face-lifts were deemed a medical necessity and "shyness" treated as a disease, while forty million went medically uninsured.

To be happy and healthy in the 1990s, one had to be, if one were to believe the media, sexually active. Whereas restraint was once preached, now it was gratification; celibacy was the new deviancy. In an age of consumption, heterosexuals were under something like a moral obligation to seek pleasure. Positive images were aimed at both sexes by the makers of movies, television and advertisements whose goal, of course, was to turn the commodification of sexuality to their own purposes. Sex was presented, like fitness, as part of healthy life style. Sexual decline was portrayed as unnatural, something that could and should be avoided. In this culture men and women rightly prided themselves on throwing off old restraints and discussing sexual issues with a new candor, but as Leonore Tiefer and others have observed, the same culture could, in narrowly defining what was sexually "normal," be unexpectedly oppressive. Some critics worried that one was moving from an age of diversity to a "new uniformity." "The last century saw a considerable increase in acceptance of diversity of sexual expression; it would be a shame if this century saw diversity replaced by uniform expectations of performance and desire." Lifestyle pills played a conservative role in this process by sustaining or reinscribing appropriate sex and gender roles. So Viagra made men sexually active again whereas the antidepressant Prozac (primarily prescribed for the female blues) made women calm. Indeed, loss of libido was one of the latter's major side effects.[54]

Viagra was only one of the forms of male enhancement on the market. In the nineteenth century it was argued that if women spent time and effort on their looks, men were largely indifferent to the appearance of their body. In twentieth-century America, such reticence was slowly cast aside as advertisers outbid each other in promising their soap or hair oil would provide a sense of well-being. By the 1990s men were spending an unprecedented amount of money on hair products and cosmetics. The seriousness with which some males groomed their bodies led observers to suggest that the importance the culture once attributed to character was now awarded to image. Men with an unfortunately receding hairline turned to Rogaine and Propecia or hair transplant operations. The next step was for men unhappy with what they regarded as a small penis to turn to surgery for help. In the 1970s doctors had offered silicon injections to increase girth; in the 1990s they claimed to be able to lengthen the penis by an operation in which the penal ligaments were released. Those who undertook such operations were driven by the "shower room syndrome," the desire to impress other men, not women. With the ligaments cut an erection could not be maintained. Length was traded for potency. In addition the price men paid for such penile enhancements could include dangerous complications like gangrene.[55] Contrasting those who were willing to go so far in the pursuit of sexual display to those who took Viagra helps puts the latter in some perspective.

"If you can have an erection naturally, you probably won't need Viagra." So stated Thomas Burnakis of the Baptist Medical Center of Jacksonville, Florida, when the little blue pill first came onto the market. Probably? The notion that a person who was not ill should nevertheless take a medication, a bizarre notion for most of the twentieth century, did not seem so by 1998. As the importance of sexuality was inflated so too were the insecurities of many men and women. Men taking Viagra could be compared to the women who had silicone breast implants. Both were doing something "unnatural" to meet an internalized ideal. Both represented in their own way medicine's abilities to manipulate the body and industry's interest in commercializing sex. The public was divided on whether such individuals were exhibiting their shallowness or their resourcefulness. They certainly manifested a fixation on the self that, Carl Elliot argues, is a key aspect of modern American culture, marked as it is by a profound ambivalence when it comes to the question of improvement. On the one hand it preaches the right to enhanced well-being, while on the other it condemns callow conformity and dependence.[56]

Did late twentieth-century urologists succeed in medicalizing impotence? The dominant approach they took to erectile dysfunctions was to regard them as problems in chemical engineering. Their discussions abounded with mechanical metaphors concerning functions, blood flows, and so on, yet when it came to the pharmaceutical corporations selling their drugs one found them still seeking to partner science with cultural valorizations of romance and marriage. The arrival of new medical explanations of impotence displaced, but did not entirely banish older beliefs in the influence of sin, guilt, bad habits, and even evil spells. A layer of biomedical reasoning was in effect added to the stock of arguments used to explain failures. We now live in a world where Wal-Mart has what one needs to deal with sexual dysfunctions. If this is in many ways a new world, Viagra has certainly not "revolutionized" sexuality. Many would argue that in being presented as a support of heterosexual marriage and traditional gender roles, it serves inherently conservative purposes. Its producers certainly implied that it would shore up traditional heterosexual relationships based on the active male and passive female, though in theory there is no reason why enhanced desire should result in such an outcome.

The drug companies may claim that the stigma of impotence has disappeared, but obviously it has not. Despite millions of men taking Viagra, the media usually only mentions it in mocking tones. The idea of an older man using it to woo young women was used to get a laugh in the film *Something's Gotta Give* (2003, dir. Nancy Meyers), and in Peter Lefcourt's novel *The Woody* (1998). In the television coverage of the run up to the invasion of Iraq in September, 2002 Saddam Hussein's ex-mistress was quoted as saying he took Viagra; when his sons Uday and Qusay Hussein were killed, the press was delighted to announce that on Uday's body was found cash, painkillers, a condom, and a supply of the diamond shaped pills.[57] Such sneering references implied that real men would not have to resort to such aids.

Viagra did not end male sexual insecurities, but to claim as some of its critics have done that it created an era of performance anxiety is wide of the mark. Such male worries can be traced far back in time. It is true that the manufacturers of erectile drugs have sought in an unprecedented fashion to create in men a sense of inadequacy. In targeting the sexually insecure, companies have declared many erstwhile normal conditions medical problems. In so doing they have followed the sellers of male remedies who over the centuries recognized that profits could only be made by making more and more men unsure of themselves. It is possible, however, that thanks to the modern media, today more men than ever before are prey to the thought that they might suffer from a sexual dysfunction. The irony is that the new

CONCLUSION

In the 1980s the world press reported that in parts of West Africa enraged mobs had killed "penis snatchers." These sorcerers, their victims claimed, had shrunk or stolen their penises as a form of blackmail. A decade later in Egypt, newspapers carried stories that Mossad, the Israeli spy agency, was surreptitiously distributing a debilitating type of chewing gum. It supposedly increased the activity of the sex glands, which in turn led to impotence; the Israeli strategy, it was believed, was to reduce Arab fertility. Around the same time impotence in China purportedly reached "epidemic" proportions. Here commentators blamed capitalism, which, by its veneration of sexuality, wealth, and modernity, had eroded an older ascetic culture.[1] Such accounts sound strikingly similar to some of the panics we have uncovered in our survey of male sexual anxieties in the Western world. A cross-cultural study that compares and contrasts notions of male incapacity would be a fascinating undertaking, though that project has to be left for another day. Here we only have time to draw to a close our history of developments in Europe and North America.

This book's goal has been to understand the main tendencies that have historically structured representations of masculine sexual inadequacy. Our key finding is that tracing concerns about impotence reveals that what it meant to be a man changed over time. In knowing more about impotence we have gained a better appreciation of shifts in the meanings given to masculinity. A large literature has been devoted to the history of women and femininity. Masculinity has until recently been taken for granted. Yet manhood, unlike womanhood, could be lost. Sexual performance was one of its proofs. It could consist of the simple demonstration of an erection in one culture or require a wife's pregnancy in another. Some men had to fail such tests to make the self-image and confidence of the majority meaningful.[2]

Depending on the ways in which a culture explained impotence, the incompetent male might feel guilty or victimized, responsible or depraved. Ambiguities always remained. The standards of manhood varied according to age, class, and race. It is not true to say that it was always the case that a man's virtues were undermined if he were revealed to be sexually inadequate.[3] Masculinity was a far more subtle and malleable ideology than many suppose. Means of remasculinization were possible. As the Romans demonstrated, one could be sexually incapacitated and yet have patriarchal power. On the other hand the oversexed male was usually regarded as uncivilized. The man who had too big a penis was, like the woman whose breasts were considered too large, subjected to ridicule. Both were usually assumed to lack intelligence.[4] Each culture sketched out its own particular collective representation of the "real man" and the sexual norms he was to meet. And as views of masculinity changed so did views of femininity, particularly the notion of the woman being the cause of the man's discomfiture, by either being too cold or too hot, too demure or too aggressive. Society's tolerance of women's sexual passions thus wax and waned.

Why did men have sex—for pleasure or as proof of competence? We found that shifting notions of masculinity reflected changing sexual ideologies and practices. Sexual potency for Christians created a marriage and also threatened it. In the modern world many of the behaviors that in the past were taken as necessary signs of virility—marrying, having many children (especially sons)—were dispensed with. The twentieth century saw the birth of "recreational sex." If sex came to have a less practical significance, it had a heightened psychological importance. It now could precede wedlock yet was seen as the basis of the happy marriage. As part and parcel of our consumer culture we believe today that that a good sex life is essential to well-being. Such cultural messages portraying sex as part of a healthy regimen can be pushed so far that they have an oppressive quality. Feminist scholars have presented women as the obvious victims of such oppression, pointing to the practice of many of faking their orgasms. The fact that men in the 1980s began to report that they too faked their orgasms was an even more striking evidence of the pressure to be pleasured.[5] Some who took Viagra were obviously bowing to the same forces. An orgasm could always be faked, but doctors long claimed that an erection could not. The pharmaceutical corporations proved such pessimists wrong.

What were the signs of male sexual failure? How erect did a man have to be? How often? Did he have to be able to penetrate and to postpone ejaculating for a certain number of minutes? Who decided what was "normal"? The evidence suggests that impotence was usually a "functional" disorder with no organic or pathological basis and the decline of potency a normal part of the aging process. Nevertheless experts were continuously redrawing the boundary drawn between "normal" and the "pathological." Male sexual problems were attributed at times to the mind and at others to the body. For over two thousand years those seeking to understand sexual fiascoes pondered its supposed psychological and psychological causes. Some cultures attributed disabilities to excesses and others to continence. But the definitions of sexual dysfunctions were always context specific and reflective of their culture.[6] To explain them in ancient times medical men fell back on magic and humoral theories; doctors of the enlightened eighteenth century blamed diet and lack of exercise; Victorian quacks targeted self-abuse; twentieth century endocrinologists sought hormonal imbalances, and urologists traced vascular blockages.

The various diagnoses—even the most "scientific"—were always part of a narrative that located a man's difficulties in his past and provided a hopeful account of his future. Impotence was culturally constructed. It was in a sense the product of social negotiations as cultural and political concerns impinged on private problems. When explanation and counsels were sought and a diagnosis given what had been a private sexual problem became a social phenomenon. A private defect that could counter the propagation of children, stable marriages, and individual well-being clearly had a public impact. We have tried to avoid fixating on medical men's search for cures for sexual dysfunctions so as not obscure the more important point that impotence was almost always perceived to be a problem for the collectivity. Those who offered aid saw as their task both to restore the health and to shore up the powers of fellow males.

What role did the category of the impotent male play? Cultures found the concept of impotence helpful to think with. That is to say, the notion of impotence performed certain cultural work. Each culture in employing it was offered the opportunity of clearly stating what it thought about masculinity and femininity. It was implicated in society's views on same sex relations, race, class, gender, and aging. The church, medicine, and the law all had to discuss it, impinging as it did on discussions of marriage, reproduction, and divorce. The notion of impotence set up a potent/impotent binary. Discussions of the disabled, the inept, and the incapacitated served to highlight the competence of the able man.

Unlike other cultural histories that plot the rise and fall of a particular issue or concern, this work has traced a preoccupation that in some ways

NOTES

INTRODUCTION

1. Robert D. Biggs, Šà.zi.ga, *Ancient Mesopotanian Potency Incantations* (Locust Valley, New York: J. J. Augustin, 1967), 22.
2. Goss and Company, *Hygeiana: A Non-Medical Analysis of the Complaints Incidental to Females* (London: Sherwood and Co., 1834), 59–60.
3. Michael Solomon, *The Literature of Misogyny in Medieval Spain: The Arcipreste de Talavera and the Spill* (Cambridge: Cambridge University Press, 1997), 11; and for a similar undertaking see Steven Angelides, *A History of Bisexuality* (Chicago: University of Chicago Press, 2001).
4. David D. Gilmore, *Manhood in the Making* (New Haven: Yale University Press, 1990); Paul R. Abrahamson and Steven D. Pinkerton, *With Pleasure: Thoughts on the Nature of Human Sexuality* (New York: Oxford University Press, 1995).
5. There is an enormous literature on this topic but one might begin with Gail Bederman, *Manliness and Civilization: A Cultural History of Gender and Race in the United States, 1880–1917* (Chicago: University of Chicago Press, 1995).
6. Charles E. Rosenberg and Janet Golden, eds., *Framing Disease: Studies in Cultural History* (New Brunswick: Rutgers University Press, 1992).
7. Ilza Veith, *Hysteria: The History of a Disease* (Chicago: University of Chicago Press, 1965); Clare Hanson, *A Cultural History of Pregnancy: Pregnancy, Medicine and Culture, 1750–2000* (London: Palgrave Macmillan, 2004); Rachel P. Maines, *The Technology of the Orgasm: "Hysteria," the Vibrator, and Women's Sexual Satisfaction* (Baltimore: Johns Hopkins Press, 1999); Marilyn Yalom, *A History of the Breast* (New York: Alfred A. Knopf, 1997); Sally Sheldon, "Reconceiving Masculinity: Imagining Men's Reproductive Bodies in Law," *Journal of Law and Society* 26 (1999): 129.
8. Thomas Laqueur, *Making Sex: Body and Gender from the Greeks to Freud* (Cambridge, Mass.: Harvard University Press, 1990), 22; but see David M. Friedman, *A Mind of Its Own: A Cultural History of the Penis* (New York: Penguin, 2001); Mels Van Driel, *The Secret Part — A Natural History of the Penis* (Oxford: Mandrake, 2001).

CHAPTER ONE

1. Ovid, *Amores*, 3.7.1–6 in *The Love Poems*, ed. A. D. Melville (Oxford: Oxford University Press, 1999), 67.
2. John M. McMahon, *Paralysin Cave: Impotence, Perception, and Text in the Satyrica of Petronius* (New York: Brill, 1998), 132.
3. McMahon, *Paralysin Cave*, 97, 200; Petronius, *Satyrica*, trans. R. Bracht Branham and Daniel Kinney (London: J. M. Dent, 1996).
4. Catullus 16, in *The Poems of Catullus*, trans. Peter Whigham (Berkeley: University of California Press, 1983).
5. Maud W. Gleason, *Making Men: Sophists and Self-Presentation in Ancient Rome* (Princeton: Princeton University Press, 1995), 59.
6. David Cohen, *Law, Sexuality and Society: The Enforcement of Morals in Classical Athens* (Cambridge: Cambridge University Press, 1991), 60–61.
7. Plato, "Timaeus," in *Plato*, trans. R. G. Bury (Cambridge, Mass.: Harvard University Press, 1961), 91c; Gleason, *Making Men*, 7; Eva C. Keuls, *The Reign of the Phallus: Sexual Politics in Ancient Athens* (New York: Harper and Row, 1985), 68; Craig Williams, *Roman Homosexuality: Ideologies of Masculinity in Classical Antiquity* (New York: Oxford University Press, 1999), 86–91.
8. Aline Rousselle, *Porneia: On Desire and the Body in Antiquity*, trans. Felicia Pheasant (Oxford: Basil Blackwell, 1988), 59; K. J. Dover, *Greek Homosexuality* (Cambridge, Mass.: Harvard University Press, 1978), 126–32; John R. Clarke, *Looking at Lovemaking: Constructions of Sexuality in Roman Art, 100 B.C.–A.D. 250* (Berkeley: University of California Press, 1998), 49.
9. A. S. F. Gow and D. L. Page, *The Greek Anthology: The Garland of Philip and Some Contemporary Epigrams* (Cambridge: Cambridge University Press, 1968), 1:171; Jeffrey Henderson, *The Maculate Muse: Obscene Language in Attic Comedy* (New York: Oxford University Press, 1991), 44, 127; Richard W. Hooper, *The Priapus Poems: Erotic Epigrams from Ancient Rome* (Urbana: University of Illinois Press, 1999).
10. Martial *Epigrams* 3.73, trans. D. R. Shackleton Bailey (Cambridge, Mass.: Harvard University Press, 1993); Jonathan Walters, "Invading the Roman Body; Manliness and Impenetrability in Roman Thought," in Judith P. Hallett and Marilyn B. Skinner, eds., *Roman Sexualities* (Princeton: Princeton University Press, 1997), 29–43; Amy Richlin, *The Garden of Priapus: Sexuality and Aggression in Roman Humor* (New Haven: Yale University Press, 1983), 59.
11. Catullus, 67.26 in *The Poems of Catullus*, trans. Peter Whigham (Berkeley: University of California Press, 1983); Petronius, *Satyrica* 130.4 from McMahon, *Paralysin Cave*, 81; Martial, *Epigrams* 11:46; 11:25; 11.61.
12. Mark Golden and Peter Toohey, eds., *Sex and Difference in Ancient Greece and Rome* (Edinburgh: Edinburgh University Press, 2003), 122.
13. Strato, *Musa Puerilis* in W. R. Paton, *Greek Anthology*, vol. 4 (Cambridge, Mass.: Harvard University Press, 1918); and see also Thomas K. Hubbard, ed., *Homosexuality in Greece and Rome: A Sourcebook of Basic Documents* (Berkeley: University of California Press 2003), 297–98.
14. Williams, *Roman Homosexuality*, 110–12; Catherine Edwards, *The Politics of Immorality in Ancient Rome* (Cambridge: Cambridge University Press, 1993), 71–73; Holt N. Parker,

"The Teratogenic Grid," in Judith P. Hallett and Marilyn B. Skinner, eds., *Roman Sexualities* (Princeton: Princeton University Press, 1997), 51.

15. Helen King, "Sowing the Field: Greek and Roman Sexology," in Roy Porter and Mikulás Teich, eds., *Sexual Knowledge, Sexual Science: The History of Attitudes to Sexuality* (Cambridge: Cambridge University Press, 1994): 29–46.

16. Eva C. Keuls, *The Reign of the Phallus: Sexual Politics in Ancient Athens* (New York: Harper and Row, 1985); Hesiod, *Theogony*, trans. M. L. West (Oxford: Oxford University Press, 1988), 580–612; Hugh Lloyd-Jones, *Females of the Species: Semonides on Women* (London: Duckworth, 1975); Demosthenes, "Against Neaera," *Private Orations*, trans. A. T. Murray (Cambridge, Mass.: Harvard University, 1939), 122; Richlin, *The Garden of Priapus*, 49.

17. S. C. Humphrey, *The Family, Women and Death: Comparative Studies* (London: Routledge, 1983).

18. Aristotle, *Politics*, ed. John Warrington (London: Dent, 1959), 7.1335b; S. G. Cole, "The Social Function of Rituals of Maturation: The Koureion and Arkteia," *Zeitschrift fur papyrologie und epigraphik*, 55 (1984): 233–44; Lesley Dean-Jones, *Women's Bodies in Classical Greek Science* (Oxford: Clarendon Press, 1994), 177; Plutarch, "Solon," in *Plutarch's Lives*, trans. Bernadotte Perrin (Cambridge, Mass.: Harvard University Press, 1959), 20.2–4.

19. Golden and Toohey, eds., *Sex and Difference*; Michel Foucault, *The Use of Pleasure*, trans. Robert Hurley (New York: Vintage Books, 1990).

20. Giulia Sissa, *Greek Virginity*, trans. Arthur Goldhammer (Cambridge, Mass.: Harvard University Press, 1990), 45; Plato, *Timaeus*, 91b–d; 86c–d; Kathleen Freeman, *The Pre-Socratic Philosophers* (Oxford: Blackwell, 1949), 283; "On Generation" in Iain M. Lonie ed., *The Hippocratic Treatises* (New York: Walter de Gruyter, 1981), 1.1.

21. Stephen R. L. Clark, *Aristotle's Man: Speculations upon Arisotelian Anthropology* (Oxford: Clarendon Press, 1975), 202; Aristotle, *Historia Animalium* in *The Works of Aristotle*, vol. 4, trans. D'Arcy Wentworth Thompson (Oxford: Clarendon Press, 1910), 586a15f; Peter Potter, "Herophilus of Chalcedon: An Assessment of His Place in the History of Anatomy," *Bulletin of the History of Medicine*, 50 (1976): 45–60.

22. Anthony Preus, "Science and Philosophy in Aristotle's *Generation of Animals*," *Journal of the History of Biology*, 3 (1970): 1–52; Prudence Allen, *The Concept of Woman: The Aristotelian Revolution, 750 BC–AD 1250* (Montreal: Eden Press, 1985); Aristotle, *Generation of Animals*, trans. A. L. Pleck (Cambridge, Mass.: Harvard University Press, 1943), 728a–b, 738a; Clark, *Aristotle's Man*, 207–10.

23. *Eumenides*, 658–62 cited in Pomeroy, *Goddesses*, 65, and see also Euripides, *Orestes*, 550–58; Plato, *Timaeus*, 91; Kathleen Freeman, *The Pre-Socratic Philosophers* (Oxford: Blackwell, 1949), 272; Aristotle, *Generation of Animals*, 763b; Plato, *Menexenus* in *The Dialogues of Plato*, trans. B. Jowett (Oxford: Clarendon Press, 1953), 1.238; and see Job, 10:10 for the metaphor: "Hast thou not poured me out as milk, and curdled me like cheese?"

24. Seneca, *Ad Lucilium Epistulae Morales*, trans. R. M. Gummere (Cambridge, Mass.: Harvard University Press, 1925), 95.18–19; Galen, *Oeuvres anatomiques, physiologiques et médicales*, trans. Dr. Ch. Daremberg (Paris: Baillière, 1856), 14, 15; Galen, *On the Affected Parts*, trans. Rudolph E. Siegel (New York: S. Karger, 1976), 6.5; Galen, *On Semen*, ed. and trans. Phillip de Lacy (Berlin; Akademie Verlag, 1992), 1.14–16, 2.2–5; Ilza Veith, *Hysteria: The History of a Disease* (Chicago: University of Chicago Press, 1965), 38; Rebecca Flemming, *Medicine and the Making of Roman Women: Gender, Nature,*

and Authority from Celsus to Galen (Oxford: Oxford University Press, 2000); Thomas Laqueur, *Solitary Sex: A Cultural History of Masturbation* (New York: Zone Books, 2003), 90–91.

25. "Whence Ariseth Barrenness in Women, and Impotency in Men?" in *The Complete Works of Plutarch* (New York: Cromwell, 1909), 3:118, and see also 196–97.

26. James George Frazer, *The Magic Art and the Evolution of Kings* in *The Golden Bough* (London: Macmillan, 1936), 1:150; Firmicus Maternus, *Mathesis*, trans. P. Monat (Paris: Les Belles Lettres, 1997), 6.31.46; McMahon, *Paralysin Cave*, 23; Homer, *Odyssey* 15.223–42; Apollodorus 1.9 in *God and Heroes of the Greeks: The Library of Apollodorus*, trans. Michael Simpson (Amherst, University of Massachusetts Press, 1976); Giulia Sissa, *Le corps virginal* (Paris: J. Vrin, 1987); Gleason, *Making Men*, 65; Horace, *Satires*, trans. Rushton Fairclough (Cambridge, Mass.: Harvard University Press, 1936), 1.8.30–32.

27. McMahon, *Paralysin Cave*, 9. See also Martial, 6.23: "You order my member, Lesbia, to be always standing for you; take my word for it, one's member is not the same as one's finger. Although you urge me with caressing hands and seductive words, your face is powerful to defeat you."

28. *The Book of Epodes*, 8 and 12 in *The Complete Works of Horace*, trans. Charles E. Passage (New York: Frederick Ungar, 1983); Herodotus, *History of the Greek and Persian Wars*, trans. George Rawlinson, ed. W. G. Forrest (London: New English Library, 1966), 2.181; Martial, *Epigram*, 3.70; and see also Lucretius, *De Rerum natura*, trans. H. A. J. Munro (London: George Bell, 1900), 4:1238–78.

29. Hippocrates, *On Airs*, 22.62–69; Aristotle, *Generation of Animals*, 725b34–35; 726a3–8.

30. Aristotle, *Generation of Animals*, 4.2.766b–c, 4.2.767a35, Aristotle, *Politics*, 7.1335b; Anthony Preus, "Biomedical Techniques for Influencing Human Reproduction in the Fourth Century BC," *Arethusa* 8 (1975): 243; Plutarch, *Moralia* 623e, 652d in *Plutarch's Moralia*, vol. 8, trans. Paul A. Clement and Herbert B. Hoffleit (Cambridge, Mass.: Harvard University Press, 1969); Pliny, *Natural History* (Cambridge, Mass.: Harvard University Press, 1940), 16.110, 24.72; Soranus, *Gynecology*, trans. Oswei Temkin (Baltimore: Johns Hopkins University Press, 1956), 1.64–65; Aelian, *On the Characteristics of Animals*, trans. A. F. Scofield (Cambridge: Harvard University Press, 1959), 15.19. On the possible effectiveness of some of these herbal potions see John M. Riddle, *Dioscorides on Pharmacy and Medicine* (Austin: University of Texas Press, 1985), 59–63, and Marie Thérèse Fontanille, *Avortement et contraception dans la médecine Greco-Romaine* (Paris: Laboratoires Searle, 1977).

31. Ovid, *Amores*, 3.7.7–14.

32. Christopher A. Faraone, *Ancient Greek Love Magic* (Cambridge, Mass.: Harvard University Press, 1999); Plutarch, "Advice to Bride and Groom," in *Plutarch's Moralia*, 140.8; and see also *The Fasti of Ovid*, trans. Sir James George Fraser (London: Macmillan, 1929), 2.425–6; Plutarch, *Antony*, in *Plutarch's Lives*, 37.

33. Aristotle, *Generation of Animals*, 725b21–22; 726a3–8; Aristotle, *Politics*, 1335a; Gow and Page, *The Greek Anthology*, 1:89.

34. Juvenal, *Satires* cited in McMahon, *Paralysin Cave*, 181.

35. Henderson, *The Maculate Muse*, 130; Richlin, *The Garden of Priapus*, 167; Martial, *Epigrams*, 11:81.

36. Cn. Cornelius Gallus [Maximianus the Etruscan], *Elegies of Old Age*, trans. Hovenden Walker (London: B. Crayle, 1688), 61–63, 64.

37. McMahon, *Paralysin Cave*, 181.

38. Dale B. Martin, "Contradictions of Masculinity: Ascetic Inseminators and Menstruating Men in Greco-Roman Culture," in Valeria Finucci and Kevin Brownlee, eds., *Generation and Degeneration: Tropes of Reproduction in Literature and History from Antiquity through Early Modern Europe* (Durham: Duke University Press, 2001), 81–108; Francis Schiller, "Venery, the Spinal Cord, and Tabes Dorsalis before Romberg: The Contribution of Ernst Horn," *Journal of Nervous and Mental Disease* 163 (July 1976): 4; Rufus d'Éphèse, *Oeuvres*, 3.8.; *Oeuvres de Rufus de Éphèse*, trans. Charles Daremberg (Paris: L'Imprimerie Nationale, 1879), 302, 318–23; Caelius Aurelianus, *On Acute Diseases and on Chronic Diseases*, trans. I. E. Drabkin (Chicago: University of Chicago Press, 1950), "Acute Diseases," 2.13.87, 3.5.48; "Chronic Diseases," 1.17, 1.127, 1.147, 1.178, 2.79, 1.182. See also Celsus, *De Medecina*, trans. W. G. Spencer (Cambridge, Mass.: Harvard University Press, 1935), 1:43–45, 67.

39. Aristotle, *Historia Animalium*, 572a30; Hesiod, *Theogony*; Anne Carson, "Putting Her in Her Place: Woman, Dirt, and Desire" in David M. Halperin, John J. Winkler, and Froma I. Zeitlin, eds., *Before Sexuality: The Construction of Erotic Experience in the Ancient Greek World* (Princeton: Princeton University Press, 1990), 140–43.

40. Carmen Priapea, CP 26, in McMahon, *Paralysin Cave*, 35.

41. Freeman, *Ancilla*, fragment 32, 99; Michel Foucault, *The Use of Pleasure*, trans. Robert Hurley (New York: Pantheon, 1985), 130; Allen, *The Concept of Woman*, 139.

42. H. N. Parker, "Love's Body Anatomized: The Ancient Erotic Handbooks and the Rhetoric of Sexuality," in Amy Richlin, ed., *Pornography and Representation in Greece and Rome* (New York: Oxford University Press, 1992), 90–111.

43. King, "Sowing the Field: Greek and Roman Sexology," 35; Hans Licht, *Sexual Life in Ancient Greece*, trans. J. H. Freeze (London: Routledge and Kegan Paul, 1932), 514–15; Ovid, *Tristia*, 2.523–524; Clarke, *Looking at Lovemaking*; Thomas A. J. McGinn, "Pompeian Brothels and Social History," *Journal of Roman Archaeology*, 42 (2002): 19–21.

44. Richlin, *The Garden of Priapus*, 50; Suetonius, *Tiberius*, 37, 42–45; Richlin, *Garden of Priapus*, 91; Ovid, *Amores*, 3.7.73–75 cited in Helen King, "Sowing the Field: Greek and Roman Sexology," 35. Note that the prudish 1919 Loeb edition of Martial only provides an Italian version of the poet's reference to youths.

45. Faraone, *Ancient Greek Love Magic*, 9–10; Suetonius, *Caligula*, 50; Plutarch, "De tuenda sanitate praecepta," in *Plutarch's Moralia*, trans. F. C. Babbitt (Cambridge, Mass.: Harvard University Press, 1928), 134.22; *Lucullus*, 43.1–2 in *Plutarch's Lives*.

46. "On the Nature of the Child," in Lonie, *The Hippocractic Treatises*, 12.4; Licht, *Sexual Life in Ancient Greece*, 364–66; Riddle, *Dioscorides on Pharmacy and Medicine*; Paulus, *The Seven Books of Paulus Aegineta*, trans. Francis Adams (London: Sydenham Society, 1844), 1:44, 46–47, 599.

47. Robert T. Gunther, ed., *The Greek Herbal of Dioscorides (1655)*, trans. John Goodyer (New York: Hafner Publishing, 1959).

48. Jerry Stannard, "Medicinal Plants and Folk Remedies in Pliny's *Historia Naturalis*," *History and Philosophy of the Life Sciences*, 4 (1982): 14–15.

49. Aristotle, *Historia Animalium*, 577a10–15.

50. Faraone, *Ancient Greek Love Magic*, 19; Dominic Montserrat, *Sex and Society in Greco-Roman Egypt* (London: K. P. International, 1966), 195; *Oeuvres d'Oribase*, trans.

Bussemaker and Daremberg (Paris: A L'Imprimerie Impériale, 1854), 8. 39; see also Aline Rousselle, *Porneia: On Desire and the Body in Antiquity*, trans. Felicia Pheasant (Oxford: Basil Blackwell, 1988), 16–17.

51. Ovid, *Amores*, 3.7. 27–36; and see also 1.14.39

52. Pliny, *Natural History*, 28.64; John J. Winkler, *The Constraints of Desire* (New York: Routledge, 1990), 81; Craig A. Williams, *Roman Homosexuality: Ideologies of Masculinity in Classical Antiquity* (New York: Oxford University Press, 1999), 92; Hooper, *The Priapus Poems*, 81.

53. Riddle, *Dioscordides on Pharmacy and Medicine*, 84.

54. Jane F. Gardner, "Sexing a Roman: Imperfect Men in Roman Law," in Lin Foxhall and John Salmon, eds., *When Men Were Men: Masculinity, Power and Identity in Classical Antiquity* (New York: Routledge, 1998), 141.

55. Susan Treggiari, *Roman Marriage: "Iusti Coniuges" from the Time of Cicero to the Time of Ulpian* (Oxford: Clarendon, 1991), 55, 167; Gardner, "Sexing a Roman," 143; see also P. E. Corbett, *The Roman Law of Marriage* (Oxford: Clarendon Press, 1930), 243–48, 53; James A. Brundage, *Law, Sex, and Christian Society in Medieval Europe* (Chicago: Chicago University Press, 1987), 36–37.

56. Seneca the Elder, *Controversiae* 2.5.14 in *Declamations*, vol. 1, trans. M. Winterbottom (Cambridge, Mass.: Harvard University Press, 1974); Juvenal, *The Satires*, trans. Niall Judd (Oxford: Clarendon Press, 1991); Sarah B. Pomeroy, *Spartan Women* (New York: Oxford University Press, 2002), 45; Plutarch, "Lycurgus and Numa" in *Plutarch's Lives*; Juvenal, *The Satires*; and see also Catullus, "Door," in *The Poems of Catullus*, 168.

57. Kathleen Freeman, *Ancilla to the Pre-Socratic Philosophers* (Cambridge, Mass.: Harvard University Press, 1984), fragment 276–77, 116; *Seneca's Morals*, ed. Roger L'Estrange (New York: J. and J. Harper, 1818), 5; Keith R. Bradley, "Child Labor in the Roman World," *Historical Reflections / Réflexions historiques* 12 (1985): 311–25.

58. McMahon, *Paralysin Cave*, 15.

CHAPTER TWO

1. R. H. Helmholtz, *Marriage Litigation in Medieval England* (Cambridge: Cambridge University Press, 1974), 89.

2. James A. Brundage, *Law, Sex, and Christian Society in Medieval Europe* (Chicago: Chicago University Press, 1987), 457; and see also 505, 566.

3. Michel Foucault, *The Use of Pleasure*, trans. Robert Hurley (New York: Pantheon, 1985), 39, and see also Catherine Rider, *Magic and Impotence in the Middle Ages* (Oxford: Oxford University Press, 2006).

4. Thomas Habinek, "The Invention of Sexuality in the World-City of Rome," in Thomas Habinek and Alessandro Schiesaro, eds., *The Roman Cultural Revolution* (Cambridge: Cambridge University Press, 1997), 23–44.

5. See also Lactantius, *The Divine Institutes*, trans. Mary F. MacDonald (Washington: Catholic University of America Press, 1964), 1.17, 6.20; Marcia L. Colish, *The Stoic Tradition from Antiquity to the Early Middle Ages*, vol. 2 (Leiden: Brill, 1985).

6. *Didache*, 2.2; *Barnabas*, 10.6–8, in Robert A. Kraft, *The Apostolic Fathers*, vol. 3 (New York: Nelson, 1965); and see also Peter Brown, "Antiquité tardive," in Philippe Ariès and Georges Duby, eds., *Histoire de la vie privée* (Paris: Seuil, 1985), 1:286–95; Ramsay

MacMullen, *Christianizing the Roman Empire AD 100–400* (New Haven: Yale University Press, 1984), 10–79.

7. Tertullian, *De spectaculis*, trans. T. R. Glover (Cambridge, Mass.: Harvard University Press, 1931), 10; St. John Chrysostom, *The Homilies of St. John Chrysostom* (Oxford: Parker, 1841), 24.414; Clemente de Alejandría, *Protréptico*, trans. Consalción Isart Hernández (Madrid: Editorial Gredos, 1994), 4.57–61; Clement of Alexandria, "The Instructor," [Paedagogus] in *The Anti-Nicene Fathers*, (Grand Rapids: Erdmans, 1951), 3.4; Saint Caesarius of Arles, *Sermons*, trans. M. M. Mueller (New York: Fathers of the Church, 1956), 51.1; 51.4.

8. Tertullian, *On the Apparel of Women* in *The Ante-Nicene Fathers* (Buffalo: Christian Literature Publishing Co., 1885), 2.1; Elaine Pagels, *Adam, Eve, and the Serpent* (New York: Random House, 1988), 17.

9. Saint Jerome, "On the Perpetual Virginity of the Blessed Mary Against Helvidius," in *Dogmatic and Polemical Works*, trans. J. N. Hritzu (Washington, D. C.: Catholic University of America, 1965), 42; Mathew Kuefler, *The Manly Eunuch: Masculinity, Gender Ambiguity, and Christian Ideology in Late Antiquity* (Chicago: University of Chicago Press, 2001), 78, 161, 177.

10. Bruce S. Thornton, *Eros: The Myth of Ancient Greek Sexuality* (Boulder, CO: Westview Press, 1997); Wayne A. Meeks, *The First Urban Christians: The Social World of the Apostle Paul* (New Haven: Yale University Press, 1983).

11. Uta Ranke-Heinemann, *Eunuchs for Heaven: The Catholic Church and Sexuality*, trans. John Brownjohn (New York: Andre Deutsch, 1990); Kathryn M. Ringrose, *The Perfect Servant: Eunuchs and the Social Construction of Gender in Byzantium* (Chicago: University of Chicago Press, 2003); Gerard E. Caspary, *Politics and Exegesis: Origen and the Two Swords* (Berkeley; University of California Press, 1979), 59.

12. Daniel Boyarin, *Carnal Israel: Reading Sex in Talmudic Culture* (Berkeley: University of California Press, 1993), 45.

13. Jeremy Cohen, *"Be Fertile and Increase, Fill the Earth and Master It": The Ancient and Medieval Career of a Biblical Text* (Ithaca: Cornell University Press, 1989), 134, 136, 177; Boyarin, *Carnal Israel*, 140–41, 197, 220–21.

14. Ringrose, *The Perfect Servant*, 113; Clement of Alexandria, *Christ the Educator*, trans. S. P. Wood (New York: Fathers of the Church, 1954), 173; Denise Kimber Buell, *Making Christians: Clement of Alexandria and the Rhetoric of Legitimacy* (Princeton: Princeton University Press, 1999), 22–26; Lanctatius, "The Workmanship of God," in *The Minor Works*, tr. M. F. McDonald (Washington, D. C.: Catholic University of America, 1965), 42; Lanctatius, *The Divine Instituites*, tr. M. F. McDonald (Washington, D. C.: Catholic University of America Press, 1964), 42, 459.

15. Augustine, *De Peccatorum Meritis et Remissione*, 2.2 cited in Pagels, *Adam, Eve, and the Serpent*, 111.

16. James Grantham Turner, *One Flesh: Paradisal Marriage and Sexual Relations in the Age of Milton* (Oxford: Clarendon Press, 1987), 43–44; Augustine, *De Civitate Dei*, 14, 19–20 cited in Pagels, *Adam, Eve, and the Serpent*, 111; Pagels, *Adam, Eve, and the Serpent*, 105; Peter Brown, *Augustine of Hippo: A Biography* (Berkeley: University of California Press, 2000), 391.

17. Brown, *Augustine of Hippo*, 502; Augustine, *Confessions*, in *Basic Writings of St. Augustine*, ed. Whitney Jones (New York: Random House, 1948), 4.2.

18. Marie-Odile Métral, *Le Mariage: Les Hésitations de l'occident* (Paris: Aubier, 1977); Dyan Elliott, *Fallen Bodies: Pollution, Sexuality, and Demonology in the Middle Ages* (Philadelphia: University of Pennsylvania Press, 1999), 104; Merry E. Wiesner-Hanks, *Christianity and Sexuality in the early Modern World: Regulating Desire, Reforming Practice* (London: Routledge, 2000), 108.

19. Percy Elwood Corbett, *The Roman Law of Marriage* (Oxford: Clarendon Press, 1930), 246–47; Brundage, *Law, Sex, and Christian Society*, 116.

20. *Hali Meidenhead*, ed. F. J. Furnivall (London: Early English Text Society, 1922), 12; Karma Lochie, *Covert Operations: The Medieval Uses of Secrecy* (Philadelphia: University of Pennsylvania Press, 1999), 199–201; Pierre J. Payer, *Sex and the Penitentials: The Development of a Sexual Code, 550–1150* (Toronto: University of Toronto Press, 1984), 33, 69; Jean Gaudemet, *Le Mariage en occident: Les Moeurs et le droit* (Paris: Les Editions du Cerf, 1987), 198; Brundage, *Law, Sex, and Christian Society*, 144–45, 164.

21. Mark Jordan, *The Invention of Sodomy in Christian Theology* (Chicago: University of Chicago Press, 1997); Brundage, *Law, Sex, and Christian Society*, 224–25, 284; Thomas G. Benedek and Janet Kubinec, "The Evaluation of Impotence by Sexual Congress and Alternatives Thereto in Divorce Proceedings," *Transactions and Studies of the College of Physicians of Philadelphia* 4 (1982): 122–33.

22. Brundage, *Law, Sex, and Christian Society*, 236, 457.

23. *The "Summa Theologica" of St. Thomas Aquinas*, trans. Fathers of the English Dominican Province (London: Burns Oates and Washbourne, 1932), Suppl. q. 58 a1.

24. Arthur T. McClory, "The Notion of Impotence in Canon Law" (Doctor of Canon Law diss., University of Laval, 1951), 2 : 294; Pierre J. Payer, *The Bridling of Desire: Views of Sex in the Later Middle Ages* (Toronto: University of Toronto Press, 1993), 73.

25. John T. Noonan, *Contraception: A History of Its Treatment by the Catholic Theologians and Canonists* (Cambridge, Mass.: Belknap Press, 1965), 284–90; John T. Noonan, *Power to Dissolve: Lawyers and Marriages in the Courts of the Roman Curia* (Cambridge, Mass.: Harvard University Press, 1972); Danielle Jacquart and Claud Thomasset, *Sexuality and Medicine in the Middle Ages*, trans. Matthew Adamson (Cambridge: Polity Press, 1988), 169.

26. Brundage, *Law, Sex, and Christian Society*, 291–92; Dyan Elliott, *Spiritual Marriage: Sexual Abstinence in Medieval Wedlock* (Princeton: Princeton University Press, 1993), 232, 286; Lynn Stanley, ed., *The Book of Margery Kempe* (New York: Norton, 2001), 17; Dyan Elliott, "Bernardino of Sienna versus the Marriage Debt," in Jacqueline Murray and Konrad Eisenbichler, eds., *Sex and Sexuality in the Premodern West* (Toronto: University of Toronto Press, 1996), 177.

27. Ranke-Heinemann, *Eunuchs for Heaven*, 207; Brundage, *Law, Sex, and Christian Society*, 415; and see also 291.

28. Jacqueline Murray, "On the Origins and Role of the 'Wise Woman' in Causes for Annulment on the Grounds of Male Impotence," *Journal of Medieval History* 16 (1990): 235–49; Elliott, *Spiritual Marriage*, 153–54; Helmholz, *Marriage Litigation in Medieval England*, 53.

29. Guy de Chauliac, *Le Guidon en français, corrigé par maitre Canappe* (Paris: Hierosme, 1550), 264–65; Michael Camille, "Manuscript Illumination and the Art of Copulation," in Karma Lochrie, Peggy McCracken, and James A. Schultz, eds., *Constructing Medieval Sexuality* (Minneapolis: University of Minnesota Press, 1997), 72; Ruth Karras, *Common*

Women: Prostitution and Sexuality in Medieval England (New York: Oxford University Press, 1996), 97; Brundage, *Law, Sex, and Christian Society,* 512.

30. McClory, "The Notion of Impotence in Canon Law," 2:318, 382–83; James E. Risk, *Marriage-Contract and Sacrament: A Manual of the Laws of the Catholic Church on Marriage for the Use of American Lawyers* (Chicago: Callaghan and Co., 1957), 61.

31. J. A. Brundage, "Matrimonial Politics in Thirteenth-Century Aragon: Moncada v. Urgel," *Journal of Ecclesiastical History,* 31 (1980): 271–82.

32. Peter Biller, *The Measure of Multitude: Population in Medieval Thought* (Oxford: Oxford University Press, 2000), 19, 39; Jacquart and Thomasset, *Sexuality and Medicine,* 171; Murray, "On the Origins and Role of the 'Wise Women,'" 235–49; Jacquart and Thomasset, *Sexuality and Medicine,* 172; Gaudemet, *Le Mariage en occident,* 248.

33. Maria Bellonci, *The Life and Times of Lucrezia Borgia,* trans. Bernard and Barbara Wall (London: Phoenix Press, 2000), 83; Ferdinand Gergorovius, *Lucretia Borgia* (New York: Appleton and Co., 1903), 108–9.

34. Guido Ruggiero, *The Boundaries of Eros: Sex Crime and Sexuality in Renaissance Italy* (New York: Oxford University Press, 1985), 146–47.

35. Lyndal Roper, *Oedipus and the Devil: Witchcraft, Sexuality, and Religion in Early Modern Europe* (London: Routledge, 1994), 95; Thomas Max Safley, *Let No Man Put Asunder: The Control of Marriage in the German Southwest: A Comparative Study, 1550–1600* (Kirksville, Missouri: The Sixteenth Century Journal Publishers, 1984), 33.

36. Safley, *Let No Man Put Asunder,* 36.

37. Safley, *Let No Man Put Asunder,* 76–77, 132.

38. Joan Cadden, *Meanings of Sex Difference in the Middle Ages* (Cambridge: Cambridge University Press, 1993), 206; Leo Steinberg, *The Sexuality of Christ in Renaissance Art and Modern Oblivion* (New York: Pantheon, 1983), 86–91; Carolyn Bynum Walker, "The Body of Christ in the Later Middle Ages: A Reply to Leo Steinberg," *Fragmentation and Redemption: Essays on Gender and the Human Body in Medieval Religion* (New York: Zone Books, 1991), 85; Martin Irvine, "Abelard and (Re)writing the Male Body: Castration, Identity, and Remasculinization" in Jeffrey Jerome Cohen and Bonnie Wheeler, eds., *Becoming Male in the Middle Ages* (New York: Garland, 1997), 87–107.

39. Madeleine Jeay, "Sexuality and Family in Fifteenth-Century France: Are Literary Sources a Mask or Mirror," *Journal of Family History* 4 (1979): 337; Jo Ann McNamara, "An Unresolved Syllogism: The Search for a Christian Gender System," in Jacqueline Murray, ed., *Conflicted Identities and Multiple Masculinities* (New York: Garland, 1999), 6; Robert Hellman and Richard O'Gorman, eds., *Fabliaux: Ribald Tales from the Old French* (New York: Cromwell, 1965), 24.

40. Michael Rocke, *Forbidden Friendships: Homosexuality and Male Culture in Renaissance Florence* (New York: Oxford University Press, 1996), 287n71; Shannon McSheffrey, "Men and Masculinities in Late Medieval London Civic Culture," in Murray, ed., *Conflicted Identities,* 265; Jacques Le Goff and Jean Schmitt, eds., *Le Charivari* (Paris: Mouton, 1981); Natalie Davis, *Society and Culture in Early Modern France* (Stanford, Calif.: Stanford University Press, 1975), 106–7.

41. Brian Spencer, *Pilgrim Souvenirs and Secular Badges, Medieval Finds from Excavations in London* (London: Stationery Office: 1998), 317–18; J. H. E. van Beuningen and A. M. Koldeweij, *Heilig en Profaan* (Den Haag: Rotterdam Papers, 1993), 254–62; Craig Williamson, *A Feast of Creatures: Anglo-Saxon Riddle Songs* (Philadelphia: University of Pennsylvania

Press, 1982), 83, 104, 105; Nancy Cotton, "Castrating (W)itches: Impotence and Magic in The Merry Wives of Windsor," *Shakespeare Quarterly*, 38 (1987), 320–26.

42. Geoffrey Chaucer, *The Canterbury Tales*, ed., J. Halverson (New York: Bobbs-Merrill, 1971), 1807–8; Paul Delaney, " 'Constantinus Africanus' *De Coitu*: A Translation," *Chaucer Review* 4 (1969): 55–65.

43. Biller, *The Measure of Multitude*, 253; Monica H. Green, *The Trotula: A Medieval Compendium of Women's Medicine* (Philadelphia: University of Pennsylvania, 2001), 122–23.

44. Patrick Singy, "Friction of the Genitals and the Secularization of Morality," *Journal of the History of Sexuality* 12 (2003): 352; Albert the Great, *Man and the Beasts: De Animalbus* [books 22–26] trans. James J. Scanlan (Binghamton, N.Y.: Medieval and Renaissance Texts and Studies, 1987).

45. Petrus Hispanus [John XXI], *The Treasury of Healthe*, trans. Humfre Lloyd (London: Lloyd, 1558), Di–ii ; Jacquart and Thomasset, *Sexuality and Medicine*, 173; Mary Frances Wack, *Lovesickness in the Middle Ages: The Viaticum and Its Commentaries* (Philadelphia: University of Pennsylvania Press, 1990), 41; Michael Solomon, *The Literature of Misogyny in Medieval Spain: The Arcipreste de Talavera and the Spill* (Cambridge: Cambridge University Press, 1997), 35; S. V. Larkey and T. Pyles, eds., *An Herbal*, (1525; New York: Scholars Press, 1942), 27; Philip Moore, *The Hope of Health* (London: J. Kingston, 1565); John Maplet, *A Greene Forest or a Natural Historie* (London: H. Denham, 1567), 38; and see also Dr. Christopher Wirtzung, *Praxis: Medicinae Universalis: or A General Practice of Physicke* (London: Bishop, 1598), 294; *Ram's Little Dodeon: A Brief Epitome of a New Herbal*, trans. Henry Lyte (London: Stafford, 1606), 138.

46. Michael Camille, "Manuscript Illumination and the Art of Copulation," in *Constructing Medieval Sexuality*, 58–90; Luke E. Maitre, *Doctor Bernard de Gordon: Professor and Practitioner* (Toronto: Pontifical Institute of Medieval Studies, 1980), 87.

47. Cadden, *Meanings of Sex Difference in the Middle Ages*, 231, 237.

48. Helen Rodnite Lemay, "Antonius Guanerius and Medical Gynecology," in Julius Kirshner and Suzanne F. Wemple, eds., *Women of the Medieval World: Essays in Honor of John H. Mundy* (Oxford: Blackwell, 1985), 323–31; Arnaldus de Villa Nova, *Here is a New Boke, called the Defence of Age and Recovery of Youth*, trans. Jonas Drummond (London: Robert Wyer, 1540), Aii.

49. Elliott, *Spiritual Marriage*, 153; Solomon, *The Literature of Misogyny in Medieval Spain*, 53, 184n11.

50. Thomas Vicary, *Profitable Treatise of the Anatomie of Mans Body* (London: Henry Bamforde, 1577) no pagination ; Thomas Cogan, *The Haven of Health* (London: Henrie Midleton, 1584), 246–47; Levine Lemnie, *The Touchstone of Complexions*, trans. Thomas Newton (London: Barth, 1581), 43; Philip Barrough, *The Method of Physick* (London: R. Field, 1617), 180; Peter Levens, *A Right Profitable Booke for All Diseases* (London: White, 1582), 102; François Rabelais, *Gargantua and Pantagruel*, trans. Burton Raffel (New York: Norton, 1990), 323–25.

51. Henry E. Sigerist, "Impotence as a Result of Witchcraft," in *Essays in Biology in Honour of Herbert M. Evans* (Berkeley: University of California Press, 1943), 539–46; Godfrid Storms, *Anglo-Saxon Magic* (Hague: Martinus Nijhoff, 1948), 83; Roper, *Oedipus and the Devil*, 188.

52. John T. McNeil and Helena M. Gamer, *Medieval Handbooks of Penance* (New York: Octagon, 1965), 119, 166, 197, 237, 291, 304, 330, 340; Georges Duby, *The Knight, the Lady*

and the Priest: *The Making of Modern Marriage in Medieval France*, trans. Barbara Bray (New York: Pantheon, 1983), 71; John T. McNeill and Helena M. Gamer, eds., *The Corrector of Burchard of Wurms* in *Medieval Handbooks of Penance* (New York: Octagon Books, 1965), 340; Jean Devisse, *Hincmar, archevêque de Reims, 845–882* (Geneva: Droz, 1975), 1:377–80, 400; Guibert, *The Autobiography of Guibert, Abbot of Nogent-sous-Coucy*, trans. C. C. Swinton Bland (London: Routledge, 1960), 40–44.

53. Lucille B. Pinto, "The Folk Practice of Gynecology and Obstetrics in the Middle Ages," *Bulletin of the History of Medicine*, 47 (1973), 513–23; Jane Bishop, "Bishops as Marital Advisors," in Kirshner and Wemple, eds., *Women of the Medieval World*, 67; Duby, *The Knight, the Lady and the Priest*, 142, 205.

54. Guibert, *The Autobiography of Guibert*, 123.

55. Dyann Elliott, "Pollution, Illusion, and Masculine Disarray: Nocturnal Emissions and the Sexuality of the Clergy," in Lochrie, McCracken, and Schultz, eds., *Constructing Medieval Sexuality*, 1–23; Elliott, *Fallen Bodies: Pollution, Sexuality, and Demonology*.

56. Ranke-Heinemann, *Eunuchs for Heaven*, 200; and see also 206–7.

57. Montague Summers, ed., *The Malleus Maleficarum of Heinrich Kramer and James Sprenger* (New York: Dover Publications, 1971), 55.

58. Summers, ed., *The Malleus Maleficarum*, 59.

59. Summers, ed., *The Malleus Maleficarum*, 60.

60. Walter Stephens, "Witches Who Steal Penises: Impotence and Illusion in *Malleus Maleficarum*," *Journal of Medieval and Early Modern Studies* 28 (1998): 495–529. Walter Stephens, *Demon Lovers* (Chicago: University of Chicago press, 2002), 312–17; Wack, *Lovesickness in the Middle Ages*, 165; Summers, ed., *The Malleus Maleficarum*, 56.

61. David Herlihy, *Medieval Households* (Cambridge, Mass.: Harvard University Press, 1985), 31–32; Jean Bodin, *On the Demon-Mania of Witches* (1580), trans. Randy A. Scott (Toronto: Centre for Reformation and Renaissance Studies, 1995), 98, 100.

62. Charles Godfrey Leland, *The Unpublished Legends of Virgil* (London: Elliot Stock, 1899), 98; and on the sexually demanding woman see Giovanni Boccaccio, *The Decameron*, trans. John Payne (New York: The Modern Libary, 1930), 288–93.

63. Jean de Coras, *Arrest memorable du Parlement de Tolose* (Lyon: Antoine Vincent, 1565), 47–48; Natalie Zemon Davis, *The Return of Martin Guerre* (Cambridge, Mass.: Harvard University Press, 1983), 19–21; Johann Weyer, *De praestigiis daemonum*, 6th ed. 1583, ed. George Mora (Binghampton: Medieval and Renaissance Texts and Studies, 1991), 464.

64. Martin, *Witchcraft and the Inquisition in Venice*, 53; Bodin, *On the Demon-Mania of Witches*, 100; James I, *Daemonologie* (1597; London: The Bodley Head, 1924), xiii.

65. Girolamo Cardano, *Opera omnia*, 2:76–77, cited in Nancy G. Siraisi, *The Clock and the Mirror: Girolamo Cardano and Renaissance Medicine* (Princeton: Princeton University Press, 1997), 221.

66. Siraisi, *The Clock and the Mirror*, 165.

67. Winfried Schleiner, "The Nexus of Witchcraft and Male Impotence in Renaissance Thought and Its Reflections in Mann's Doktor Faustus," *Journal of English and Germanic Philology* 84 (April 1985): 175; Weyer, *De praestigiis daemonum*, 334–35; Reginald Scot, *Discoverie of Witchcraft*, 1584 (New York: Da Capo Press, 1971), 77, 80.

68. Michel de Montaigne, "On the Powers of the Imagination," in *The Essays of Michel de Montaigne*, trans. M. A. Screech (London: Allen Lane, 1991), 112, 114.

69. Montaigne, "On the Powers of the Imagination," 115.

CHAPTER THREE

1. "Son dada demeura court à Lérida" was a line in a song about the Prince de Condé's failure to perform in an amorous engagement. Frances Mossiker, *Madame de Sévigné: A Life and Letters* (New York: Knopf, 1983), 95; Madame de Sévigné, *Correspondance* (Paris: Gallimard, 1925), 1:1047.

2. David Lindley, *The Trials of Frances Howard: Fact and Fiction at the Court of King James* (New York: Routledge, 1993), 99; Ramble Cotgrave, *A Dictionarie of the French and English Tongues* (London: Adam Islip, 1611); Thomas Middleton, *The Witch*, ed. Elizabeth Schafer (New York: N. N. Norton, 1994), 20 (text references are to this edition).

3. Robert Burton, *The Anatomy of Melancholy* (Oxford: Lichfield and Short, 1621), 287, and see also Vincent Tagereau, *Discours sur l'impuissance de l'homme et de la femme* (Paris: Brayet and Rousset, 1612), 142; Ruth Martin, *Witchcraft and the Inquisition in Venice, 1550–1650* (Oxford: Basil Blackwell, 1989), 107, 127.

4. John Nada, *Carlos the Bewitched: The Last Spanish Hapsburg, 1661–1700* (London: Jonathan Cape, 1962), 222, 235.

5. John Pechey, *The Compleat Midwife's Practice Enlarged* (London: Rhodes, 1698), 243; Nicholas Culpeper, *A Directory for Midwives* (London: Peter Cole, 1660), 89; Jane Sharp, *The Complete Midwife's Companion; or the Art of Midwifery Improved* (London: Simon Miller), 101; and see also Thomas Lupton, *A Thousand Notable Things of Sundry Sortes* (London: Hughe Spooner, 1579), 20; Abbé Jean Baptiste Thiers, *Traité des superstitions anciennes et modernes* (1679; Amsterdam: Bernard, 1723), 324; Keith Christiansen, "Lorenzo Lotto and the Tradition of Epithalmic Paintings," *Apollo* (September 1986): 166–73.

6. John Webster, *The Displaying of Supposed Witchcraft* (London: S. M., 1677), 246; Joseph Bajada, *Sexual Impotence: The Contribution of Paolo Zacchia ,1584–1659* (Rome: Editrice Pontifica Universita Gregorianà, 1988), 121; Thiers, *Traité des superstitions anciennes et modernes*, 2:319–34; Giancarlo Carabelli, *In the Image of Priapus* (London: Duckworth, 1996); Julia Peakman, *Mighty Lewd Books: The Development of Pornography in Eighteenth-Century England* (New York: Palgrave Macmillan, 2003), 109–10.

7. *Works of Robert Herrick*, ed., Alfred Pollard (London: Lawrence and Bullen, 1891), 1:10.

8. Daniel Defoe, *Conjugal Lewdness: or, Matrimonial Whoredom—A Treatise Concerning the Use and Abuse of the Marriage Bed* (London: J. Warner, 1727), 152; Robert Burns, "Address to the Deil," *The Poems and Songs of Robert Burns*, ed., James Kinsley (Oxford: Clarendon Press, 1968), 1:170, lines 61–62, "crouse" meaning cocksure; and see also Emmanuel Le Roy Ladurie, *Jasmin's Witch* (Aldershot: Scholar Press, 1987).

9. Levinus Lemnius, *The Secret Miracles of Nature in Four Books* (1658), cited in Alexandra Shepherd, *Meanings of Manhood in Early Modern England* (Oxford: Oxford University Press, 2003), 60; Burton, *The Anatomy of Melancholy*, 317; John Downame, *Foure Treatises Tending to Diswade All Christians* (London: Hall, 1613), 151.

10. Angus McLaren, *Reproductive Rituals: The Perception of Fertility in England from The Sixteenth Century to the Nineteenth Century* (London: Methuen, 1984), 19–20; Winfried Schleiner, *Medical Ethics in the Renaissance* (Washington, D.C.: Georgetown University Press, 1995), 135–36; Ambroise Paré, *Oeuvres complètes*, ed. J.-F. Malgaigne (Paris: J.-B. Baillière, 1841), 1:161; 2:636.

11. Louys de Serres, *Discours de la nature, causes, signes, & empechemens de la conception, & de la Sterilité des femmes* (Lyon: Antoine Chard, 1625), 93–94.

12. De Serres, *Discours de la nature*, 225; see also Alain Molinier, "Pérenniser et concevoir," in Jean Delumeau et Daniel Roche, eds., *Histoire des Pères et de la paternité* (Paris: Larousse, 2000), 93.

13. Anthony Fletcher, *Gender, Sex and Subordination in England 1500–1800* (New Haven: Yale University Press, 1995), 55; and see also Kathleen M. Crowther-Heyck, "'Be Fruitful and Multiply': Genesis and Generation in Reformation Germany," *Renaissance Quarterly* 55 (2002): 904–35.

14. Sinibaldus, *Rare Verities: The Cabinet of Venus Unlocked* (London: P. Briggs, 1657), 39–43; Michael Ettmüller, *Etmullerus Abridg'd: or, A Compleat System of the Theory and Practice of Physic, Being a Description of All Diseases Incident to Men, Women and Children* (London: E. Harris 1699), 572–74; Philip Barrough, *The Method of Physick* (London: R. Field, 1617), 180.

15. Helkiah Crooke, *Microcosmographia* (London: R. C., 1651), 156; John Pechey, *The Compleat Midwife's Practice Enlarged* (London: Rhodes, 1698), 22, 26.

16. Sharp, *The Complete Midwife's Companion*, 18; Anon., *Compleat Midwifes Practice* (London: Nathaniel Brooke, 1656), 1:24, 26, 39; 2:67; John Sadler, *The Sick Woman's Private Looking-Glasse* (London: Griffin, 1636), 119.

17. Anon., *Compleat Midwifes Practice*, 20; *Aristotle's Master-Piece* (London: Booksellers, 1694); *Aristotle's Masterpiece* (London: D. P., 1740?), 11; *Aristotle's Last Legacy* (London: Booksellers, 1776), 26–28; *The Works of Aristotle the famous philosopher containing his Complete Masterpiece* (Derby: Thomas Richardson, c.1840), 5.

18. A Physician [Nicolas de Venette], *Conjugal Love Reveal'd*, 7th ed. (London: Thomas Hinton, 1720?), 117; Nicolas de Venette, *Conjugal Love; or, The Pleasures of the Marriage Bed* (London: The Booksellers, 1770?), 50, 105, 154–55, 184.

19. Edward Ward, *The Whole Pleasures of Marriage* (London: Norris, 1710), 61; *The Works of William Shakespeare* (New York Oxford University Press, 1904), 866.

20. Robert T. Gunther, ed., *The Greek Herbal of Dioscorides*, trans. John Goodyer (1655) (New York: Hafner Publishing, 1959); Nicholas Culpeper, *Galen's Art of Physick* (London: P. Cole, 1652), 41–44; Nicholas Culpeper, *The English Physician Enlarged* (London; J. Churchill, 1714), 25, 85, 90, 91, 160, 214, 215, 227; and see also Anon., *Complete Midwife's Practice Enlarged* (London: Nathaniel Brook, 1663), 254, 312–13.

21. *Now or Never: Or, A New Parliament of Women* (London: George Norton, 1656), 6; Thomas Otway, *The Soldier's Fortune* in *The Works of Thomas Otway*, ed. J. C. Ghosh (Oxford: Clarendon Press, 1932), act 5, lines 599–601; Elizabeth Blackwell, *A Curious Herbal* (London: Harding, 1737), 2:102; Sir George Etherege, *She Would If She Could*, ed. Charlene M. Taylor (Lincoln: University of Nebraska Press, 1971).

22. Susan Dwyer Amussen, *An Ordered Society: Gender and Class in Early Modern England* (Oxford: Basil Blackwell, 1988), 99–105.

23. Bernard Capp, *When Gossips Meet: Women, Family, and Neighbourhood in Early Modern England* (Oxford: Oxford University Press, 2003), 198; Peter M. Moogk, "'Thieving Buggers' and 'Stupid Sluts': Insults and Popular Culture in New France," *William and Mary Quarterly* 26 (1979): 536; Roger Thompson, *Unfit for Modest Ears: A Study of Pornographic, Obscene, and Bawdy Works Written or Published in England in the Second Half of the Seventeenth Century* (London: Macmillan, 1979), 103.

24. Charles Sedley, "The Happy Pair" (1702), lines 267–71, in *The Poetical and Dramatic Works of Sir Charles Sedley*, ed. V. de Sola Pinto (London: Constable and Company, 1928), 1:63–73.

25. Thompson, *Unfit for Modest Ears*, 106; Sinibaldus, *Rare Verities*, 19.

26. John Henry Meibomius, *A Treatise of the Use of Flogging in Medicine and Venery* (Paris: Isidore Lisieux, 1898); *Fifteen Real Comforts of Matrimony* (London: Benjamin Alsop, 1683), 46; Anon. [John Armstrong], *The Oeconomy of Love: A Poetical Essay* (London: T. Cooper, 1737), lines 529–31; and see also Thompson, *Unfit for Modest Ears*, 105; Schleiner, *Medical Ethics in the Renaissance*, 140–47.

27. "A Satyr on Charles II" (circa 1673), in David M Vieth, ed., *The Complete Poems of John Wilmot, Earl of Rochester* (New Haven: Yale University Press, 1968), 61, lines 28–31.

28. Katherine B. Crawford, "The Politics of Promiscuity: Masculinity and Heroic Representation at the Court of Henry IV," *French Historical Studies* 26 (2003): 225–52.

29. John Ehrman, *The Younger Pitt* (New York: Dutton, 1969), 1:108.

30. *The Women's Petition against Coffee, Representing to Public Consideration the Grand Inconveniencies Accruing to their Sex from the Excessive Use of that Drying, Enfeebling Liquor* (London, 1674), 3; *Aristotle's Last Legacy, Unfolding the Mysteries of Nature in the Generation of Man* (London, 1741), 90; and see also Judith C. Mueller, "Imperfect Enjoyment at Market Hill: Impotence, Desire, and Reform in Swift's Poems to Lady Acheson," *English Literary History* 66 (1999): 51–70.

31. *Polly Peachum's Jests* (London: J. Roberts, 1728), 43; P. M. Zall, *A Nest of Ninnies: And Other English Jestbooks of the Seventeenth Century* (Lincoln: University of Nebraska Press, 1979), xv, 260; and see also *The Puzzle: Being a Choice Collection of Conundrums* (London: Jonathan Carpenter, 1745); *Cambridge Jests: Being Wit's Recreation* (Newcastle, 1750), 6, 16–17; *A Whetstone for Dull Wits* (Newcastle, 1765), 1, 8; *Wit Newly Revived, Being a Book of Riddles* (Newcastle, 1775), 7; *The Trial of Wit, or, A New Riddle-Book* (Glasgow, 1782), 2, 8; *The Merry Andrew; or, Macaroni Jester* (London, 1786), 6, 12, 16, 28.

32. Laurence Sterne, *The Life and Opinions of Tristram Shandy* (London: Penguin, 1976), and see also R. F. Brissenden, *Virtue in Distress: Studies in the Novel of Sentiment from Richardson to Sade* (London: Macmillan, 1974), 208–9; Felicity A. Nussbaum, *The Limits of the Human: Fictions of Anomaly, Race, and Gender in the Long Eighteenth Century* (Cambridge: Cambridge University Press, 2003), 101–5; Judith C. Mueller, "Fallen Men: Representations of Male Impotence in Britain," *Studies in Eighteenth-Century Culture* 28 (1999): 85–102; Karen Harvey, *Reading Sex in the Eighteenth Century: Bodies and Gender in English Erotic Culture* (Cambridge: Cambridge University Press, 2005), 137–39.

33. Gordon Williams, *A Dictionary of Sexual Language and Imagery in Shakespearean and Stuart Literature* (London: Athlone Press, 1994), 1:125, 173–74, 395, 551–52, 566–67; Julie Coleman, *Love, Sex, and Marriage: A Historical Thesaurus* (Amsterdam: Rodopi, 1999), 200–201; P. J. Leroux, *Dictionnaire comique, satyrique, critique, burlesque, libre et proverbial* (Paris: [A Pampelune] 1786); Thompson, *Unfit for Modest Ears*, 106–7; Roger Thompson, ed., *Samuel Pepy's Penny Merriments* (London: Constable, 1976), 260–63; Edward Ward, *Nuptial Dialogues and Debates: or, An Useful Prospect of the Felicities and Discomforts of a Marry'd Life, Incident to all Degrees, from the Throne to the Cottage* (London: T. Norris, 1710), 43. On July 26, 1664, Samuel Pepys confided to his diary that he sought the advice of women "of my not getting children" and they merrily gave many suggestions concerning warming drinks and advantageous positions. Henry B. Wheatley, ed., *The Diary of Samuel Pepys* (New York: Random House, 1946), 1:942.

34. Anon., *The Ten Pleasures of Marriage* (London: 1682), 50, 51, 68; *Grand dictionnaire universel du XIXe siècle* (Paris: Pierre Larousse, 1866–90), 9:61; and see also Raymond

Stephanson, *The Yard of Wit: Male Creativity and Sexuality, 1650–1750* (Philadelphia: University of Pennsylvania Press, 2004), 207–10, 250n103.

35. Anon., *Roxburghe Ballads* (London, 1774), 1:28–29; Lisa Jardine, *Still Harping on Daughters: Women and Drama in the Age of Shakespeare* (Brighton: Harvester Press, 1983), 123; Fletcher, *Gender, Sex and Subordination*, 5–11; Kenneth A. Lockridge, *On the Sources of Patriarchal Rage: The Commonplace Books of William Byrd and Thomas Jefferson and the Gendering of Power in the Eighteenth Century* (New York: New York University Press, 1992), 6–19; Thompson, *Unfit for Modest Ears*, 109.

36. Niccolò Machiavelli, *Mandragola*, trans. Anne and Henry Paolucci (New York: Bobbs-Merrill, 1957); Sinibaldus, *Rare Verities*, 16–17; Elizabeth A. Foyster, *Manhood in Early Modern England: Honour, Sex and Marriage* (London: Longman, 1999), 68–71; Daniel Defoe, *Conjugal Lewdness: or, Matrimonial Whoredom—A Treatise Concerning the Use and Abuse of the Marriage Bed* (London: Warner, 1727), 131; John Marten, *A Treatise of All the Degrees and Symptoms of the Venereal Disease* (London: S. Crouch, 1708), 424–25; Charles Ancillon, *Eunuchism Display'd* (London: E. Curll, 1718), 168–69, 216, 219, 220.

37. Anon., *Roxburghe Ballads*, 8:190–91; and see Joy Wiltenburg, *Disorderly Women and Female Power in the Street Literature of Early Modern England and Germany* (Charlottesville: University Press of Virginia, 1992), 148–51.

38. Anon., *Roxburghe Ballads*, 2:447; J. Woodfall Ebsworth, ed., *Roxburghe Ballads* (Hertford: Ballad Society, 1871–99), 8:670.

39. Ebsworth, *Roxburghe Ballads*, 8.3:679–81.

40. Marjorie Garber, "Out of Joint," in David Hillman and Carla Mazzio, eds., *The Body in Parts: Fantasies of Corporeality in Early Modern Europe* (London: Routledge, 1997), 27; *Aristotle's Masterpiece* (London: D. P., 1740?), 43; Anon., *Roxburghe Ballads*, 1:46–47.

41. *Fifteen Real Comforts of Matrimony* (London: Benjamin Alsop, 1683), 37, 42, 45, 48.

42. David M. Turner, *Fashioning Adultery: Gender, Sex and Civility in England, 1660–1740* (Cambridge: Cambridge University Press, 2002), 88; *An Essay Upon Improving and Adding to the Strength of Great Britain and Ireland by Fornication Justifying the Same from Scripture and Reason* (Dublin, 1735), 16.

43. Anon., *Roxburghe Ballads*, 2:410.

44. *Fifteen Real Comforts of Matrimony*, 79.

45. Anon., *Roxburghe Ballads*, 3:196; Ebsworth, *Roxburghe Ballads*, 8.1:197.

46. John Garfield, *The Wandering Whore (1660–1661)* (University of Exeter: The Rota, 1977), 13; *Polly Peachum's Jests* (London: J. Roberts, 1728), 12.

47. *The Fumbler's Rant* (Glasgow: J and M Robertson, 1808), 2.

48. Thomas Hamilton, Earl of Haddington, *A Select Choice of Humorous Poems in the Lucious Taste* (London: P. Wicks, 1770), 15.

49. Robert Gould, *A Satyr Against Wooing: With a View of the Ill Consequences that attend it* (London, 1698), 8.

50. *The Works of Mr. Robert Gould* (London: Lewis, 1709), 2:53. Gould noted the use of spas by those in search of sexual rejuvenation in "To My Lord Chamberlain at Bath."

51. George Etherege, "The Imperfect Enjoyment," in *The Works of George Etherege*, ed. A. Wilson Verity (London: Nimmo, 1888), 397–99; and see earlier examples drawn from Thomas Campion and Thomas Nashe in Lindley, *The Trials of Frances Howard*, 100–102.

52. Vieth, ed., *The Complete Poems of John Wilmot, Earl of Rochester*, 38.

53. William Wycherley, *The Complete Works of William Wycherley*, ed. Montague Summers (London: Nonesuch Press, 1924), 3:201–2; 4:249–50.

54. Cited in Angeline Goreau, "Two English Women in the Seventeenth Century," in Philippe Ariès and André Béjin, eds., *Western Sexuality: Practice and Precept in Past and Present Times*. trans. Anthony Forster (Oxford: Basil Blackwell, 1985), 111; and see also Brandford K. Mudge, *The Whore's Story: Women, Pornography, and the British Novel, 1684–1830* (Oxford University Press, 2000), 133.

55. Felicity A. Nussbaum, *The Brink of All We Hate: English Satires on Women, 1660–1750* (Lexington: University Press of Kentucky, 1984), 57–76; Leo Braudy, "Remembering Masculinity: Premature Ejaculation Poetry of the Seventeenth Century," *Michigan Quarterly Review* 33 (1994): 177–201; Crébillon fils (Claude-Prosper Jolyot de Crébillon), *The Sofa* (1742), in Michel Feher, ed., *The Libertine Reader: Eroticism and Enlightenment in Eighteenth-Century France* (New York: Zone Books, 1997), 255.

56. Thomas Hamilton, Earl of Haddington, *A Select Choice of Humorous Poems in the Lucious Taste* (London: P. Wicks, 1770), 43, 168–69, 196–97.

57. *The Whore: A Poem. Written by A Whore of Quality* (1782?), cited in Fiona Pitt-Kethley, *The Literary Companion to Sex* (New York: Random House, 1992), 252.

58. Mary de la Rivière Manley, *The Royal Mischief* (London: R. Bentley, F. Saunders, J. Knapton and R. Wellington, 1696), 46.

59. Ben Jonson, *Epicoene*, ed. Edward Partridge (New Haven: Yale University Press, 1971), 164–65. For a French comedy of impotence, see Claude-Prosper Jolyot de Crébillon, *L'Ecumoire (Tanzaï and Néardané)* (Paris: Le Devin, 1930), 66–68.

60. William Wycherley, *The Country Wife*, ed. James Ogden (New York: Norton, 1991).

61. Turner, *Fashioning Adultery*, 102; Giles Slade, "The Two-Backed Beast: Eunuchus and Priapus in *The Country Wife*," *Restoration and Eighteenth-Century Theatre Research* 7 (1992): 23–34. Somewhat similar is Mme de Beauharnais' *L'Abélard supposé* (1780) cited in Angelica Goodden, *The Complete Lover: Eros, Nature, and Artifice in the Eighteenth-Century French Novel* (Oxford: Clarendon Press, 1989), 18–19.

62. William Gouge, *Of Domestical Duties: Eight Treatises* (London: Edward Brewster, 1634), 182–83.

63. Edmund S. Morgan, *Religion and Domestic Relations in Seventeenth-Century New England* (Westport, CT: Greenwood, 1980), 34–35; John Demos, *A Little Commonwealth: Family Life in Plymouth Colony* (New York: Oxford University Press, 1970), 94; Richard Godber, *Sexual Revolution in Early America* (Baltimore: Johns Hopkins University Press, 2002), 58–61; Martin Duberman, "Male Impotence in Colonial Pennsylvania," *Signs* 4 (1978): 401; Thomas A. Forster, "Deficient Husbands: Manhood, Sexual Incapacity, and Male Marital Sexuality in Seventeenth-Century New England," *William and Mary Quarterly* 56 (1999): 727; Lyle Koehler, *A Search for Power: The "Weaker Sex" in Seventeenth-Century New England* (Urbana: University of Illinois Press, 1980), 78–84; Anne S. Lombard, *Making Manhood: Growing Up Male in Colonial New England* (Cambridge: Harvard University Press, 2003).

64. Antonia Fraser, *The Weaker Vessel: Woman's Lot in Seventeenth-Century England* (New York: Random House, 1985), 296; Martin Ingram, *Church Courts, Sex and Marriage in England, 1570–1640* (Cambridge: Cambridge University Press, 1987), 172–73; Lindley, *The Trials of Frances Howard*, 98–104.

65. Anon., *Cases of Divorce for Several Causes* (London: E. Curll, 1723), 9; George Abbot, *The*

Case of Impotency, As Debated in England, in that Remarkable Tryal, 1613, between Robert Earl of Essex, and Lady Frances Howard, who, After Eight Years Marriage, commenc'd a Suit Against him for Impotency (London: Curll, 1719), 2 vols.

66. Anon., *Cases of Divorce for Several Causes*, 55; John Crawfurd, *The Cases of Impotency and Virginity Fully Discuss'd* (London: Thomas Gammon, 1732); Peter Wagner, "The Pornographer in the Courtroom: Trial Reports About Cases of Sexual Crimes and Delinquencies as a Genre of Eighteenth-Century Erotica," in Paul-Gabriel Boucé, ed., *Sexuality in Eighteenth-Century England* (Manchester: Manchester University Press, 1982), 125; and see also Peter Wagner, *Eros Revived: Erotica of the Enlightenment in England and America* (London: Paladin, 1990).

67. A. D. Harvey, *Sex in Georgian England: Attitudes and Prejudices from the 1720s to the 1820s* (London: Duckworth, 1994), 152; Laura Gowing, *Common Bodies: Women, Touch and Power in Seventeenth-Century England* (New Haven: Yale University Press, 2003), 43; Cynthia B. Herrup, *A House in Gross Disorder: Sex, Law, and the 2nd Earl of Castlehaven* (New York: Oxford University Press, 1999), 137–38; Ralph Strauss, *The Unspeakable Curll* (London: Chapman and Hall, 1927), 40–41.

68. Anon., *The Cases of Impotency Debated in the late Famous Tryal at Paris* (London: E. Curll, 1714), vol. 1, appendix, x2.

69. Mueller, "Fallen Men: Representations of Male Impotence in Britain," 87.

70. Herrup, *A House in Gross Disorder*, 138; Lawrence Stone, *Broken Lives: Separation and Divorce in England, 1660–1857* (Oxford: Oxford University Press, 1993), 132, 133.

71. Joseph Bajada, *Sexual Impotence: The Contribution of Paolo Zacchia, 1584–1659* (Rome: Editrice Pontifica Universita Gregorianà, 1988), 104; Adrien de Bussy De Lamer and Germain Fromageau, *Le Dictionnaire des cas de conscience* (Paris: Coignard, 1733), 2: cols. 42, 66.

72. Jean Verdier, *La jurisprudence de la médecine, de la chirurgie, et de la pharmacie , en France* (1762–63; Paris: J. B. Baillière, 1834), 101; Pierre Darmon, *Damning the Innocent: A History of the Persecution of the Impotent in pre-Revolutionary France*, trans. Paul Kean (New York: Viking, 1986), 54.

73. Darmon, *Damning the Innocent*, 60, 63.

74. Anon. (Jean Bouhier?), *Traité de la dissolution du mariage pour cause d'impuissance* (Luxembourg: Kragt, 1735), 20, 95.

75. Darmon, *Damning the Innocent*, 197–98.

76. David Hunt, *Parents and Children in History: The Psychology of Family Life in Early Modern France* (New York: Basic Books, 1970), 162, 170.

77. Peter Cryle, *Geometry in the Bedroom: Configurations of French Erotic Narrative* (Ithaca: Cornell University Press, 1994), 100.

78. Molinier, "Pérenniser et concevoir," 93.

79. *A Merry Allegorico-Botanico-Vadinical Piece: or, The Natural History of the Arbor Vitæ: or The Tree of Life* (London: Gardeners, 1732); *Dn__Sw__t's Medley* (Dublin: The Booksellers, 1749).

80. Laura Gowing, *Common Bodies: Women, Touch and Power in Seventeenth-Century England* (Yale University Press, 2003), 114–16; Elizabeth Foyster, "A Laughing Matter? Marital Discord and Gender Control in Seventeenth-Century England" *Rural History* 4 (1993): 5–21; Norman N. Holland, *Laughing: A Psychology of Humor* (Ithaca: Cornell University Press, 1982), 17.

CHAPTER FOUR

1. On Marten see Ralph Strauss, *The Unspeakable Curll* (London: Chapman and Hall, 1927), 26–28.

2. John Marten, *A Treatise of All the Degrees and Symptoms of the Venereal Disease* (London: S. Crouch, 1708), 165; John Marten, *Gonosologium Novum; or, A New System of All the Secret Infirmities and Diseases, Natural, Accidental, and Venereal in Men and Women* (London: N. Crouch, 1709), 21, 55.

3. Marten, *Gonosologium Novum,* 33, 39, 40, 61.

4. Marten, *Gonosologium Novum,* 33, 38, 39, 40, 61.

5. Marten, *Gonosologium Novum,* 42, 50–51, 59.

6. Marten, *Gonosologium Novum,* 34; Michael Ettmüller, *Etmullerus Abridg'd: or, A Compleat System of the Theory and Practice of Physic, Being a Description of All Diseases Incident to Men, Women and Children* (London: E. Harris 1699), 567; Marten, *A Treatise of All the Degrees,* 418; Thomas W. Laqueur, *Solitary Sex: A Cultural History of Masturbation* (New York: Zone Books, 2003), 29.

7. David Stevenson, "Recording the Unspeakable: Masturbation in the Diary of William Drummond," *Journal of the History of Sexuality* 9 (2000): 223–39; James A. Brundage, *Law, Sex, and Christian Society in Medieval Europe* (Chicago: Chicago University Press, 1987), 26; Roy Porter, "Mixed Feelings: The Enlightenment and Sexuality in Eighteenth-Century Britain," in Paul Gabriel Boucé, ed., *Sexuality in Eighteenth-Century Britain* (Manchester: Manchester University Press, 1982), 17; Jean Stegers and Anne van Neck, *Masturbation: The History of a Great Terror,* trans. Kathryn A. Hoffman (New York; Palgrave, 2001); Michael Stolberg, "Self-Pollution, Moral Reform, and the Venereal Trade: Notes on the Sources and Historical Context of Onania (1716)," *Journal of the History of Sexuality* 9 (2000): 37; Michael Stolberg, "An Unmanly Vice: Self-Pollution, Anxiety, and the Body in the Eighteenth Century," *Social History of Medicine* 13 (2000): 1–21.

8. *Onania; or the Heinous Sin of Self-Pollution,* 8th ed. (London: Thomas Crouch, 1723), 18–19.

9. Anon. [Louis de la Caze], *L'Idée de l'homme physique et moral* (Paris: Guérin and Delatour, 1755), 292–300; Mr **** [Jean-Philippe Dutoit-Mambrini], *De l'Onanisme; ou discours philosophique et moral sur la luxure artificielle & sur tous les crimes relatifs* (Lausanne: Antoine Chapuis, 1760), 35, 43.

10. S. A. D. Tissot, *Onanism. Or, a Treatise upon the Disorders produced by Masturbation: or, the Dangerous Effects of Secret and Excessive Venery* (London: B. Thomas, 1766), 80; and see also Tissot's "Manstupration ou Manustupration," *Encyclopédie ou dictionnaire raisonné des sciences, des arts, et de métiers par une société des gens de lettres* (Genève, 1772), 10:51–54.

11. Anne C. Vila, *Enlightenment and Pathology: Sensibility in the Literature and Medicine of Eighteenth-Century France* (Baltimore: Johns Hopkins University Press, 1998), 94–107; Jesse Foot, *Observations upon the New Opinions of John Hunter in his late Treatise on the Venereal Disease* (London: T. Beckett, 1786), 138, 200.

12. G. Archibald Douglas, *The Nature and Causes of Impotence in Men, and Barrenness in Women Explained* (London: P. Brett, 1772), 18, 21; *Domestic Medicine* cited in Ludmilla Jordanova, "Interrogating the Concept of Reproduction in the Eighteenth Century," in Faye D. Ginsberg and Rayna Rapp, eds., *Conceiving the New World Order: The Global Politics of Reproduction* (Berkeley: University of California Press, 1995), 380; William

Buchan, *Observations Concerning the Prevention and Cure of the Venereal Disease* (London: T. Chapman, 1796), 220, 221; Christopher William Hufeland, *The Art of Prolonging Human Life* (London: J. Bell, 1797), 1:168; 2:13, 16.

13. David Stevenson, *The Beggar's Benison: Sex Clubs of Enlightenment Scotland* (East Linton: Tuckwell Press, 2001).

14. John Floyer, *The History of Cold Bathing Both Ancient and Modern with appendix by Dr. Edward Baynard* (London: William and John Innys, 1722), 26.

15. John Archer, *Every Man His Own Doctor* (London: Peter Lillicrap, 1671), 103; A Physician, *The Ladies Physical Directory* (London: By the author, 1739), 60, 61, 63, 65, 67.

16. William Brodum, *A Guide to Old Age, or, A Cure for the Indiscretions of Youth* (London: Myers, 1795), 2 vols.; "Collection of Advertisements of Patent and Proprietary Medicines," circa 1790–1810 (British Library); Ebenezer Sibley in *The Medical Mirror or, Treatise on the Impregnation of the Human Female* (London: 1794); Samuel Solomon, *A Guide to Health* (West Derby: J. Speed, 1817), 167, 168. And see also William H. Helfand, "Samuel Solomon and the Cordial Balm of Gilead," *Pharmacy in History* 31.4 (1989): 151–59.

17. James Hodson, *Nature's Assistant to the Restoration of Health* (London: J. Matthews, 1794), 123.

18. Dr. James Graham, *A Lecture on the Generation, Increase and Improvement of the Human Species* (London: Smith, 1783), 58; Roy Porter, *Health for Sale* (Manchester: Manchester University Press, 1989), 146–82.

19. *The Works of William Harvey*, trans. Robert Willis (London: Sydenham Society, 1965), 362.

20. Howard Adelman, *Marcello Malpighi and the Evolution of Biology* (Ithaca: Cornell University Press, 1966), 2:861; Clara Pinto-Correia, *The Ovary of Eve: Egg and Sperm and Preformation* (Chicago: University of Chicago Press, 1997), 43; Regnier de Graaf. *On the Human Reproductive Organs*, trans. H. D. Jocelyn and B. P. Setchell (Oxford: Blackwell, 1972), 12, 15, 29, 31–32, 44. And see also H. D. Joycelin and B. P. Setchell, eds., "Regnier de Graaf on the Human Reproductive Organs," *Journal of Reproduction and Fertility*, suppl. 17 (1972): 47–50.

21. Edward G. Ruestow, "Images and Ideas: Leeuwenhoek's Perception of the Spermatozoa," *Journal of the History of Biology* 16 (1983): 189; Peter J. Bowler, "Preformation and Pre-Existence in the Seventeenth Century: A Brief Analysis," *Journal of the History of Biology* 4 (1971): 221–44; Albrecht von Haller, *First Lines of Physiology* (Edinburgh: Charles Elliot, 1786), 1:428, 2:176, 177, 178, 181; and see also Sander Gilman, *Sexuality: An Illustrated History* (New York: John Wiley and Sons, 1989), 194–97.

22. Monsieur Pomet, *A Compleat History of Druggs* (London: R. Bonwicke, 1712), 79; A Physician, *Speculations on the Mode and Appearances of Impregnation in the Human Female* (Edinburgh, 1789), 43; F. E. Fodéré cited in Michael Ryan, *The Philosophy of Marriage* (London: Churchill, 1837), 331; F. E. Fodéré, "Impuissance," *Traité de médecine légale* (Paris: Mame, 1813), 366; F. N. L. Poynter, "Hunter, Spallanzani, and the History of Artificial Insemination," in G. L. Stevenson and R. P. Multhauf, eds., *Medicine, Science and Culture: Historical Essays in Honor of Oswei Temkin* (Baltimore: Johns Hopkins University Press, 1968); and see also Jean A. Mainil, "Dans les regles du plaisir: Médecine et obscenité au siècle des lumières," (Ph.D. diss., University of Michigan, 1994); Mary Fissell, "Gender and Generation: Representing Reproduction in Early Modern England," *Gender and History* 7 (1995): 433–56.

23. Estelle Cohen, "The Body as a Historical Category: Science and Imagination, 1660–1760," in Mary Winkler and Letha B. Cole, eds., *The Good Body: Asceticism in Contemporary Culture* (New Haven: Yale University Press, 1994), 67–90.

24. John Cleland, *Memoirs of a Woman of Pleasure* (1749; New York: Putnam's, 1963), 55–56; Marquis de Sade, *Justine or the Misfortunes of Virtue*, trans. Helen Weaver (New York: Bell Publishing, 1966), 18.

25. Cleland, *Memoirs of a Woman of Pleasure*, 51; De Sade, *Justine or the Misfortunes of Virtue*, 188–89.

26. Antoine Hotman, *Traicté de la dissolution du mariage par l'impuissance & froideur de l'homme ou de la femme* (Paris: Mamert Patisson, 1581); Ambroise Paré, *Oeuvres complètes*, ed. J.-F. Malgaigne (Paris: J.-B. Baillière, 1841) 3:668; and see also Thomas G. Benedek and Janet Kubinec, "The Evaluation of Impotence by Sexual Congress and Alternatives Thereto in Divorce Proceedings," *Transactions and Studies of the College of Physicians of Philadelphia* 4 (1982): 134–53; Monique Cuillieron, "Les causes matrimoniales des officialités de Paris au Siècle des Lumières, 1726–1789," *Revue historique de droit français et étranger* 66 (1988): 527–35.

27. Vincent Tagereau, *Discours sur l'impuissance de l'homme et de la femme* (Paris: Brayet and Rousset, 1612), 32, 91, 124, 192; and on de Langey see *Grand dictionnaire universel du XIXe siècle* (Paris: Pierre Larousse, 1866–90), 9:611.

28. Erasmus Darwin, *The Temple of Nature* (1803; London: Scolar Press, 1973), 33; Porter, "Mixed Feelings: The Enlightenment and Sexuality in Eighteenth-Century Britain," 6; Linda Walsh, "'Arms to Be Kissed a Thousand Times': Reservations About Lust in Diderot's Art Criticism," in Gill Perry and Michael Rossington, eds., *Feminity and Masculinity in Eighteenth-Century Art* (Manchester University Press, 1994).

29. Pierre Bayle, "Quellenec," in *The Dictionary Historical and Critical of Mr. Peter Bayle* (London: Midwinter, 1737), 4:799.

30. *Encyclopédie ou dictionnaire raisonné*, 8:333; and see William Harvey's earlier assertion: "Desire, indeed, without fulfilment wastes away so that in those who practise abstinence and chastity the testicles are meagre or the penis retracted into the belly, and they are completely frigid." Gweneth Whitteridge, ed., *The Anatomical Lectures of William Harvey* (London: Livingstone, 1964), 185; Antoine Gaspard Boucher d'Argis, *Principes sur la nullité du mariage pour cause d'impuissance* (London, 1756), 120–42; Voltaire, *A Philosophical Dictionary* (New York: E. R. Dumont, 1901), 1:182, 185, 187.

31. "Congrès aboli," *Causes célèbres et intéressantes*, ed. François Gayot de Pitaval (Amsterdam: J. F. Bassompierre, 1775), 8:191–270; "Réfutation de l'apologie du congrès," *Causes célèbres et intéressantes*, ed. François Gayot de Pitaval (Amsterdam: J. F. Bassompierre, 1775), 11:204–371. Examinations proved more than impotence; one carried out in 1765 revealed that mademoiselle Grand Jean was a woman, not a man, and therefore her marriage to another woman was void. *Grand dictionnaire universel du XIXe siècle* (Paris: Pierre Larousse, 1866–90), 9:611.

32. *Encyclopédie ou dictionnaire raisonné*, 8:334; Daniel Teysseire, *Obèse et impuissant: Le dossier médicale d'Elie-de-Beaumont, 1765–1776* (Grenoble: Editions Jérôme Millon, 1995), 29, 43, 120.

33. Teysseire, *Obèse et impuissant*, 60–61.

34. *Encyclopédie ou dictionnaire raisonné*, 8:333.

35. Thomas A. Forster, "Deficient Husbands: Manhood, Sexual Incapacity, and Male

Marital Sexuality in Seventeenth-Century New England," *William and Mary Quarterly* 56 (1999): 740; "Congrès aboli," 8:191–270.

36. *Boswell's London Journal, 1762–1763*, ed. Frederick A. Pottle (New York: McGraw-Hill, 1950), 117, 139; Jean-Jacques Rousseau, *Confessions*, trans. Christopher Kelly in *Collected Writings of Rousseau*, (Hanover: University Press of New England, 1995), 269.

37. John Hunter, *A Treatise on the Venereal Disease* (London: The author, 1786), 200–203. Hunter suggested a week's abstinence usually provided a cure; William Buchan, *Observations Concerning the Prevention and Cure of the Venereal Disease* (London: T. Chapman, 1796), 228.

38. Michael McKeown, "Historicizing Patriarchy: The Emergence of Gender Difference in England, 1660–1760," *Eighteenth-Century Studies* 28 (1995): 295–322; Michael Stolberg, "An Unmanly Vice: Self-Pollution, Anxiety, and the Body in the Eighteenth Century," *Social History of Medicine* 13 (2000): 19; Joanne Bailey, *Unquiet Lives: Marriage and Marriage Breakdown in England, 1660–1800* (Cambridge: Cambridge University Press, 2003), 163–66.

39. "Factum D****, Marie-Anne P.," *Recueil de pièces et mémoires pour les maîtres en l'art & science de chirurgie*, 10 (1771): 6, 8; François Fodéré, "Impuissance," *Traité de médecine légale* (Paris: Mame, 1813), 1:359–93; Jean Verdier, *La jurisprudence de la médecine, de la chirurgie, et de la pharmacie en France* (1762–63; Paris: J. B. Baillière, 1834), 102; Jeffrey Merrick, "Impotence in Court and at Court," *Studies in Eighteenth-Century Culture* 25 (1996): 188–93.

40. Pierre Roussell, *Système physique et morale de la femme* (Paris: Vincent, 1775); P. G. Cabanis, *Rapports du physique et du moral de l'homme* (Paris: Crapart, Caille, et Ravier, 1802); Ludmilla Jordanova, *Sexual Visions: Images of Gender in Science and Medicine Between the Eighteenth and Twentieth Centuries* (Madison: University of Wisconsin Press, 1989), 27; and see also Marlene Legates, "The Cult of Womanhood in Eighteenth-Century Thought," *Eighteenth-Century Studies* 10 (1976): 21–39; Katherine M. Rogers, *The Troublesome Helpmate: A History of Misogyny in Literature* (Seattle: University of Washington Press, 1966); Sarah Maza, *Private Lives and Public Affairs: The Causes Célèbres of Prerevolutionary France* (Berkeley: University of California Press, 1993).

41. Tim Hitchcock, *English Sexualities, 1700–1800* (London: St. Martin's Press, 1997), 39–40; Robert B. Shoemaker, *Gender in English Society, 1650–1850: The Emergence of Separate Spheres?* (London: Longman, 1998), 68–71.

42. William Byrd, *The London Diary (1717–1721) and Other Writings*, ed. Louis B. Wright and Marion Tinling (New York: Oxford University Press, 1958), 182; and see also 221, 250, 253, 324; Shawn Lisa Maurer, *Proposing Men: Dialectics of Gender and Class in the Eighteenth-Century Periodicals* (Stanford: Stanford University Press, 1998); George E. Haggerty, *Men in Love: Masculinity and Sexuality in the Eighteenth Century* (New York: Columbia University Press, 1999).

43. *The Poems of John Wilmot, Earl of Rochester*, ed. Keith Walker (Oxford: Basil Blackwell, 1984), 41–42; Nicholas Murray, *World Enough and Time: The Life of Andrew Marvell* (Boston: Little, Brown and Co., 1999), 196–97; A. D. Harvey, *Sex in Georgian England: Attitudes and Prejudices from the 1720s to the 1820s* (London: Duckworth, 1994), 137.

44. Philip Carter, "Men About Town: Representations of Foppery and Masculinity in Early Eighteenth-Century Urban Society," in Hannah Barker and Elaine Chalus, eds., *Gender in Eighteenth-Century England: Roles, Representations and Responsibilities* (London:

Longman, 1997), 39; G. J. Barker-Benfield, *The Culture of Sensibility: Sex and Society in Eighteenth-Century Britain* (Chicago: University of Chicago Press, 1992), 340–41; S. A. D. Tissot, *De la santé des gens de lettres* (Lausanne: Grasset, 1769); Marten, *Gonosologium Novum*, 39; Ettmüller, *Etmullerus Abridg'd*, 571.

45. David M. Turner, *Fashioning Adultery: Gender, Sex and Civility in England, 1660–1740* (Cambridge: Cambridge University Press, 2002).

46. Joseph wrote his brother that Louis had erections and emissions when alone but "never when on the job." Derek Beales, *Joseph II: In the Shadow of Maria Theresa, 1741–1780* (Cambridge: Cambridge University Press, 1987), 1:374; Lawrence Brockliss and Colin Jones, *The Medical World of Early Modern France* (Oxford: Clarendon Press, 1997), 632.

47. Antoine de Baecque, *Le Corps de l'histoire: métaphors et politique, 1770–1800* (Paris: Calmann-Lévy, 1993), 46, 47, 58, 67, 68; Merrick, "Impotence in Court and at Court," 194–98; Lynn Hunt, *The Family Romance of the French Revolution* (Berkeley: University of California Press, 1992), 50; Antoine de Baecque, "The 'Livres remplis d'horreur': Pornographic Literature and Politics at the Beginning of the French Revolution," in P. Wagner, ed., *Erotica and the Enlightenment* (New York: Peter Lang, 1991), 123–65; Joan Landes, *Visualizing the Nation: Gender, Representation, and Revolution in Eighteenth-Century France* (Ithaca: Cornell University Press, 2001), 66.

48. James Thomas Flexner, *Washington: The Indispensable Man* (Boston: Little, Brown, 1974), 42, 367; Richard Brookhiser, *Founding Father: Rediscovering George Washington* (New York: Free Press, 1996), 164.

CHAPTER FIVE

1. Mary Luytens, *Millais and the Ruskins* (London: John Murray, 1967), 230; see also 156, 193, 218, 229, 260–63; and see also Phyllis Rose, *Parallel Lives: Five Victorian Marriages* (New York: Knopf, 1983); Jennifer M. Lloyd, "Conflicting Expectations in Nineteenth-Century British Matrimony: The Failed Companionate Marriage of Effie Gray and John Ruskin," *Journal of Women's History* 11 (1999): 86–109.

2. Frederick Kirchhoff, *William Morris: The Construction of a Male Self, 1856–1872* (Athens: Ohio University Press, 1990), 66, 74, 148; Susan Chitty, *The Beast and the Monk: A Life of Charles Kingsley* (London: Hodder and Stoughton, 1974), 86; Luytens, *Millais and the Ruskins*, 263: Trev Lynn Broughton, *Men of Letters, Writing Lives: Masculinity and Literary Auto/Biography in the Late Victorian Period* (New York: Routledge, 1999), 144–45.

3. Peter Gay, *The Bourgeois Experience: Education of the Senses* (Oxford: Oxford University Press, 1984); M. Jeanne Peterson, *Family, Love, and Work in the Lives of Victorian Gentlewomen* (Bloomington: Indiana University Press, 1989), 41–45.

4. Michael Mason, *The Making of Victorian Sexuality* (Oxford: Oxford University Press, 1994), 126.

5. Ben Barker-Benfield, "The Spermatic Economy: A 19th Century View of Sexuality" in Michael Gordon, ed., *The American Family in Social-Historical Perspective* (New York: St. Martin's Press, 1978), 374–402; Karen Dubinsky, *The Second Greatest Disappointment: Honeymooning and Tourism at Niagara Falls* (Toronto: Between the Lines, 1999).

6. Joan Scott, "Statistical Representations of Work: The Politics of the Chamber of Commerce's Statistique de l'industrie à Paris, 1847–48," in Steven Lawrence Kaplan and Cynthia J. Koepp, eds., *Work in France: Representations, Meaning, Organization and*

Practice (Ithaca: Cornell University Press, 1986), p. 361n83; Alain Corbin, *Le Temps, le désir et l'horreur* (Paris: Aubier, 1991), 91–105.

7. Kim Townsend, *Manhood at Harvard: William James and Others* (New York: Norton, 1996), 59.

8. William Acton, *The Functions and Disorders of the Reproductive Organs* (London: John Churchill, 1857), 84; William Acton, *The Functions and Disorders of the Reproductive Organs*, 3rd ed. (London: John Churchill, 1862), 102–3.

9. James George Beaney, *The Generative System and Its Functions in Health and Disease* (Melbourne: F. F. Bailliere Publisher, 1875), 358; Walter Hamilton Acland Jacobson, *The Diseases of the Male Organs of Generation* (London: J. and A. Churchill, 1893), 489; Harry Campbell, *Differences in the Nervous Organization of Man and Woman* (London: Lewis, 1891), 153, 201–2; R. W. Shufeldt, "The Treatment of Psychological Impotency," *New Albany Medical Herald*, (Nov., 1898): 308.

10. Robert Ultzmann, *The Neuroses of the Genito-Urinary System in the Male*, trans. Gardner W. Allen (Philadelphia: F. A. Davis Co., 1902), 152.

11. Eugene Fuller, *Disorders of the Male Sexual Organs* (London: Young J. Pentland, 1895), 135.

12. R. J. Culverwell, *Medical Counsellings* (London: Sherwood and Co., 1841), 255; William A. Hammond, *Sexual Impotence in the Male and Female* (Detroit: George S. Davis, 1887). 82, 83; Shufeldt, "The Treatment of Psychological Impotency," 308, 309.

13. Pierre Garnier, *Impuissance physique et morale* (1883) cited in Stephen Kern, *Anatomy and Destiny: A Cultural History of the Human Body* (New York: Bobbs-Merrill, 1975), 106–7; Carl Degler, *At Odds: Women and the Family in America from the Revolution to the Present* (New York: Oxford University Press, 1980), 259–61.

14. William Buchan, *A Treatise on the Prevention and Cure of the Venereal Disease* (London: T. Cadell and W. Davies, 1808), 285; Louis Seraine, *De la santé des gens mariés* (Paris: F. Savy, 1865), 248; Hammond, *Sexual Impotence in the Male and Female*, 236, 237.

15. Charles Knowlton, *Fruits of Philosophy* (Mount Vernon: Peter Pauper Press, 1937), 89; Sylvester Graham, *A Lecture to Young Men on Chastity* (1834; London: Strange, 1843), xix; J. L. Curtis, *Manhood: The Causes of its Premature Decline with Directions for its Perfect Restoration* (London: Author, 1840), and its French translations *De la Virilité* (Paris, 1847) and *Guide médical du mariage* (Paris: F. Brachet, 1868); *L'ami discret* (Paris: R. and L. Parry, 1854), 44; George M. Beard, *Sexual Neurasthenia* (New York: E. B. Treat, 1884), 103; F. R. Sturgis, *Sexual Debility in Men*, (London: Rebman, 1901), 285, 287; Richard J. Ebbard, *How to Restore Life-Giving Energy* (London: Modern Medical Publishing Company, 1903), 80.

16. *Lexicon Balatronicum: A Dictionary of Buckish Slang, University Wit, and Pickpocket Eloquence* (London: C. Chappel, 1811); *The Letters of William Hazlitt*, ed. Hersche Moreland Sikes (London: Macmillam, 1978), 116; S. M. Waddams, *Sexual Slander in Ninteenth-Century England: Defamation in the Ecclesiastical Courts, 1815–1855* (Toronto: University of Toronto Press, 2000), 140.

17. *The Ri-tum Ti-Tum Songster* (London: West, 1837), 3–5, 44–46, 29–30; *The Rambler's Flash Songster* (London: West, 1865), 12, 23–24. In the British Library this volume is bound in with *The Flash Chaunter, The Cuckold's Nest*, and *The Cockchafer*; J. S. Bratton, *The Victorian Popular Ballad* (London: Macmillan, 1975), 159, 161, 184; Marie-Véronique Gauthier, *Chanson, sociabilité et grivoiserie au XIXe siècle* (Paris: Aubier, 1992), 248; Martine Segalen, *Mari et femme dans la société paysanne* (Paris: Flammarion, 1980), 138.

18. Auguste Debay, *Hygiène et physiologie du mariage* (Paris: E. Dentu, 1881), 261–62; John Cowan, *The Science of a New Life* (New York: Cowan and Co., 1880), 103; Léon Roger-Milès, *Nos Femmes et nos enfants: Choses sanglantes et criminalité* (Paris: E. Flammarion, 1893), 10–11 cited in Ann Louis Shapiro, *Breaking the Codes: Female Criminality in Fin-de-Siècle Paris* (Stanford: Stanford University Press, 1996), 200; Robert W. Taylor, *A Practical Treatise on Sexual Disorders* (London: Henry Kimpton, 1897), 96.

19. Cowan, *The Science of a New Life*, 369; Auguste Debay, *Histoire naturelle de l'homme et de la femme* (Paris: E. Dentu, 1868), 322; Bram Djikstra, *Evil Sisters: The Threat of Female Sexuality and the Cult of Manhood* (New York: Knopf, 1996); Cyndy Hendershot, *The Animal Within: Masculinity and the Gothic* (Ann Arbor: University of Michigan Press, 1998), 25.

20. Dr. L. J. Kahn, *Nervous Exhaustion: Its Cause and Cure* (New York: Kahn, 1870), 19–20; William H. Parker, *The Science of Life; or, Self-Preservation* (Boston: Peabody Medical Institute, 1881), 162; Albert H. Hayes, *The Science of Life, or, Self Preservation* (Boston: Peabody Medical Institute, 1868), 180, 181; and see also the *Lancet* 96 (August 13, 1870): 22–225.

21. Richard von Krafft-Ebing, *Psychopathia Sexualis*, 12th ed. (1903) in Lucy Bland and Laura Doan, eds., *Sexology Uncensored: The Documents of Sexual Science* (Cambridge: Polity Press, 1998), 46; Alexandre Parent-Duchâtelet, *De la prostitution dans la ville de Paris* (Paris: Baillière, 1836), 2 vols.

22. Frederick Hollick, *The Male Generative Organs in Health and Disease* (New York: T. W. Strong, 1851), 215.

23. Michael Ryan, *Lectures on Population, Marriage, and Divorce* (London: Renshaw and Rush, 1831), 13; Thomas Laycock, *Mind and Brain, or, The Correlations of Consciousness and Organization* (Edinburgh, Sutherland and Knox, 1860), 2:303–4.

24. Taylor, *A Practical Treatise on Sexual Disorders*, 78–79; Debay, *Hygiène et physiologie du mariage*, 263; Seraine, *De la santé des gens mariés*, 293.

25. Shufeldt, "The Treatment of Psychological Impotency," 310.

26. R. W. Shufeldt, "Impotency; Medically and Legally Considered" *Pacific Medical Journal* 48 (Jan., 1905): 5.

27. James Richard Smyth, "Impotence and Sterility," *Lancet* 36 (Aug. 23, 1841): 783.

28. O. S. Fowler, *Amativeness; or, Evils and Remedies of Excessive and Perverted Sexuality* (Manchester: John Heywood, 1851), 10, 12; Debay, *Histoire naturelle de l'homme et de la femme*, 321.

29. James G. Kiernan, "Sex Transformation and Psychic Impotence," *American Journal of Dermatology* (1905): 68, 70; Hammond, *Sexual Impotence in the Male and Female*, 14, 40; 67; Jean Lorrain, *Monsieur de Phocas*, trans. Francis Amery (London: Dedalus/Hippocrene, 1994), 35, 57; Sturgis, *Sexual Debility in Men*, 265, 313; and see also Jay Hatheway, *The Gilded Age Construction of Modern American Homophobia* (London: Palgrave Macmillan, 2003).

30. Alfred Binet, "Fétichisme dans l'amour," *Revue philosophique* 24 (1887): 143–67, 252–74; Hammond, *Sexual Impotence in the Male and Female*. 41, 80–81; Paolo Mantegazza, *Hygiène de l'amour* (Paris: A La Librairie Illustrée, 1887), 154–55; Robert A. Nye, "The Medical Origins of Sexual Fetishism," in Emily Apter and William Pietz, eds., *Fetishism as Cultural Discourse* (Ithaca: Cornell University Press, 1993), 13–30.

31. Richard von Krafft-Ebing, *Psychopathia Sexualis: A Medico-Forensic Study* (New York: Pioneer Publications, 1945), 13; and see also Jean-Martin Charcot and Valentin Magnan, "Inversion du sens génital," *Archives de neurologie* 3 (1882): 54–57.

32. Kiernan, "Sex Transformation and Psychic Impotence," 70; Hippolyte Bernheim, "De la psychothérapie dans les impotences et aberrations génésiques" *Revue médicale de l'est* 35 (1903): 225–29.

33. Chandak Sengoopta, "'A Mob of Incoherent Symptoms'? Neurasthenia in British Medical Discourse, 1860–1920," in Marijke Gijswijt-Hofstra and Roy Porter, eds., *Cultures of Neurasthenia: From Beard to the First World War* (New York: Rodopi, 2001), 97–116; Janet Oppenheimer, *"Shattered Nerves": Doctors, Patients, and Depression in Victorian England* (New York: Oxford University Press, 1991), 142, 143, 144; and see also Barbara L. Marshall, "Snips and Snails and Theorists' Tales: Classical Sociological Theory and the Making of 'Sex,'" *Journal of Classical Sociology* 2 (2002): 135–55.

34. Gail Bederman, *Manliness and Civilization: A Cultural History of Gender and Race in the United States, 1880–1917* (Chicago: University of Chicago Press, 1995); see also C. K. Mills, *Mental Overwork and Premature Disease Among Public and Professional Men* (Washington: Smithsonian Misc. Collections, 1885); David Frisby, *Fragments of Modernity: Theories of Modernity in the Work of Simmel, Kracauer, and Benjamin* (Cambridge: MIT Press, 1986), 72–74; William T. Belfield, *Diseases of the Urinary and Male Sexual Organs* (New York: William Wood and Company, 1884), 335.

35. George M. Beard, *American Nervousness: Its Causes and Consequences* (New York: G. P. Putnam's Sons, 1881), 153–54; George M. Beard, *Sexual Neurasthenia* (New York: E. B. Treat, 1884); Irving C. Rosse, "Sexual Incapacity in its Medico-Legal Relations," in R. A. Witthaus and Tracy C. Becker, eds., *Medical Jurisprudence: Forensic Medicine and Toxicology* (New York: William Wood, 1894), 2:395; A. Bassett Jones and Llewellyn J. Llewellyn, *Malingering or the Simulation of Disease and Mental Disease* (London: Heinemann, 1917), 532.

36. Beard, *Sexual Neurasthenia*, 26; C. H. F. Routh, *On Overwork and Premature Mental Decay: Its Treatment* (London: Baillière, Tindall, and Cox, 1886), 24; S. A. K. Strahan, *Marriage and Disease* (London: Kegan Paul, Trench, Trübner and Co., 1892); Biswanger cited in Doris Kaufman, "Neurasthenia in Wilhelmine Germany: Culture, Sexuality, and the Demands of Nature," in Marijke Gijswijt-Hofstra and Roy Porter, eds., *Cultures of Neurasthenia from Beard to the First World War* (Amsterdam: Rodopi, 2001), 167; Hammond, *Sexual Impotence in the Male and Female*, 23; Fernand Levillain, *La Neurasthénie* (Paris: Maloine, 1891), 98–99.

37. G. Frank Lydston, *Impotence and Sterility with Aberrations of the Sexual Function and Sex-Gland Implementation* (Chicago: Riverton Press, 1917), 122; Victor G. Vecki, *Sexual Impotence* (Philadelphia and London: W. B. Saunders Company, 1912), 91.

38. Richard Quain, *A Dictionary of Medicine* (London: Longmans, Green and Co., 1885), 690; Hayes, *The Science of Life, or, Self Preservation*, 170; Taylor, *A Practical Treatise on Sexual Disorders*, 96; Charles Féré, *The Evolution and Dissolution of the Sexual Instinct* (Paris: Carrington, 1904) cited in Robert A. Nye, *Sexuality* (Oxford: Oxford University Press, 1999), 174; Raymond Gamel cited in Frank Proschan, "'Syphilis, Opiomania, and Pederasty': Colonial Constructions of Vietnamese (and French) Social Diseases," *Journal of the History of Sexuality* 11 (2002): 625; and see also Ruth Bernard Yeazell, *Harems of the Mind: Passages of Western Art and Literature* (New Haven: Yale University Press, 2000); Ann Stoler, "Making Empire Respectable: The Politics of Race and Sexual Morality in Twentieth-Century Colonial Cultures," *American Ethnologist* 16 (1989): 54–55; Anne McClintock, *Imperial Leather: Race, Gender and Sexuality in Colonial*

Conquest (New York: Routledge, 1995); Mrinalini Sinha, *Colonial Masculinity: The 'Manly Englishman' and the 'Effeminate Bengali' in the Late Nineteenth Century* (Manchester: Manchester University Press, 1995).

39. Maurice de Fleury, *Les grands symptômes neurasthéniques: Pathogénie et traitement* (Paris: Alcan, 1901), 199–210.

40. Claudia Durst Johnson, "Impotence and Omnipotence in *The Scarlet Letter*," *New England Quarterly* 66 (1993): 594–612; D. A. Miller, "1839: Body *Bildung* and Textual Liberation," in Denis Holier, ed., *A New History of French Literature* (Cambridge, Mass.: Harvard University Press, 1989), 681–83.

41. Claire de Duras, *Olivier ou le secret*, ed. Denise Virieux (Paris: José Corti, 1971). Anka Muhlstein, *A Taste for Freedom: The Life of Astolphe de Custine*, trans. Theresa Waugh (New York: Helen Marx Books, 1996), 163–65. Custine, a homosexual, later married and had a son.

42. Stendhal [Henri Beyle], *Armance, or, Scenes from a Parisian Salon in 1827* (London: Merlin Press, 1960), 212–13, 214, 215; Stendhal, *Correspondance*, eds. Henri Martineau and V. del Litto (Paris: Bibliothèque de la Pléiade, 1967), 2:96–98. "Babilan," from Babilano Pallavicini, a seventeenth-century Italian, known for the scandal caused by the dissolution of his marriage.

43. Paul Désalmand, *Cher Stendhal: Un pari sur la gloire* (Charenton-Le-Pont: Presses de Valmy, 1999), 217–222; Stendhal, *De l'amour*, ed. Henri Martineau (Paris: Le Divan, 1927), 168–75.

44. Michel Folman, *Les impuissants de génie* (Paris: Debresse, 1956), 84; Honoré de Balzac, *Massimilla Doni* (Libraire José Corti, 1964), 92; Jean Lorrain, *Dans l'oratoire* (Paris: Dalou, 1888), 45.

45. Jean-Pierre Bertrand, Michel Biron, Jacques Dubois, and Jeannine Paque, *Le Roman célibataire: D'A Rebours à Paludes* (Paris: José Corti, 1996); Marie Bonaparte, *The Life and Works of Edgar Allan Poe* (London: Imago Publishing, 1949), 79, 219, 397, 656.

46. Gabrielle Houbre, *La discipline de l'amour: L'éducation sentimentale des filles et des garçons à l'âge du romantisme* (Paris: Plon, 1997), 113; Charles Bernheimer, *Figures of Ill Repute: Representing Prostitution in Nineteenth-Century France* (Cambridge, Mass.: Harvard University Press, 1989); Gustave Flaubert, *Correspondance*, ed. Jean Bruneau (Paris: Gallimard, 1973), 3:409; Maurice Le Blond, *Essai sur le naturisme* (Paris: Mercure de France, 1896) quoted in Jean Pierrot, *L'Imaginaire décadent, 1880–1900* (Paris: Presses Universitaires de France, 1977); and on Baudelaire's English counterpart Algernon Charles Swinburne see Jean Overton Fuller, *Swinburne: A Critical Biography* (Chatto and Windus, 1968), 178–79; Théophile Gautier, *Romans, contes et nouvelles*, ed. Pierre Laubriet (Paris: Gallimard, 2002), 1017; Pierrot, *L'Imaginaire décadent, 1880–1900*, 158; see also Barbara Spackman, *Decadent Genealogies: The Rhetoric of Sickness from Baudelaire to D'Annunzio* (Ithaca: Cornell University Press, 1989); Folman, *Les impuissants de génie*, 40.

47. Ernest Raynaud, in *La Mêlée symboliste* (Paris: La Renaissance du Livre, 1918), 1:65; Jacques de Nittis, *Vénus ennemie* (Paris: Editions de la Revue Blanche, 1900); Henri Stofft, "Une impuissance érectile en 1900," *Histoire des sciences médicale* 26 (1992): 179–87; Alfred Vallette, *Le Roman d'un homme sérieux* (Paris: Mercure de France, 1994), 46.

48. Cazals cited in Auriant [Alexandre Hadjivassiliou], *Souvenirs sur Madame Rachilde* (Paris: A l'Ecart, 1989), 9; Frank Wedekind, *Diary of an Erotic Life*, ed. Gerhard Hay,

trans. W. E. Yuill (Oxford: Basil Blackwell, 1990), 67; Joseph Gérard, *La Grande névrose* (Paris: Flammarion, 1889), 437.

49. Paul Bourget, *Essais de psychologie contemporaine*, 99–106; Emily Apter, introduction to Octave Mirbeau's "Selections" in Asti Hustvedt, ed., *The Decadent Reader: Fiction, Fantasy, and Perversion from Fin-de-Siècle France* (New York: Zone Books, 1998), 974; Richard Noël, *A l'aube du symbolisme; hydropathes, fumistes et décadents* (Paris: Nizet, 1961), 256–57; Max Nordau, *Degeneration* (1895; London: Heineman, 1913), 18; Robert Baldick, *La vie de J. K. Huysmans* (Paris: Editions Denoël, 1958), 89.

50. Regenia Gagnier, *Idylls of the Marketplace: Oscar Wilde and the Victorian Public* (Stanford: Stanford University Press, 1986), 160; Leon Edel, *Henry James: The Untried Years: 1843–1870* (Philadelphia, New York: J. B. Lippincott Company: 1953), 175–76, 183; Elaine Showalter, *Sexual Anarchy: Gender and Culture at the Fin de Siècle* (New York: Penguin, 1990), 148.

51. Margaret Waller, *The Male Malady: Fictions of Impotence in the French Romantic Novel* (New Brunswick: Rutgers University Press, 1993), 3.

52. Sally Peters, *Bernard Shaw: The Ascent of the Superman* (New Haven: Yale University Press, 1996), 118; Eugène Terraillon, *L'Honneur, sentiment et principe moral* (Paris: Alcan, 1912), 171–78; Carolyn A. Conley, *The Unwritten Law: Criminal Justice in Victorian Kent* (New York: Oxford University Press, 1991), 91n71.

53. John Glaister, "The Medico-Legal Aspects of Impotency in the Sexes," *The Practitioner*, 45 (1915): 23–30; Irving C. Rosse, "Sexual Incapacity in its Medico-Legal Relations," Witthaus and Becker, *Medical Jurisprudence*, 2:393; Marcellin-Casimir Michal, *Considérations médico-légales sur l'impuissance* (Montpellier: Martel, 1814); Jean-Paul Branlard, *Le Sexe et l'état des personne: aspects historique, sociologique et juridique* (Paris: Librairie Générale de Droit et de Jurisprudence, 1993), 299–300.

CHAPTER SIX

1. J. A. Murray, "Ligation of the Dorsal Vein of the Penis for Functional Impotence, with a Report of Five Cases" *Journal of the American Medical Association* (hereafter *JAMA*) 29 (Oct. 9, 1897): 733.

2. Ornella Moscucci, *The Science of Women; Gynaecology and Gender in England, 1800–1929* (Cambridge: Cambridge University Press, 1990), 1. Urologists at the 1891 Congress of American Physicians did create an andrology section, but nothing came of it. See *JAMA*, 17 (1891): 63.

3. Toronto *Daily Mail*, Oct. 20, 1892; John F. Kasson, *Houdini, Tarzan, and The Perfect Man: The White Male Body and the Challenge of Modernity in America* (New York: Hill and Wang, 2001), 49; Harvey Green, *Fit for America: Health, Fitness, Sport, and American Society* (New York: Pantheon Books, 1986), 252; *Le Sourire*, Aug. 25, 1899; F. B. Courtenay, *Revelations of Quacks and Quackery* (London: H. Baillière, 1865), 8.

4. R. and L. Perry and Co., *Silent Friend* (London: By the Authors, 1847); Goss and Company, *Hygeiana: A Non-Medical Analysis of the Complaints Incidental to Females* (London: Sherwood and Co., 1834), 59–60; Goss and Company, *The Aegis of Life: A Non-Medical Commentary on the Indiscretions Arising from Human Frailty* (London: Goss and Company, 1830); Sylvester Graham, *A Lecture to Young Men on Chastity* (London: Strange, 1843), 54; Walter De Roos, *The Medical Adviser* (London: By the Author, 1850), 30–38; Samuel La'Mert,

Self-preservation : A Medical Treatise on Nervous & Physical Debility, Spermatorrhœa, Impotence & Sterility with Practical Observations on the use of the Microscope in the Treatment of the Diseases of the Generative System (London: Reynell & Weight, 1855), *La Préservation personnelle: traité médicale sur les maladies des organes de la génération* (Paris: Ledoyen and Laroque, 1848); Samuel La'Mert *La Préservation personnelle*, traduit de l'anglais par M. J. M. et D. D. M. (Paris: Laroque Jeune, 1860); William H. Parker, *The Science of Life; or, Self-Preservation* (Boston: Peabody Medical Institute, 1881), 110; Albert H. Hayes, *The Science of Life, or, Self Preservation* (Boston: Peabody Medical Institute, 1868), 206.

5. William Acton, *The Functions and Disorders of the Reproductive Organs in Childhood, Youth, Adult Age, and Advanced Life Considered in their Physiological, Social and Moral Relations*, 3rd ed. (London: John Churchill, 1862), 209; *Handbook of Dr. Kahn's Museum* (London: W. Snell, 1863); L. J. Kahn, *Nervous Exhaustion: Its Cause and Cure* (New York: Kahn, 1870).

6. *Lancet* 36 (Sep. 25, 1841): 923–24; 41 (Dec. 9, 1843): 329; John Corry, *The Detector of Quackery* (London: Crosby, 1802), 58; Golding Bird, *Urinary Deposits, Their Diagnosis, Pathology, and Therapeutical Indications* (London; John Churchill, 1857), 379; Reginald Harrison, *Lectures on the Surgical Disorders of the Urinary Organs* (London: Churchill, 1887), 530; Olive Anderson, *Suicide in Victorian and Edwardian England* (Oxford: Clarendon Press, 1987), 187.

7. Harrison, *Lectures*, 529; Homer Bostwick, *A Treatise on the Nature and Treatment of Seminal Diseases, Impotency, and Other Kindred Affections* (New York: Burgess, Stringer and Co., 1848), 10; Acton, *The Functions and Disorders of the Reproductive Organs*, 1st ed. (1857), 92.

8. Michael Ryan, *Lectures on Population, Marriage, and Divorce* (London: Renshaw and Rush, 1831), 10, 13; R. J. Culverwell, *Medical Counsellings* (London: Sherwood and Co., 1841), 243–285; Acton, *The Functions and Disorders of the Reproductive Organs* (1875, 6th ed.), 87; Frederick Hollick, *The Male Generative Organs in Health and Disease* (New York: T. W. Strong, 1851), 199; James George Beaney, *The Generative System and Its Functions in Health and Disease* (Melbourne: F. F. Bailliere Publisher, 1875), 212.

9. Augustus Gardner, *The Causes and Curative Treatment of Sterility* (New York: De Witt and Davenport, 1856), 59; Acton, *The Functions and Disorders of the Reproductive Organs*, 1st ed. (1857), 72; Félix Roubaud, *Traité de l'impuissance et de la stérilité chez l'homme et chez la femme* (Paris: J.-B. Baillière, 1855), 256; Louis Seraine, *De la santé des gens mariés* (Paris: F. Savy, 1865), 249.

10. Dr. Rauland (Félix Roubaud), *Le Livre des époux* (Paris: La Librairie Nouvelle, 1852), 114–35; Beaney, *The Generative System*, 218; George Harley, *The Urine and Its Derangements* (London: Churchill, 1872), 276; R. W. Shufeldt, "Impotency; Medically and Legally Considered" *Pacific Medical Journal* 48 (Jan. 1905): 6.

11. William A. Hammond, *Sexual Impotence in the Male and Female* (Detroit: George S. Davis, 1887), 129; Auguste Debay, *Histoire naturelle de l'homme et de la femme* (Paris: E. Dentu, 1868), 328; Robert W. Taylor, *A Practical Treatise on Sexual Disorders* (London: Henry Kimpton, 1897), 96; Thomas Low Nichols, *Esoteric Anthropology (The Mysteries of Man)* (Malver: T. L. Nichols, 1873), 89; B. G. Jefferis and J. L. Nichols, *Search Lights on Health* (Naperville, Ill.: J. K. Nichols, 1894), 305, 390; and see also Kevin J. Mumford, "'Lost Manhood' Found: Male Sexual Impotence and Victorian Culture in the United States," *Journal of the History of Sexuality* 3 (1992): 39.

12. James H. Dunn, "Impotence in the Male and Its Treatment," *Northwestern Lancet* 5 (Nov. 1, 1885): 445; Walter cited in Michael Mason, *The Making of Victorian Sexuality* (Oxford: Oxford University Press, 1994), 47; Roubaud, *Traité de l'impuissance*, 1:311.

13. R. J. Culverwell, *Lecture to Young Men on Chastity and Its Infringements* (London: Sherwood, 1847), 36; Jean Stengers and Anne van Neck, *Histoire d'une grande peur: La masturbation* (Brussels: Editions de l'Université de Bruxelles, 1984), 27; Jayme A. Sokolow, *Eros and Modernization: Sylvester Graham, Health Reform, and the Origins of Victorian Sexuality in America* (Rutherford: Fairleigh Dickinson University Press, 1983), 77–99; Ed Cohen, *Talk on the Wilde Side: Toward a Genealogy of a Discourse on Male Sexualities* (London: Routledge, 1993), 35–68.

14. Samuel W. Gross, *A Practical Treatise on Impotence, Sterility, and Allied Disorders of the Male Sexual Organs* (London: Henry Kimpton, 1881), 64; Ryan, *Lectures on Population*, 14; James Richard Smyth, *Miscellaneous Contributions to Pathology and Therapeutics* (London: Simpkin, Marshall, and Co., 1844), 208; Hollick, *The Male Generative Organs*; Hammond, *Sexual Impotence*, 94; Robert Ultzmann, *The Neuroses of the Genito-Urinary System in the Male*, trans. Gardner W. Allen (Philadelphia: F. A. Davis, 1890), 154; W. Frank Glenn, "Impotence in the Male," *Southern Practitioner*, June 1892, 240.

15. François Lallemand, *On the Causes, Symptoms and Treatment of Spermatorrhoea*, trans. Henry J. McDougall (London: John Churchill, 1851); Richard Dawson, *An Essay on Spermatorrhoea and Urinary Deposits* (London: Aylotte and Jones, 1851); Beaney, *The Generative System*, 231; George Drysdale, *The Elements of Social Science* (London: Truelove, 1875), 99; and see also Thésée Pouillet, *La Spermatorrhée* (Paris: Delahaye, 1877).

16. William Buchan, *A Treatise on the Prevention and Cure of the Venereal Disease* (London: T. Cadell and W. Davies, 1808), 292; John L. Milton, *Practical Remarks on the Treatment of Spermatorrhoea and some forms of Impotence* (London: S. Highley, 1854).

17. Samuel Solomon, *A Guide to Health* (West Derby: J. Speed, 1817), 167, 168; Henry Beasley, *The Druggist's General Receipt Book* (London: John Churchill, 1850), 150; E. Senate, *The Medical Monitor, Containing Observations on the Effects of Early Dissipation* (London: By the author, 1810); Walter De Roos, *The Medical Adviser* (London: By the author, 1850), 48, 54.

18. Sylvester Graham, *A Lecture to Young Men on Chastity* (London: Strange, 1843), 61–62.

19. Harvey Green, *Fit for America: Health, Fitness, Sport, and American Society* (New York: Pantheon Books, 1986), 266; Courtenay, *Revelations of Quacks and Quackery*, 18; M. H. Utley, *Didactic Elucidations, respecting the Original Sin, or the Sin of Imagination, and its Consequences, Morally, Physically and Mentally* (Montreal, 1874).

20. Acton and Maudsley cited in Trev Lynn Broughton, *Men of Letters, Writing Lives: Masculinity and Literary Auto/Biography in the Late Victorian Period* (New York: Routledge, 1999), 149–50, 191n13; Dawson, *An Essay on Spermatorrhoea*, 125; Hayes, *The Science of Life*, 183; Nichols, *Esoteric Anthropology*, 290.

21. Acton, *The Functions and Disorders of the Reproductive Organs*, 2nd ed. (1867), 160–62; Culverwell, *Lecture to Young Men*, 89; Seraine, *De la santé des gens mariés*, 302; Jean-Alexis Belliol, *Conseils aux hommes affaiblis* (Paris: Dentu, 1877); Auguste Debay, *Hygiène et physiologie du mariage* (Paris: E. Dentu, 1881), 272.

22. Jefferis and Nichols, *Search Lights on Health*, 401–2; Nichols, *Esoteric Anthropology*, 181; John Cowan, *The Science of a New Life* (New York: Cowan and Co., 1869); Bernarr Macfadden, *The Virile Powers of Superb Manhood* (New York: Physical Culture Publishing Company, 1900), 15.

23. Hollick, *The Male Generative Organs*, 302–20; Joseph Morel de Rubempré, *Les Secrets de la génération* (Paris: Roy-Terry, 1830), 293–97; Glenn, "Impotence in the Male," 242.

24. William T. Belfield, *Diseases of the Urinary and Male Sexual Organs* (New York: William Wood and Company, 1884), 339; Stead cited in Judith R. Walkowitz, *City of Dreadful Delight: Narratives of Sexual Danger in Late-Victorian London* (Chicago: University of Chicago Press, 1992), 100; Roubaud, *Traité de l'impuissance*, 213; and see also Debay, *Hygiène et physiologie du mariage*, 268–87.

25. Rauland, *Le Livre des époux*, 224; Hollick, *The Male Generative Organs*, 216; John J. Caldwell, "Impotence and Sterility—Their Causes and Treatment by Electricity and Damiana, etc.," *Virginia Medical Monthly*, 1879, 441; Julius Althus, *On Impotency and Its Treatment by Electricity* (London: Longmans, Green and Co., 1896); Ultzmann, *The Neuroses of the Genito-Urinary System*, 153; Hammond, *Sexual Impotence in the Male and Female*, 200–201, 207; and on the vacuum pump see Seraine, *De la santé des gens mariés*, 307.

26. T. B. Curling, *A Practical Treatise on the Diseases of the Testis* (London: John Churchill and Sons, 1866), 399; Culverwell, *Lecture to Young Men*, 54–55; George Drysdale, *The Elements of Social Science* (London: Truelove, 1875), 81; Paolo Mantegazza, *Hygiène de l'amour* (Paris: A La Librairie Illustrée, 1887); Joseph W. Howe, *Excessive Venery, Masturbation, and Continence* (New York: Bermingham, and Co., 1883), 184; Gross, *A Practical Treatise on Impotence*, 64.

27. Dawson, *An Essay on Spermatorrhoea*, 48; Hammond, *Sexual Impotence in the Male and Female*, 26, 96; Charles E. Rosenberg, "Sexuality, Class and Role in Nineteenth-Century America," in Elizabeth H. Pleck and Joseph H. Pleck, eds., *The American Man* (Englewood Cliffs, NJ: Prentice-Hall, 1980), 230; Freddy Mortier, Willem Colen, and Frank Simon, "Inter-Scientific Reconstructions in the Discourse on Masturbation, 1760–1950," *Paedagogica Historica* 30 (1994): 839–40.

28. James Paget, *Clinical Lectures and Essays* (London: Longman Green, 1875), 268–92; Gross, *A Practical Treatise on Impotence*, 28.

29. George G. Gascoyen, "On Spermatorrhoea and Its Treatment," *British Medical Journal* 1 (Jan.–June, 1872): 67–69, 95–96; William A. Roberts, *A Practical Treatise on Urinary and Renal Diseases* (London: Smith, Elder and Co., 1885), 169–71.

30. Dunn, "Impotence in the Male and Its Treatment," 446; E. R. Palmer, "A Contribution to the Physiology of Sexual Impotence" *New York Medical Journal* 10 (July 2, 1892): 5.

31. James Richard Smyth, "Impotence and Sterility," *Lancet* 36 (Aug. 23, 1841): 783; Hammond, *Sexual Impotence in the Male and Female*, 182; Debay, *Hygiène et physiologie du mariage*, 260; Acton, *The Functions and Disorders of the Reproductive Organs*, 2nd ed. (1867), 149; M. E. Descourtilz, *De l'impuissance et de la stérilité* (Paris: Masson et Yonet, 1831), 2:130–33; Roubaud, *Traité de l'impuissance*, 1:186; and see also Gail Pat Parsons, "Equal Treatment for All: Medical Remedies for Male Sexual Problems," *Journal of the History of Medicine* 32 (1977): 55–71; Ellen Bayuk Rosenman, "Body Doubles: The Spermatorrhea Panic," *Journal of the History of Sexuality* 12 (2003): 392–93.

32. Roubaud, *Traité de l'impuissance*, 1:144; Acton, *The Functions and Disorders of the Reproductive Organs*, 6th ed. (1875), 86; Glenn, "Impotence in the Male," 239; Hollick, *The Male Generative Organs*, 200.

33. Bransford Lewis, "A Materialistic View of Sexual Impotence," *Medical News* 61 (Nov. 19, 1892): 571–72.

34. Hammond, *Sexual Impotence in the Male and Female*, 183; Gilbert Ballet, *Neurasthenia*, trans. P. Campbell Smith (London: Kimpton, 1911), 364; Henry M. Lyman, *The Practical Home Physician* (1893), 531, cited in John S. and Robin Haller, *The Physician and Sexuality in Victorian America* (Urbana: University of Illinois Press, 1974), 231; and see also Richard Quain, *A Dictionary of Medicine* (London: Longmans, Green and Co., 1885), 690–91.

35. Ultzmann cited in Ballet, *Neurasthenia*, 365; Ryan, *Lectures on Population*, 34; Mason, *The Making of Victorian Sexuality*, 184.

36. Maurice M. Tinterow, *Foundations of Hypnosis from Mesmer to Freud* (Springfield, Ill.: Charles C. Thomas, 1970), 556, 564; Hippolyte Bernheim, "De la psychothérapie dans les impotences et aberrations génésiques," *Revue Médicale de l'est*, 35 (1903): 225–29.

37. Ryan, *Lectures on Population*, 14, 26; Descourtilz, *De l'impuissance*, 1:328.

38. Austin Flint, *A Treatise on the Principles and Practices of Medicine* (Philadelphia: Henry Lea, 1881), 940–41; Gross, *A Practical Treatise on Impotence*, 62, 65, 66; George M. Beard, *Sexual Neurasthenia* (New York: E. B. Treat, 1884), 90–91; Belfield, *Diseases of the Urinary and Male Sexual Organs*, 339.

39. Gross, *A Practical Treatise on Impotence*, 32; Acton, *The Functions and Disorders of the Reproductive Organs*, 1st ed. (1857), 90; Ultzmann, *The Neuroses of the Genito-Urinary System in the Male*, 149; Lewis, "A Materialistic View of Sexual Impotence," 570–73.

40. Stephen Kern, *Anatomy and Destiny: A Cultural History of the Human Body* (New York: Bobbs-Merrill, 1975), 105; Christopher David O'Shea, "Visions of Masculinity: Home-Health Advice Literature, Medical Discourse and Male Sexuality in English-Canada, 1870–1914," (Ph.D. diss., University of Guelph, 2003), 183–201; Angela Gugliotta, "'Dr. Sharp and His Little Knife,': Therapeutic and Punitive Origins of Eugenic Vasectomy—Indiana, 1892–1921," *Journal of the History of Medicine* 53 (1998): 373.

41. F. R. Sturgis, "On the Physical Causes of Sexual Debility in the Male, as Distinguished from the Psychical Causes," *Canada Lancet* 26 (1893–94): 260; Ultzmann, *The Neuroses of the Genito-Urinary System in the Male*, 148; Eugene Fuller, *Disorders of the Male Sexual Organs* (London: Young J. Pentland, 1895); J. S. Wooten, "Ligation of the Dorsal Vein of the Penis as a Cure for Atonic Impotence," *Texas Medical Journal* 18 (1902–3): 325–28; and see also G. Frank Lydston, "The Surgical Treatment of Impotence," *American Journal of Medicine* 15 (1903): 1571; Murray, "Ligation of the Dorsal Vein of the Penis," 733.

42. Glenn, "Impotence in the Male," 241; Gross, *A Practical Treatise on Impotence*, 41; Taylor, *A Practical Treatise*, 83–84; P. C. Remondino, *History of Circumcision* (Philadelphia: F. A. Davis Co., 1900), 206–13, 327n79; and see David L. Gollaher, *Circumcision: The World's Most Controversial Surgery* (New York: Basic Books, 2000); Robert A. Darby, *Surgical Temptation: The Demonization of the Foreskin and the Rise of Circumcision in Britain* (Chicago: University of Chicago Press, 2005).

43. G. Frank Lydston, *Impotence and Sterility* (Chicago: Riverton Press, 1917), 90.

44. Gross, *A Practical Treatise on Impotence*, 87; Ultzmann, *The Neuroses of the Genito-Urinary System in the Male*, 140; Mantegazza, *Hygiène de l'amour*, 129–30.

CHAPTER SEVEN

1. Ernest Hemingway, *The Sun Also Rises* (New York: Charles Scribner's Sons, 1926), 15, 17. On Hemingway's interest in the subject, and his own organ ("Mr. Scrooby"), see

Kenneth Lynn, *Hemingway* (New York: Simon and Schuster, 1987), 327–29, 398–401, 457–61, 513, 519.

2. Gabriel Chevallier, *La Peur* (1930; Paris: Le Livre Club du Libraire, 1951), 96; Jean-Yves Le Naour, *Misères et tourments de la chair durant la Grande Guerre: les moeurs sexuelles des français, 1914–1918* (Paris: Aubier, 2002), 311–19; Ernst Toller, *Hinkemann* (1923) in *Seven Plays* (New York: Liveright Publishing, 1936); Patrice Petro, *Joyless Streets: Women and Melodramatic Representation in Weimar Germany* (Princeton: Princeton University Press, 1989); Richard W. McCormick, *Gender and Sexuality in Weimar Modernity: Film, Literature, and "New Objectivity"* (New York: Palgrave, 2001).

3. Joanna Bourke, *Dismembering the Male: Men's Bodies, Britain and the Great War* (London: Reaktion Books, 1996); Kevin White, *The First Sexual Revolution: The Emergence of Male Heterosexuality in Modern America* (New York: New York University Press, 1993); Maurizia Boscagli, *Eye on the Flesh: Fashions of Masculinity in the Early Twentieth Century* (Boulder, Colo.: Westview, 1996); Michael Kane, *Modern Men: Mapping Masculinity in English and German Literature, 1880–1930* (London: Cassell, 1999); James Joyce, *Ulysses* (London: Bodley Head, 1937), 687; and on Lawrence's own impotence and his belief in male menopause, see, Jeffrey Meyers, *D. H. Lawrence: A Biography* (London: Macmillan, 1990), 331–32, 341; David Ellis, *D. H. Lawrence, Dying Game, 1922–1930* (Cambridge: Cambridge University Press, 1998), 355–56, 507–8.

4. Charles A. Mercier, "A Problem in Diagnosis" *Lancet* 167 (Mar. 10, 1906): 670–71.

5. Sigmund Freud, "On the Universal Tendency to Debasement in the Sphere of Love," (1912), *Standard Edition of the Complete Psychological Works of Sigmund Freud*, ed. James Strachey (London: Hogarth Press, 1953) (hereafter *SE*), 11:179.

6. Freud, "On the History of the Psycho-Analytic Movement," (1914), *SE*, 14:15.

7. Freud, "Observations on Transference-Love," cited in Paul Roazen, *Freud and His Followers* (New York: Knopf, 1975), 54.

8. Elisabeth Roudinesco, *Histoire de la psychanalyse en France* (Paris: Seuil, 1986), 1:32.

9. Freud, review of Maxim Steiner's *The Psychical Disorders of Male Potency* (1913), *SE*, 12:345; "Inhibitions, Symptoms and Anxiety" (1926), *SE*, 20:88.

10. Freud, "Extracts from Fliess Papers" (1892–1899), *SE*, 1:180, 181, 198–99.

11. Freud, "On the Universal Tendency to Debasement in the Sphere of Love" (1912), *SE*, 11:183.

12. Freud, "On the Universal Tendency to Debasement in the Sphere of Love," *SE*, 11:182, 185; Wilhelm Reichs, *Early Writings*, trans. Philip Schmitz (New York: Farrar, Straus and Giroux, 1975), 77.

13. Freud, "On the Universal Tendency to Debasement in the Sphere of Love," *SE*, 11: 184–85, 188.

14. Freud, "Some Psychical Consequences of the Anatomical Distinction Between the Sexes" (1925), *SE*, 19: 257; "Fetishism" (1927), *SE*, 21:154; "Three Essays on the Theory of Sexuality" (1905), *SE*, 7:195; "Leonardo da Vinci and a Memory of Childhood" (1910), *SE*, 11:96; but see also Karen Horney, "Dread of Women," in *Feminine Psychology* (New York: Norton, 1967), 133–46; Sarah Kofman, *L'Enigme de la femme, la femme dans les textes de Freud* (Paris: Galilée, 1980).

15. Freud, "Obsessive Actions and Religious Practices" (1907), *SE*, 9:121 (but see Ovid, *Amores*, 3.7.83–84 in *The Love Poems*, ed. A. D. Melville [Oxford: Oxford University Press, 1999] for a suspiciously similar story of a young woman whose lover could not

perform: "And lest her maids should know of this disgrace / To cover it, spilt water on the place"); "The Interpretation of Dreams" (1900), *SE*, 4:187, 291; and on the rarity of analysts being explicitly told of the problem see Wilhelm Stekel, *Impotence in the Male*, trans. Oswald H. Boltz (1923; New York: Liveright, 1927), 1:42.

16. Freud, "Fragment of an Analysis of a Case of Hysteria" (1905), *SE*, 7:47.

17. Freud, "Psychopathology of Everyday Life" (1901), *SE*, 6:206.

18. Freud, "The Interpretation of Dreams," *SE*, 5:364, 472–73.

19. Freud, "Extracts from the Fliess Papers," *SE*, 1:262. Following Fliess's belief in male sexual cycles, Freud declared himself to be impotent every twenty-eight days. Jeffrey Moussaieff Masson, ed., *The Complete Letters of Sigmund Freud to Wilhelm Fliess* (Cambridge, Mass.: Harvard University Press, 1985), 215. Stekel agreed that examination dreams were related to fear of failure: "The examination anxiety of the neurotic often reveals itself as sexual dread. . . . Mostly these people are also impotent. Fear of the woman corresponds to their fear of the examiner" (*Conditions of Nervous Anxiety and Their Treatment*, trans. Rosalie Gabler [1923; London: Routledge and Kegan Paul, 1950], 245); Ernest Jones, *Sigmund Freud, Life and Work* (London: Hogarth Press, 1955), 2:431; Freud to Fleiss, October 31, 1897, "Extracts from the Fliess Papers," *SE*, 1:267; Emma Jung to Freud, November 6, 1911, in *The Freud/Jung Letters*, ed. William McGuire (Princeton: Princeton University Press, 1974), 456.

20. Freud, "'Civilized' Sexual Morality and Modern Nervousness" (1908), *SE*, 9:201.

21. Reich, *Early Writings*, 201–2; and see also Stekel, *Conditions of Nervous Anxiety*, 249; Karl Abraham, *Clinical Papers and Essays on Psycho-Analysis*, trans. Hilda C. Abraham (London: Hogarth Press, 1955), 63.

22. Stekel, *Impotence in the Male*, 1:11; and on the fetishes some men needed in order to perform see, Wilhelm Stekel, *Sexual Aberrations: The Phenomena of Fetishism in Relation to Sex*, trans. S. Parker (1923; New York: Liveright, 1930), 1:202, 312–13; and for his treatment of women see Stekel's *Frigidity in Woman* (New York: Boni and Liveright, 1926).

23. Paul E. Stepansky, *In Freud's Shadow: Adler in Context* (London: Analytic Press, 1983), 90, 116; Henry V. Dicks, *Clinical Studies in Psychopathology* (London: Edward Arnold, 1947), 167.

24. Otto Fenichel, *The Psychoanaltyic Theory of Neurosis* (New York: Norton, 1945), 170, 172.

25. Ernest Jones, *Papers on Psycho-Analysis* (London: Baillière, Tindall and Cox, 1918), 550; Theodor Reik, *Of Love and Lust* (New York: Farrar, Strauss and Co., 1941), 430, 434.

26. Reik, *Of Love and Lust*, 431; Israel S. Wechsler, *The Neuroses* (Philadelphia; W. B. Saunders, 1929), 267; and see also John F. W. Meagher, *A Study of Masturbation and the Psychosexual Life* (London: Bailliere, Tindall and Cox, 1929).

27. Freud, "On the Universal Tendency to Debasement in Love," *SE*, 11:187.

28. Wilfred Harris, "Impotence in Men," *Practitioner* 95 (July, 1915): 9; Wechsler, *The Neuroses*, 208; Jones, *Papers on Psycho-Analysis*, 552–53; Meagher, *A Study of Masturbation*, 45; Dicks, *Clinical Studies in Psychopathology*, 163–64.

29. Stekel, *Impotence in the Male*, 2:183, 250–51; and see also Wilhelm Stekel, *Compulsion and Doubt*, trans. Emil Gutheil (1927; London: Peter Nevill Ltd., 1950), 392–97; Wilhelm Stekel, *Marriage at the Crossroads*, trans. Allen D. Garman (New York: William Godwin, 1931), 95; Stekel, *Technique of Analytical Psychotherapy*, trans. Eden and Cedar Paul (New York: W.W. Norton, 1940), 159; Wilhelm Stekel, *The Homosexual Neurosis*, trans. James S. van Teslaar (1921; New York: Emerson Books, 1945).

30. Sandor Ferenczi, "De l'impuissance psycho-sexuelle," *Psychoanalyse I. Oeuvres complètes 1908-1912* (Paris: Payot, 1968).

31. Wilhelm Stekel, *The Autobiography of Wilhelm Stekel* (New York: Liveright, 1950), 107–8, 123; Stekel, *Conditions of Nervous Anxiety*, 248, 254; Stekel, *Marriage at the Crossroads*, 48; Stekel, *Technique of Analytical Psychotherapy*, 62; Stekel, *Impotence in the Male*, 1:11, 46.

32. Stekel, *Technique of Analytical Psychotherapy*, 39; Wilhelm Stekel, *Auto-Erotism: A Psychiatric Study of Onanism and Neurosis*, trans. James S. Teslaar (1921; New York: Liveright Publishing, 1950); Stekel, *Impotence in the Male*, 1:56, 116.

33. R. G. Gordon, *The Neurotic Personality* (London: Kegan Paul, Trench, Trubner, and Co., 1927), 218–19; T. A. Ross, *The Common Neuroses* (London: Edward Arnold, 1937), 116, 117.

34. Stekel, *Impotence in the Male*, 1:205.

35. Stekel, *Impotence in Male*, 1:38; Thomas Szasz, *Karl Kraus and the Soul Doctors* (Baton Rouge: Louisiana State University Press, 1976), 103. Reich confessed to rendering a patient completely impotent by suggesting that when he had sex with his wife he was actually aroused by homosexual fantasies (Reich, *Early Writings*, 205).

36. André Tridon, *Sex Happiness* (New York: Boni and Liveright, 1922); Ira S. Wile and Mary Day Winn, *Marriage in the Modern Manner* (New York: Century Co., 1929); Charles Clinton, *Married Sweethearts: The Rôle of Sex Behavior in Marriage* (New York; Macfadden Book Co., 1933); Michael Hau, *The Cult of Health and Beauty in Germany: A Social History, 1890-1930* (Chicago: University of Chicago Press, 2003), 78.

37. June Rose, *Marie Stopes and the Sexual Revolution* (London: Faber and Faber, 1992), 76–78; Ruth Hall, *Passionate Crusader: The Life of Marie Stopes* (New York: Harcourt Brace Jovanovich, 1977), 38, 89–95; and for a sympathetic portrayal of Stopes, see Keith Briant, *Passionate Paradox: The Life of Marie Stopes* (New York: Norton, 1962).

38. On the annulment of the novelist Antonia White's 1921 marriage see Susan Chitty, *Now to My Mother: A Very Personal Memoir of Antonia White* (London: Weidenfeld and Nicolson, 1985), 14–18.

39. Marie Carmichael Stopes, *Married Love: A New Contribution to the Solution of Sex Difficulties* (London: G. P. Putnam's Sons, 1920), 18; Marie Stopes to Alfred Sutro, November 7, 1927, in Lewis Sawin, "Alfred Sutro, Marie Stopes, and her *Vectia*," *Theatre Research International*, 10 (85): 66–67.

40. Professor of genetics at King's College, London, Gates was at Harvard University from 1942 to 1957. See Ruggles Gates Papers, King College, London; *Dictionary of National Biography, 1961-1970* (Oxford: Oxford University Press, 1981), 424–25; Elazar Barkan, *The Retreat of Scientific Racism* (Cambridge: Cambridge University Press, 1992), 168–76; Nancy Stepan, *The Idea of Race* (London: Macmillan, 1982), 168–69; unidentified correspondent to Gates, April 3, 1936, Ruggles Gates Papers.

41. Paul B. Rich, *Race and Empire in British Politics* (Cambridge: Cambridge University Press, 1986), 112–13.

42. Gates letter, April 24, 1962, Stopes Papers, British Museum, Add Ms 59848.

43. Rose, *Marie Stopes*, 79.

44. Orson S. Fowler, *Creative and Sexual Science* (Philadelphia: National Publishing Co., 1870), 70; J. B. Keswick, *Woman: Her Physical Culture* (Scarborough: L. N. Fowler, 1895), 2:68; and see also Peter Gay, *The Bourgeois Experience, Victoria to Freud*, vol. 1 (New York: Oxford University Press, 1984); Carl N. Degler, "What Ought To Be and What Was: Women's Sexuality in the Nineteenth Century," *American Historical Review*, 79 (1974):

1467–90; Helen Lefkowitz Horowitz, *Rereading Sex: Battles over Sexual Knowledge and Suppression in Nineteenth-Century America* (New York: Knopf, 2002), 111–12.

45. Marie Stopes, *Enduring Passion* (London: G. P. Putnam's Sons, 1928), 39; Marie Stopes, *Marriage in My Time* (London: Rich and Cowan, 1935), 57. Despite finding Stopes's romanticism laughable, Dora Russell admitted that the average wife found her husband sexually "stuffy." Her marriage to Bertrand Russell was ended partly due to his impotence. See Dora Russell, *The Tamarisk Tree* (London: Elek, 1975), 168; Dora Russell, *Hypatia or Woman and Knowledge* (London: Kegan Paul, Trench, Trebner and Co., 1925), 74; Stephen Brooke, "The Body and Socialism: Dora Russell in the 1920s," *Past and Present* 189 (November 2005), 149.

46. Stopes, *Married Love*, 80; Stopes, *Enduring Passion*, 91; Marie Stopes, *The Human Body* (New York: Blue Ribbon Books, 1926), 222. In Berlin, Iwan Boch cited interviews to claim that up to 40 percent of women were frigid and that wives' lack of sexual appetite was due to their husbands' incompetence. Ute Frevert, *Women in German History: From Bourgeois Emancipation to Sexual Liberation* (Oxford: Berg, 1989), 132.

47. Stopes, *The Human Body*, 226; Stopes, *Enduring Passion*, 40, 41, 43, 52, 65. Stopes suggested that some women, including the unmarried, might be treated by glandular extracts in capsule form.

48. Edward Carpenter, *Love's Coming of Age* (1896; London: George Allen and Unwin, 1948), 30; Jessamyn Neuhaus, "The Importance of Being Orgasmic: Sexuality, Gender, and Marital Sex Manuals in the United States, 1920–1963," *Journal of the History of Sexuality* 9 (2000): 447–73.

49. Savory cited in Michael Gordon, "From an Unfortunate Necessity to a Cult of Mutual Orgasm: Sex in American Marital Education Literature, 1830–1940," in James M. Henslin, ed., *Studies in the Sociology of Sex* (New York: Appleton Century Crofts, 1971), 53–77; W. F. Robie, *Rational Sex Ethics: Further Investigations* (Boston: Gorham Press, 1919); Charles William Malchow, *The Sexual Life* (St. Louis: C. V. Mosby, 1907), 176; Tridon, *Sex Happiness*, 171; C. B. S. Evans, *Man and Woman in Marriage* (London: John Lane the Bodley Head Ltd., 1932), 49.

50. Evans, *Man and Woman in Marriage*, 61; Tridon, *Sex Happiness*, 167.

51. Bernard Bernard, *Sex Conduct in Marriage* (Chicago: Health and Life Publications, 1926); and see also G. Courtney Beale, *Wise Wedlock: The Complete Treatise on Birth Control and Marriage* (London: Health Promotion Ltd., 1921), 76, 85–88; Le Mon Clark, *Emotional Adjustment in Marriage* (London: Henry Kimpton, 1937), 125; Joseph Collins, *A Doctor Looks at Love and Life* (London: Brentano's, 1926), 33–35; Helena Wright, *The Sex Factor in Marriage* (London: Noel Douglas, 1930), 17, 31–32. According to Margaret Sanger, "He alone can accomplish this. For the desire of the wife can be awakened by her loved one only." Margaret Sanger, *Happiness in Marriage* (New York: Brentano's, 1926), 125; and see also Leland Foster Wood, *Foundations of Happiness in Marriage* (Providence, R.I.: The Roger Williams Press, 1934).

52. R. L. Dickinson and L. Beam, *A Thousand Marriages: A Medical Study of Sex Adjustment* (London: Williams and Norgate, 1932), 126; Sanger, *Happiness in Marriage*, 93; Peter Laipson, "'Kiss without Shame, for She Desires It': Sexual Foreplay in American Marital Advice Literature, 1900–1925," *Journal of Social History*, 3 (1996): 507–12.

53. Isabel E. Hutton, *Hygiene of Marriage* (London: William Heinemann, 1923), 32–33; M. J. Exner, *The Sexual Side of Marriage* (London: George Allen and Unwin, 1932), 86, 122;

Evans, *Man and Woman in Marriage*, 58; Tridon, *Sex Happiness*, 158; Wright, *The Sex Factor in Marriage*, 72; Th. H. van de Velde, *Fertility and Sterility in Marriage: Their Voluntary Promotion and Limitation* (London: Heinemann, 1931), 225. Stopes and Sanger agreed that a woman required at least twenty to thirty minutes to be sexually satisfied.

54. Stekel, *Marriage at the Crossroads*, 2; Sanger, *Happiness in Marriage*, 27; Stopes, *Enduring Passion*, 33.

55. Marie Stopes to Alfred Sutro, November 7, 1927, in Sawin, "Alfred Sutro," 66–67.

56. Stopes, *Enduring Passion*, 55–56; James Robinson and Leo Jacobi, *Sex Morality: Past, Present and Future* (New York: Critic and Guide Company, 1912), 27.

57. Stopes, *Enduring Passion*, 58, 60, 76; V. S. Whitehead and C. A. Hoff, *Ethical Sex Relations or the New Eugenics* (Chicago: John A. Hertel Co.,1928), 109; Sanger, *Happiness in Marriage*, 32, 153, 167–69.

58. In her late fifties Stopes had her second husband sign a statement in which he accepted her right to take lovers. She subsequently began an affair with the twenty-five-year-old Keith Briant. See Hall, *Passionate Crusader*, 277–78; Stopes, *Married Love*, 84; and see also Leslie D. Weatherhead, *The Mastery of Sex through Psychology and Religion* (London: Student Christian Movement, 1934), 230.

59. Stopes, *Enduring Passion*, 81, 111, 189; and on Stopes's advice to male correspondents see Lesley A. Hall, *Hidden Anxieties: Male Sexuality, 1900–1950* (Oxford: Polity Press, 1991) and Lesley A. Hall, "Perspective: The Age-old and Hidden Torments of Impotence," *British Journal of Sexual Science* 22, no. 6 (Nov.–Dec. 1995): 24–26.

60. Rose, *Marie Stopes*, 76; Dr. Eynon, *Manuel de l'amour conjugal* (Paris: Librairie Artistique et Médicale, 1909), 128–144; Havelock Ellis, *Psychology of Sex* (New York: Emerson, 1933), 260.

61. W. F. Robie, *Rational Sex Ethics* (Boston: Gorham Press, 1916), 220; Hutton, *Hygiene of Marriage*, 56–59; and see Havelock Ellis' assertion that "such unions are by no means below the average in happiness." Havelock Ellis, *Psychology of Sex*, 259; Phyllis Grosskurth, *Havelock Ellis: A Biography* (Toronto: McClelland and Stewart, 1980), 286.

62. Oppenheim cited in White, *The First Sexual Revolution*, 71; Joseph Tennenbaum, *The Riddle of Sex* (London: George Routledge and Sons, 1930), 237; Katharine Bement Davis, *Factors in the Sex Life of Twenty-two Hundred Women* (New Yorker: Harper and Brothers, 1929), 78; Dickinson and Beam, *A Thousand Marriages*, 68; G. V. Hamilton, *A Research in Marriage* (New York: Albert and Charles Boni, 1929), 387; Kenneth Walker, *Physiology of Sex* (Harmondsworth: Penguin Books, 1940), 88–89.

63. Van de Velde, *Fertility and Sterility in Marriage*, 234, 243.

64. Van de Velde, *Fertility and Sterility in Marriage*, 228–29; and see also Floyd Dell, "The Anti-Birth Control Neuroses," *Birth Control Review* 12 (Sept 1928): 254–54; George Ryley Scott, *Scott's Encyclopedia of Sex* (London: T. Werner Laurie, 1939), 167; and see also Whitehead and Hoff, *Ethical Sex Relations*, 106; Bernard. S. Talmey, *Love: A Treatise on the Science of Sex-Attraction* (New York: Practitioner's Publishing Company, 1916), 192.

65. Eustace Chesser, *Love without Fear* (1941; London: Arrow Books, 1966), 11; Leslie D. Weatherhead, *Mastery of Sex: Through Psychology and Religion* (1931; London: SCM Press, 1964), 179; Bernard S. Talmey, *Woman: A Treatise on the Normal and Pathological Emotions of Feminine Love* (New York: Practitioner's Publishing Company, 1912), 94, 96, 195, 214.

66. Paul Popenoe, *Problems of Human Reproduction* (Baltimore: Williams and Wilkins, 1926), 130, 132.

67. Beale, *Wise Wedlock*, 86–87; Gregorio Marañón, *The Evolution of Sex*, trans. Warren B. Wells (London: Allen and Unwin, 1932), 74; Sanger, *Happiness in Marriage*, 123; J. F. Tuthill, "Impotence," *Lancet* 265 (Jan. 15, 1955): 126.

68. Antony M. Ludovici, *Man: An Indictment* (London: Constable, 1927), 119–36; M. Palazzoli, *L'Impuissance sexuelle chez l'homme* (Paris: Masson, 1935), 110–11; Tennenbaum, *The Riddle of Sex*, 230, 239–40; Eynon, *Manuel de l'amour conjugal*, 128–44; Van de Velde, *Fertility and Sterility in Marriage*, 229–30; and see also Robinson, *Sex Morality*, 28–30.

69. Joseph Dülberg, *Sterile Marriages* (London: T. Werner Laurie, 1920), 54, 73, 232; Max von Gruber, *Hygiene of Sex* (Baltimore: Williams and Wilkins, 1928), 108; Th. H. van de Velde, *Ideal Marriage: Its Physiology and Technique*, tr. Stella Browne (1926; New York: Random House, 1961), 271.

70. Abraham Buschke and Friedrich Jacobson, *Sex Habits; a Vital Factor in Well-Being*, trans. Eden and Cedar Paul (New York: Emerson Books, 1936), 136, 149.

71. Max Hodann, *A History of Modern Morals*, trans. Stella Browne (London : Heinemann, 1937), 144.

72. Samuel D. Schmalhausen, "The Sexual Revolution," in V. F. Calverton and Samuel D. Schmalhausen, eds. *Sex in Civilization* (Garden City, N.Y.: Garden City Publishing Company, 1929), 380.

CHAPTER EIGHT

1. Peter Schmidt, *The Conquest of Old Age*, trans. Eden and Cedar Paul (London: Routledge, 1931), 108, 117, 119, 123, 124, 136.

2. Adele Clarke, *Disciplining Reproduction: Modernity, American Life Sciences, and "the Problems of Sex"* (Berkeley: University of California Press, 1998).

3. Frank P. Davis, *Impotency, Sterility and Artificial Impregnation* (St. Louis: C. V. Mosby Company, 1917), 69.

4. Victor G. Vecki, *Sexual Impotence* (Philadelphia and London: W. B. Saunders Company, 1912), 341; Davis, *Impotency, Sterility and Artificial Impregnation*, 68; and see also Gregorio Marañón, *The Evolution of Sex and Intersexual Conditions*, trans. Warren B. Wells (London: George Allen and Unwin, 1932), 27, 68, 70, 250; Oswald Swinney Lowsley and Thomas Joseph Kirwin, *Clinical Urology* (Baltimore: Williams and Wilkins Co., 1944), 351–57; Frank Hinman, *The Principles and Practice of Urology* (Philadelphia: W. B. Saunders, 1935), 836; and see also Kenneth Walker and Eric B. Strauss, *Sexual Disorders in the Male* (London: Hamish Hamilton, 1944), 132–33; J. Shah, "Erectile Dysfunction through the Ages," *BJU International* 90, no. 4 (2002): 437.

5. BMA (British Medical Association), *More Secret Remedies: What They Cost & What They Contain* (London: BMA, 1912); Wellcome Library, CMCS file no. SA/BMA/box 119/C. 426 Patent Medicines; William J. Robinson, *A Practical Treatise on the Causes, Symptoms, and Treatment of Sexual Impotence* (New York: Critic and Guide, 1923), 176; Davis, *Impotency, Sterility and Artificial Impregnation*, 51, 67; *Journal of the American Medical Association* (hereafter *JAMA*) 91 (1928): 1823–24; 94 (1930), 1619–20.

6. Vecki, *Sexual Impotence*, 353; Joseph Loewenstein, *The Treatment of Impotence: With Special Reference to Mechanotherapy* (London: Hamish Hamilton, 1947), 16, 24, 26.

7. Stanislas Higier, *Les Fonctions sexuelles mâles et leurs troubles* (Paris: G. Doin, 1932); Diane Long Hall, "Biology, Sex Hormones and Sexism in the 1920s," *Philosophical Forum*,

5 (1973–74): 81–96; and for an overview see Chandak Sengoopta, *The Most Secret Quintessence of Life: Sex, Glands, and Hormones, 1850–1950* (Chicago: University of Chicago Press, 2006).

8.   Dr. Brown-Sequard, "The Effects Produced on Man by Subcutaneous Injections of a Liquid Obtained From the Testicles of Animals," *Lancet* 134 (July 20, 1889): 105–6; Merriley Borell, "Brown-Séquard's Organotherapy and its Appearance in America at the End of the Nineteenth Century," *Bulletin of the History of Medicine* 50 (1976) 309–20; Chandak Sengoopta, "Transforming the Testicle; Science, Medicine and Masculinity, 1800–1950," *Medicina nei Secoli Arte e Scienza* 13 (2001): 637–55.

9.   Victor D. Lespinasse, "Transplantation of the Testicle," *JAMA* 61 (1913): 1869–70; G. Frank Lydston, *Impotence and Sterility with Aberrations of the Sexual Function and Sex-Gland Implementation* (Chicago: Riverton Press, 1917), 225, 226–51; and see also G. Frank Lydston, "Sex Gland Implantation: Additional Cases and Conclusions to Date," *JAMA* 66 (1916): 1540–43.

10. L. L. Stanley, "An Analysis of One Thousand Testicular Substance Implantations," *Endocrinology* 6 (1922): 787–94; Robinson, *A Practical Treatise*, 411; and see also Walker and Strauss, *Sexual Disorders in the Male*, 45.

11. Serge Voronoff and George Alexandrescu, *Testicular Grafting from Ape to Man*, trans. Theodore C. Merrill (London: Brentano's, 1928), 27, 28; David Hamilton, *The Monkey Gland Affair* (London: Chatto and Windus, 1986); Serge Voronoff, *The Conquest of Life* (London: Williams and Norgate, 1933), 45; *New York Times*, Oct. 3, 1921, 28:3; and see also Max Hodann, *History of Modern Morals*, trans. Stella Browne (London: Heinemann, 1937), 29; Paul Kammerer, *Rejuvenation and the Prolongation of Human Efficiency* (London: Methuen, 1924), 63.

12. Benjamin E. Dawson, *Orificial Surgery* (Kansas City, Mo.: Western Baptist Publishing Company, 1925); Eric S. Juhnke, *Quacks and Crusaders: The Fabulous Careers of John Brinkley, Norman Baker, and Harry Hoxsey* (Lawrence: University of Kansas Press, 2002); R. Alton Lee, *The Bizarre Careers of John R. Brinkley* (Lexington: University Press of Kentucky, 2002).

13. "You Can't Do What My Last Man Did," transcribed from vocals by Ethel Waters and Slow Kid Thomas, recorded August 25, 1925; Lee, *The Bizarre Careers of John R. Brinkley*, 241; Brett A. Berliner, "Mephistopheles and Monkeys: Rejuvenation, Race, and Sexuality in Popular Culture in Interwar France," *Journal of the History of Sexuality*, 13 (2004): 306–25; Italo Svevo, *Further Confessions of Zeno*, trans. Ben Johnson and P.N. Furbank (Berkeley: University of California Press, 1969), 145.

14. George Ryley Scott, *Three Hundred Sex, Marriage and Birth Control Questions Answered* (London: T. Werner Laurie, 1941), 49; Sir Arthur Conan Doyle, *The Penguin Complete Sherlock Holmes* (London: Penguin, 1981), 1082–83; and see Joseph A. Kester, *Sherlock's Men: Masculinity, Conan Doyle, and Cultural History* (Aldershot: Ashgate, 1997), 59; Charles Percy Snow, *New Lives for Old* (London: Gollancz, 1933); Mikhail Bulgakov, *Heart of a Dog*, trans. Mirra Ginsburg (New York: Grove Press, 1968).

15. Eugen Steinach and Josef Loebel, *Sex and Life: Forty Years of Biological and Medical Experiments* (London: Faber and Faber, 1940), 21.

16. *London Times*, May 14, 1921, 7c; Hamilton, *Monkey Gland*, 46–47; "Gland Treatment Spreads in America," *New York Times*, Apr. 8, 1923, ix.2.7; Eden Paul and Norman Haire, *Rejuvenation: Steinach's Researches on the Sex Glands* (London: British Society for

the Study of Sex Psychology, 1923); Sarah Wright, "Gregorio Marañón and 'The Cult of Sex': Effeminacy and Intersexuality in 'The Psychopathology of Don Juan' (1924)," *Bulletin of Spanish Studies* 81 (2004): 726; George F. Corners (George Sylvester Viereck), *Rejuvenation: How Steinach Makes People Young* (New York: Thomas Seltzer, 1923), vii; Robinson, *A Practical Treatise*, 424; and see Chandak Sengoopta, "The Modern Ovary: Constructions, Meanings, Ideas," *History of Science* 28 (2000): 455–60.

17. "Gland Operation to Retard Senility" *New York Times*, November 20, 1921, ii.10:3; and on ultraviolet rays for diminished desire and potency see also Arnold Lorand, *Life Shortening Habits and Rejuvenation* (Philadelphia: F. A. Davis, 1922), 240; Harry Benjamin, "Steinach Therapy Against Old Age," *American Medicine* 38 (1932): 467–72, 492; Ernest Jones, *The Life and Work of Sigmund Freud* (New York: Basic Books, 1957), 3:104; Diana Wyndham, "Versemaking and Lovemaking: W. B. Yeats' 'Strange Second Puberty': Norman Haire and the Steinach Rejuvenation Operation," *Journal of the History of the Behavioral Sciences* 39 (2003): 25–50; Tim Armstrong, *Modernism, Technology and the Body: A Cultural Study* (Cambridge: Cambridge University Press, 1998), 155.

18. Susan Merrill Squier, *Babies in Bottles: Twentieth-Century Visions of Reproductive Technology* (New Brunswick: Rutgers University Press, 1994), 37–38; George Ryley Scott, *The Quest for Youth: A Study of All Available Methods of Rejuvenation and of Retaining Physical and Mental Vigor in Old Age* (London: Torchstream, 1953), 9; Benjamin, "Steinach Therapy Against Old Age," 467; Chandak Sengoopta, "'Dr. Steinach Is Coming to Make Old Young': Sex Glands, Vasectomy and the Quest for Rejuvenation in the Roaring Twenties," *Endeavour* 27, no. 3 (2003): 122–26; Kammerer, *Rejuvenation and the Prolongation of Human Efficiency*, 101. A believer in acquired characteristics, Kammerer's career was destroyed when evidence of his faking test results came to light.

19. Corners, *Rejuvenation*, 15; Kammerer, *Rejuvenation and the Prolongation of Human Efficiency*, 181, 185; Schmidt, *The Conquest of Old Age*, 218; Walker and Strauss, *Sexual Disorders in the Male*, 63.

20. Norman Haire, *Rejuvenation: The Work of Steinach, Voronoff and Others* (New York: Macmillan Company, 1925), 205; Benjamin Harrow, *Glands in Health and Disease* (London: George Routledge and Sons, 1922), 104–5; Kenneth M. Walker, "The Internal Secretion of the Testis," *Lancet* 203 (Jan. 5, 1924): 16–21; Kenneth M. Walker and J. A. Lumsden, "Steinach's Rejuvenation Operation," *Lancet* 203 (Feb. 2, 1924): 223–26; Morris Fishbein, *The Medical Follies* (New York: Boni and Liveright, 1925), 161–71; Jessica Jahiel, "Rejuvenation Research and the American Medical Association in the Early Twentieth Century: Paradigms in Conflict," (Ph.D. diss., Boston University, 1992).

21. Kenneth M. Walker, *Male Disorders of Sex* (New York: W. W. Norton & Co., 1930), 76, 77; Jean Paul Pratt, "Sex Functions in Man," in Edgar Allen, ed., *Sex and Internal Secretions: A Survey of Recent Research* (London: Baillière, Tindall and Cox, 1939), 1269, 1276; Henry R. Harrower, *An Endocrine Handbook* (Glendale, Calif.: Harrower Laboratory, 1939), 103.

22. Paul Niehans, *Introduction to Cellular Therapy: Lectures* (La Tour-de-Peilz: By the Author, 1959); Patrick M. McGrady, *The Youth Doctors* (New York: Coward-McCann, 1968), 59–68.

23. *Lancet* 217 (May 2, 1931): 95; and for a specialist who carried out Steinach operations while admitting hormones remained mysterious substances, see Charles H. Chetwood, *Practice of Urology and Syphology* (London: Oxford University Press, 1928), 552.

24. Gerhard J. Newerla, "The History and Isolation of the Male Hormone," *New England Journal of Medicine* 228 (1943): 39–47; Anne Fausto-Sterling, *Sexing the Body: Gender Politics and the Construction of Sexuality* (New York: Basic Books, 2000), 181–84.

25. Benjamin Harrow and Carl P. Sherwin, *The Chemistry of the Hormones* (London: Ballière, Tindall and Cox, 1934), 152; Paul de Kruif, *The Male Hormone* (New York: Harcourt, Brace and Co., 1945), 94, 177, and see also James B. Hamilton, *Endocrinology* 21 (1937): 649; "Doctors Report Synthetic Drug Restores Not Youth but Energy for Business," *New York Times*, April, 24, 1939, 19.3; August A. Werner, "The Male Climacteric," *JAMA* 132 (1946): 188–94.

26. Steinach and Loebel, *Sex and Life*, 268–27; Nelly Oudshoorn, *An Archeology of Sex Hormones* (London: Routledge, 1994), 108.

27. Robinson, *A Practical Treatise*, 406; Dan Healey, *Homosexual Desire in Revolutionary Russia: The Regulation of Sexual and Gender Dissent* (Chicago: University of Chicago Press, 2001), 180, fig. 13. On Magnus Hirschfeld's Institute for Sexual Science and the sale of pharmaceuticals, see *http://www.hirschfeld.in-berlin.de/institut/en/theorie/theo_19.html* (accessed February 1, 2006); and see Alfred Döblin, *Alexanderplatz Berlin: The Story of Franz Biberkopf*, trans. Eugene Jolas (New York: Frederick Ungar Publishing, 1931), 33–35; Ernst Toller, *Hinkemann* (1923) in *Seven Plays* (New York: Liveright Publishing, 1936), 183.

28. G. W. Carnick Co., *Dependable Gland Products Price List* (c.1923), Wellcome Institute; Henry R. Harrower, *A Manual of Pluriglandular Therapy* (London: Endocrines Limited, 1924), 239; see also Henry R. Harrower, *Practical Organotherapy: The Internal Secretions in General Practice* (Glendale, Calif.: The Harrower Laboratory, 1922); Middlesex Laboratory of Glandular Research, Ltd., *The Treatment of Impotence* (London: Middlesex Laboratory of Glandular Research, Ltd., c. 1930); Harrower, *An Endocrine Handbook*, 104–5.

29. Nelly Oudshoorn, "On Bodies, Technologies, and Feminisms," in Angela N. H. Creager, Elizabeth Lunbeck, and Londa Schiebinger, eds., *Feminism in Twentieth-Century Science, Technology, and Medicine* (Chicago: University of Chicago Press, 2002), 205; Sheila M. Rothman and David J. Rothman, *The Pursuit of Perfection: The Promise and the Perils of Medical Enhancement* (New York: Pantheon, 2003); J. D. Pratt, "Endocrine Disorders in Sex Function in Man," in Edgar Allen and Edward A. Doisy, eds., *Sex and Internal Secretions* (Baltimore: Williams and Wilkins, 1932), 880–913.

30. Harry Benjamin, "The Story of Rejuvenation," *American Mercury*, Dec. 1935, 480–83.

31. Edward Lawrence Keyes and Edward Lawrence Keyes, Jr., *The Surgical Diseases of the Genito-Urinary Organs* (New York: Appleton and Co., 1906), 798; Armstrong, *Modernism, Technology and the Body*; Kevin White, *The First Sexual Revolution: The Emergence of Male Heterosexuality in Modern America* (New York: New York University Press, 1993), 19.

32. Christopher William Hufeland, *The Art of Prolonging Human Life* (London: J. Bell, 1797), 1:168; 2:13; and see also Jean-Martin Charcot, *Clinical Lectures of the Diseases of Old Age*, trans. Leigh H. Hunt (New York: William Wood and Company, 1881); Haire, *Rejuvenation*, 8.

33. Davis, *Impotency, Sterility and Artificial Impregnation*, 74; Max Hühner, *A Practical Treatise on Disorders of the Sexual Function in the Male and Female* (Philadelphia: F. A. Davis, 1923), 94; Keyes and Keyes, *The Surgical Diseases of the Genito-Urinary Organs*, 799.

34. Max Thorek, "Male Climacterium," *Medical Journal and Record*, 119 (1924) sup. 47; Irvin S. Koll, *Diseases of the Male Urethra* (Philadelphia: W. B. Saunders, 1918), 117; Gregorio Marañón, *The Climacteric (The Critical Age)* trans. K. S. Stevens (St. Louis: C. V. Mosby, 1929), 349–72; Chandak Sangoopta, "Revuvenation and the Prolongation of Life: Science or Quackery?" *Perspectives in Biology and Medicine*, 37 (1993): 55–66.

35. G. Stanley Hall, *Senescence: The Last Half of Life* (London: Appleton and Co., 1922), 309; and see Aldred Scott Warthin, *Old Age: The Major Involution* (New York: Paul B. Hoeber, 1929), 172–74.

36. Jack London, "The Rejuvenation of Major Rathbone" (1899) in *The Complete Short Stories of Jack London*, ed. Earl Lasbor, Robert C. Leitz III, and I. Milo Shephard, (Stanford: Stanford University Press, 1993), 1:273–82; Corners, *Rejuvenation*, 14; Margaret Morganroth Gullette, "Creativity, Aging, Gender: A Study of Their Intersections, 1910–1935," in Anne M. Wyatt-Brown and Janice Rossen, eds., *Aging and Gender in Literature: Studies in Creativity* (Charlottesville: University Press of Virginia, 1993), 19–48.

37. Italo Svevo, *Further Confessions of Zeno*, trans. Ben Johnson and P. N. Furbank (Berkeley: University of California Press, 1969), 29, 256, 269; Aldous Huxley, *Brave New World* (New York: Harper and Row, 1946), 66–67; Gertrude Atherton, *Black Oxen* (New York: A. L. Burt, 1923); Gertrude Atherton, *Adventures of a Novelist* (London: Jonathan Cape, 1932), 537–40; Julie Prebel, "Engineering Womanhood: The Politics of Rejuvenation in Gertrude Atherton's *Black Oxen*," *American Literature* 76, no. 2 (2004): 307–37; Mary Scharlieb, *Change of Life: Its Difficulties and Dangers* (London: Scientific Press, 1941), 35.

38. Voronoff and Alexandrescu, *Testicular Grafting from Ape to Man*, table 1; Kammerer, *Rejuvenation and the Prolongation of Human Efficiency*, 132.

39. Lydston, *Impotence and Sterility*, 21; Marañón, *The Evolution of Sex*, 209, 210, 217, 220; Walker and Strauss, *Sexual Disorders in the Male*, 102, 103.

40. Sengoopta, "The Modern Ovary," 463; Susan Squier, "Incubabies and Rejuvenates: The Traffic Between Technologies of Reproduction and Age-Extension" in Kathleen Woodward, ed., *Figuring Age: Women, Bodies, Generations* (Bloomington: Indiana University Press, 1999), 89; Laura Davidow Hirshbein, "The Glandular Solution: Sex, Masculinity, and Aging in the 1920s," *Journal of the History of Sexuality* 9 (2000): 277–304; Julia E. Rechter, "'The Glands of Destiny': A History of Popular, Medical and Scientific Views of the Sex Hormones in 1920s America," (Ph.D. diss., University of California at Berkeley, 1997).

41. Edred M. Corner, *Male Diseases in General Practice* (London: Hodder and Stoughton, 1910), 228; Lydston, "Sex Gland Implantation," 1541.

42. Schmidt, *The Conquest of Old Age*, 50; Adele Clarke, "Money, Sex, and Legitimacy in Chicago, circa 1892–1940: Lillie's Center of Reproductive Biology," in *Perspectives on Science* 1 (1993): 404; Francis H. A. Marshall, *The Physiology of Reproduction* (London: Longmans, Green and Co., 1922), 658.

43. Benjamin, "Steinach Therapy Against Old Age," 471; Corners, *Rejuvenation*, 23, 49–50; G. Frank Lydston, *That Bogey Man the Jew* (Kansas City, Mo., Burton Publishing Company, 1921); Hunter McGuire and G. Frank Lydston, *Sexual Crimes Among the Southern Negroes* (Louisville, Ky.: Renz and Henry, 1893); G. Frank Lydston, "Further Observations on Sex Gland Implantation," *JAMA* 72 (1919): 396–98.

44. Louis Berman, *The Glands Regulating Personality* (1921) cited in Margaret Sanger, *The Pivot of Civilization* (New York: Brentano's, 1922), 223; *New York Times*, Oct. 2, 1921, ii,

4:1; Oct. 6, 1921, 11:1; Oct. 19, 21:2; Oct. 22, 9:1; Dec. 4, viii, 4:1; Dec. 8, 21:7; Feb. 5, 1922, iii, 9:1; Feb. 6, 6:1; Feb. 8, 12:2; Feb. 11, 1:2; Aug. 8, 40:2; Aug. 25, 4:6; Nov. 28, 12:1; Dec. 1, 2:7; Dorothy L. Sayers, *The Unpleasantness at the Bellona Club* (1928; London: Harper and Brothers, 1956), 215.

45. A. J. Ochsner, "Surgical Treatment of Habitual Criminals," *JAMA* 32 (April 22, 1899): 867–68; and see also the article by the influential urologist William Belfield, "Race Suicide for Social Parasites," *JAMA* 50 (1908), 55; Angela Gugliotta, "'Dr. Sharp and His Little Knife': Therapeutic and Punitive Origins of Eugenic Vasectomy—Indiana, 1892–1921," *Journal of the History of Medicine* 53 (1998): 371–406; Philip R. Reilly, *The Surgical Solution; A History of Involuntary Sterilization in the United States* (Baltimore: Johns Hopkins University Press, 1991), 30–33; G. S. Gosney and Paul Popenoe, *Sterilization for Human Betterment* (New York: Macmillan, 1929), 24; and see also J. H. Landman, *Human Sterilization* (Macmillan, 1932), 235–38.

46. Robert Reid Rentoul, *Proposed Sterilization of Certain Mental and Physical Degenerates* (London: Walter Scott, 1903), 17; Lydston, *Impotence and Sterility*, 90; and see also Bernard S. Talmey, *Love: A Treatise on the Science of Sex-Attraction* (New York: Practitioner's Publishing Company, 1916), 344–45.

47. W. S. Baring-Gould, *The Lure of the Limerick* (London: Rupert Hart-Davis, 1969), 87; and for less amusing accounts of hormones used to cure homosexuality and increase productivity in Eastern Europe see Healey, *Homosexual Desire in Revolutionary Russia: The Regulation of Sexual and Gender Dissent*, 134–36; Eric Naiman, "Discourse Made Flesh: Healing and Terror in the Construction of Soviet Subjectivity," in Igal Halfin, ed., *Language and Revolution: Making Modern Political Identities* (London: Frank Cass, 2002), 287–316.

48. Lydston, "Sex gland implantation," 1540; Corners, *Rejuvenation*, 23; Steinach and Loebel, *Sex and Life*, 116–18; Marañón, *The Evolution of Sex*, 168–69

49. Haire, *Rejuvenation*, 139–43.

50. Magnus Hirschfeld, *Sexual Pathology: A Study of Derangements of the Sexual Instinct*, trans. Jerome Gibbs (New York: Emerson Books, 1947), 310–13; and see Chandak Sengoopta, "Glandular Politics: Experimental Biology, Clinical Medicine, and Homosexual Emancipation in Fin-de-Siècle Central Europe," *Isis* 89 (1998), 448, 456; *JAMA* 75 (1920): 755; Haire, *Rejuvenation*, 139–46; Walker, *Male Disorders of Sex*, 76; Niehans, *Introduction to Cellular Therapy*, 20.

51. Gunnar Broberg and Nils Roll-Hansen, *Eugenics and the Welfare State: Sterilization Policy in Norway, Sweden, Denmark, and Finland* (East Lansing: Michigan State University Press, 1996), 38, 42; on Sand see Carl R. Moore, "Biology of the Mammalian Testis and Scrotum," *Quarterly Review of Biology* 1, no.1 (1926): 4–50; and on Vaernet see Richard Plant, *Pink Triangle: The Nazi War Against Homosexuals* (New York: Henry Holt, 1986) 175–78.

52. Paul Kammerer, *The Inheritance of Acquired Characteristics*, trans. A. Paul Maeker-Branden (New York: Boni and Liveright, 1924), 340–41; Alexis Carrel, *Man the Unknown* (New York: Harper and Brothers, 1935), 299, 303; A. H. Reggiani, "Alexis Carrel the Unknown: Eugenics and Population Research under Vichy," *French Historical Studies* 25 (Spring 2002): 331–56.

53. On Hitler's use of invigorating glandular preparations and hormones see Hugh Trevor-Roper, *The Last Days of Hitler* (London: Macmillan, 1978), 67–74; David Irving, *The Secret Diaries of Hitler's Doctor* (New York: Macmillan, 1983), 67–74.

CHAPTER NINE

1. Philip Nobile, "What Is the New Impotence, and Who's Got It?" *Esquire* (Oct. 1972): 98; and see also George L. Ginsberg, "The New Impotence," *Archives of General Psychiatry*, March 1972, 218–20; Sam Julty, *Male Sexual Performance* (New York: Grosset and Dunlap, 1975).

2. David Riesman with Nathan Glazer and Reuel Denney, *The Lonely Crowd: A Study of the Changing American Character* (New Haven: Yale University Press, 1950), 123; K. A. Cuordileone, "'Politics in an Age of Anxiety': Cold War Political Culture and the Crisis in American Masculinity, 1949–1960," *Journal of American History* 87, no. 2 (2000); Ferdinand Lundberg and Marynia Farnham, *Modern Women: The Lost Sex* (New York: Harper and Brothers, 1947); Beth L. Bailey, *From Front Porch to Back Seat: Courtship in Twentieth-Century America* (Baltimore: Johns Hopkins University Press, 1988), 103–8. On similar responses in Europe see Dagmar Herzog, *Sex after Fascism: Memory and Morality in Twentieth-Century Germany* (Princeton: Princeton University Press, 2005).

3. Alfred C. Kinsey, Wardell B. Pomeroy, and Clyde E. Martin, *Sexual Behavior in the Human Male* (Philadelphia: W. B. Saunders and Co., 1948), 325; and see Paul Robinson, *The Modernization of Sex: Havelock Ellis, Alfred Kinsey, William Masters, and Virginia Johnson* (New York: Harper and Row, 1976); Jonathan Gathorne-Hardy, *Alfred C. Kinsey: Sex the Measure of All Things: A Biography* (London: Pimlico, 1998); James H. Jones, *Alfred C. Kinsey: A Public/Private Life* (New York: Norton, 1997).

4. Kinsey, *Sexual Behavior in the Human Male*, 323.

5. Kinsey, *Sexual Behavior in the Human Male*, 235–37; and see Paul H. Gebhard and Alan B. Johnson, *The Kinsey Data* (Bloomington: Indiana University Press, 1979), table 78.

6. Alfred C. Kinsey, Wardell B. Pomeroy, Clyde E. Martin, and Paul H. Gebhard, *Sexual Behavior in the Human Female* (Philadelphia: W. B. Saunders, 1953), 171–73; Kinsey, *Sexual Behavior in the Human Male*, 307, 325, 580. As a follow up to his report, Kinsey also made the deflating discovery that in ejaculating, men were more likely to "dribble" than to "squirt" (see Jones, *Alfred C. Kinsey*, 605–6).

7. Robert O. Blood, *Marriage* (New York: Free Press, 1962), 370–71; Harvey Kaye, *Male Survival: Masculinity without Myth* (New York: Grosset and Dunlop, 1974), 87; Robert Bahr, *The Virility Factor: Masculinity Through Testosterone, the Male Sex Hormone* (New York: G. P. Putnam's Sons, 1976); John Johnson, *Disorders of Sexual Potency in the Male* (London: Pergamon Press, 1968).

8. Donald W. Hastings, *Impotence and Frigidity* (London: J. and A. Churchill, 1963), vii; Isadore Rubin, *Sexual Life after Sixty* (New York: Basic Books, 1965), 78–84; "Bimini Fué Descubierta!! Is 'Pega Palo' the Answer?" *JAMA* 165 (1957): 695–96.

9. Janet Sayers, *Mothers of Psychoanalysis: Helene Deutsche, Karen Horney, Anna Freud, Melanie Klein* (New York: Norton, 1991), 47–48; Philip Wylie, *Generation of Vipers* (1942; New York: Rinehart and Company, 1955), 194, 208; Edward A. Strecker, *Their Mothers' Sons: The Psychiatrist Examines an American Problem* (New York: Lippincott, 1951).

10. Edmund Bergler, *Counterfeit-Sex* (New York: Grune and Stratton, 1958), 61, 74.

11. Rudolf Brun, *General Theory of Neuroses* (New York: International Universities Press, 1951), 272; Edmund Bergler, *Divorce Won't Help* (New York: Harper and Brothers, 1948), 88; Bergler, *Counterfeit-Sex*, xiv; Edmund Bergler, *The Revolt of the Middle-Aged Man* (London: Bernard Hanison, 1958), 23, 150; Kinsey, *Sexual Behavior in the Human Male*, 206–7.

12. Leonard J. Friedman, *Virgin Wives: A Study of Unconsummated Marriages* (London: Tavistock Publications, 1962), 144.

13. Herman H. Rubin, *Glands, Sex and Personality* (1952) cited in Jessamyn Neuhaus, "The Importance of Being Orgasmic: Sexuality, Gender, and Marital Sex Manuals in the United States, 1920–1963," *Journal of the History of Sexuality* 9 (2000): 465; John Thomas Gill, *How to Hold Your Husband: A Frank Psychoanalysis for Happy Marriage* (Philadelphia: Dorrance & Company, 1951).

14. Charles W. Socarides, *Homosexuality* (New York: Jason Aronson, 1978), 42.

15. Bergler, *Counterfeit-Sex*, xxiv; Lawrence M. Hatterer, *Changing Homosexuality in the Male: Treatment for Men Troubled by Homosexuality* (New York: McGraw-Hill, 1970), 36; Helen Meyer Hacker, "The New Burdens of Masculinity," *Marriage and Family Living*, 19 (1957): 227–33; Socarides, *Homosexuality*, 97.

16. John R. Cavanagh, *Counseling the Invert* (Milwaukee: Bruce Publishing Company, 1966), 139; George W. Henry, *All the Sexes: Studies of Masculinity and Femininity* (Toronto: Rinehart & Co., 1955), 149; Eustace Chesser, *Sexual Behavior: Normal and Abnormal* (London: Medical Publications Ltd, 1949), 135; Dr. Joan Graham [Joan Malleson], *Any Wife or Any Husband: A Book for Couples Who Have Met Sexual Difficulties and for Doctors* (London: William Heinemann, 1955), 119, 124, 136; Hatterer, *Changing Homosexuality in the Male*, 342.

17. Allan Berubé, *Coming Out Under Fire: The History of Gay Men and Women in World War Two* (New York: Free Press, 1990), 259; Cavanagh, *Counseling the Invert*, 180; Patricia Kayo Sexton, *The Feminized Male: Classrooms, White Collars and the Decline of Manliness* (New York: Random House, 1969), 3–4, 198, 201; Estelle B. Freedman, "'Uncontrolled Desires': The Response to the Sexual Psychopath, 1920–1960," in Kathy Peiss and Christina Simmons with Robert A. Padgug, eds., *Passion and Power: Sexuality in History* (Philadelphia: Temple University Press, 1989), 203–16.

18. Jeffrey Weeks, *Sex, Politics and Society: The Regulation of Sexuality since 1800* (London: Longman, 1989), 237; E. F. Griffith, *Modern Marriage* (London: Gollancz, 1934); David R. Mace, *Marriage Counselling* (London: J. A. Churchill, 1948), 50; and see also Walter R. Stokes, *Modern Pattern for Marriage* (London: Reinhardt and Evans, 1949).

19. Emily H. Mudd, "A Case Study in Marriage Counseling," *Marriage and Family Living* 7 (1945): 52–54; Helena Wright, *Sex Fulfillment in Married Women* (London: Williams and Norgate, 1947), 11, 54–55; S. Leonard Simpson, "Impotence," *British Medical Journal* (Mar. 25, 1950): 692; Hannah and Abraham Stone, *A Marriage Manual* (London: Victor Gollancz, 1952), 236–39.

20. Alex Comfort, *The Biology of Senescence* (1956; New York: Elsevier, 1979), 169, 170; and see also George Ryley Scott, *The Quest for Youth: A Study of All Available Methods of Rejuvenation and of Retaining Physical and Mental Vigor in Old Age* (London: Torchstream, 1953), 61; Isadore Rubin, *Sexual Life After Sixty* (New York: Basic Books, 1965); Helmut J. Ruebsaat and Raymond Hill, *The Male Climacteric* (New York; Hawthorn Books, 1975); Elaine Cumming and William E. Henry, *Growing Old: The Process of Disengagement* (New York: Basic Books, 1961), 22; Blood, *Marriage*, 370–71.

21. Michael Gordon and Penelope J. Shankweiler, "Different Equals Less: Female Sexuality in Recent Marriage Manuals," *Journal of Marriage and the Family* 33 (1971): 459–76; Marcus Collins, *Modern Love: An Intimate History of Men and Women in Twentieth-Century Britain* (London; Atlantic Books, 2003), 98; Graham, *Any Wife or Any Husband*,

75; J. H. Wallis and H. S. Booker, *Marriage Counseling* (London: Routledge and Kegan Paul, 1958), 40.

22. Edwin W. Hirsch, *Sex Power* (Chicago: Research Publications of Chicago, 1947), 27; Thurman B. Rice, *Sex, Marriage, and Family* (New York: J. B. Lippincott, 1946), 88.

23. Hastings, *Impotence and Frigidity*, 109; Henry, *All the Sexes*, 136.

24. Maxine Davis, *The Sexual Responsibility of Woman* (London: William Heinemann, 1957), 21, 31, 83, 149; Hirsch, *Sex Power*, 111; and see the reference to the wife's "defective provocation" in John E. Eichenlaub, *The Marriage Art* (London: Mayflower-Dell, 1961), 169; Mary Macaulay, *Art of Marriage* (London: Delisle, 1952), 47; Graham, *Any Wife or Any Husband*, 74, 85; Rebecca Liswood, *A Doctor Speaks Her Mind About Sex* (London: Frederick Muller, 1961), 129.

25. Ernest R. Groves, Gladys Hoagland Groves and Catherine Groves, *Sex Fulfillment in Marriage* (New York: Emerson Books, 1942), 224; Helen Meyer Hacker, "The New Burdens of Masculinity," *Marriage and Family Living* 19 (1957): 231.

26. J. F. Tuthill, "Impotence," *Lancet* 265 (Jan. 15, 1955): 126; 265 and (Jan. 29, 1955): 251–52; Vance Packard, *The Sexual Wilderness: The Contemporary Upheaval in Male-Female Relationships* (New York: David McKay Company, 1968), 276.

27. Barbara Ehrenreich, Elizabeth Hess, and Gloria Jacobs, *Re-Making Love: The Feminization of Sex* (New York: Doubleday, 1986); Robert Bell, *Premarital Sex in a Changing Society* (Englewood Cliffs, N.J.: Prentice Hall 1966), 137; David Mace, *Sexual Difficulties in Marriage* (London: National Marriage Guidance Council, 1983), 6; Leslie H. Farber, "I'm Sorry, Dear," *Commentary* (Nov. 1964): 47–54; B. Lyman Stewart "Is Impotence Increasing?" *Medical Aspects of Human Sexuality* 5 (Oct. 1971): 35; Karl Miller, "The Sisterhood," *New York Review of Books*, April 20, 1972, 22; and see also Marc Feigen Fasteau, *The Male Machine* (New York: Dell, 1975), 28–30.

28. Scott, *The Quest for Youth*, 70; Clifford Allen, *A Textbook of Psychosexual Disorders* (New York: Oxford University Press, 1962), 281–82; Davis, *The Sexual Responsibility of Woman*, 149; Packard, *The Sexual Wilderness*, 122; Herbert A. Otto "Is Impotence Increasing?" *Medical Aspects of Human Sexuality* 5 (Oct. 1971): 36; Lara Marks, *Sexual Chemistry: A History of the Contraceptive Pill* (New Haven: Yale University Press, 2001), 193.

29. William H. Masters and Virginia E. Johnson, *Human Sexual Response* (Boston: Little, Brown, 1966); and *Human Sexual Inadequacy* (Boston: Little, Brown, 1970); and on Masters's carrying on of the rejuvenators' view of aging as a disease see his "Sex Steroid Influence on the Aging Process," *American Journal of Obstetrics and Gynecology* 4 (October 1957): 733–42.

30. Masters and Johnson, *Human Sexual Response*, 51–90; Masters and Johnson, *Human Sexual Inadequacy*, 159.

31. The same argument had been made earlier in Joseph Wolpe, *Psychotherapy by Reciprocal Inhibition* (Stanford: Stanford University Press, 1958), 131–35.

32. Masters and Johnson, *Human Sexual Inadequacy*, 107; and on Dr. A. H. Kegel's suggestion that women strengthen their vaginal sphincter muscles, see Eichenlaub, *The Marriage Art*, 169; Albert Ellis, *The Art and Practice of Love* (London: Souvenir Press, 1961), 208–9; and on the continuing employment of hypnosis see Frank Caprio, *How to Solve Your Sex Problems with Self-Hypnosis* (North Hollywood: Wilshire Book Company, 1964); David Reuben, *Everything You Always Wanted to Know About Sex But were Afraid to Ask* (London: Pan, 1971), 107.

33. Masters and Johnson, *Human Sexual Inadequacy*, 209; Edward M. Brecher, *The Sex Researchers* (London: Panther, 1972), 314.

34. Masters and Johnson, *Human Sexual Inadequacy*, 137–51.

35. Albert Ellis, *Sex and the Liberated Man* (Secaucus, N.J.: Lyle Stuart, Inc., 1976), 16; William E. Hartman and Marilyn A. Fithian, *Treatment of Sexual Dysfunction: A Basic Approach* (Northvale, N.J.: Jason Aronson, 1983); Helen Singer Kaplan, *The New Sex Therapy: Active Treatment of Sexual Dysfunctions* (New York: Quadrangle, 1974), 263, 270; Patricia and Richard Gillan, *Sex Therapy Today* (London: Open Books, 1976), 203; see also Vern L. Bullough, *Science in the Bedroom: A History of Sex Research* (New York: Basic Books, 1994), 196–205; Janice M. Irvine, *Disorders of Desire: Sex and Gender in Modern American Sexology* (Temple University Press, Philadelphia, 1990), 67–94; 192–203; Leonore Tiefer, *Sex Is Not a Natural Act and Other Essays* (Boulder: Westview Press, 1994); John Heidenry, *What Wild Ecstasy: The Rise and Fall of the Sexual Revolution* (New York: Simon and Schuster, 1997).

36. Masters and Johnson, *Human Sexual Inadequacy*, 164–66, 175; and see also Bernie Zilbergeld, *Men and Sex: A Guide to Sexual Fulfilment* (Boston: Little, Brown and Co., 1978); Lionel S. Lewis and Dennis Brisset, "Sex as Work: A Study of Avocational Counseling," *Social Problems* 15 (1967): 8–18; Dennis Brisset and Lionel S. Lewis, "Guidelines for Marital Sex: An Analysis of Fifteen Popular Marriage Manuals," *Family Coordinator* 19 (1970); 41–48; André Béjin, *Le Nouveau temperament sexuel: Essai sur la rationalisation et la démocratisation de la sexualité* (Paris: Editions Kime, 1990).

37. Edwin W. Hirsch, *Impotence and Frigidity* (New York: Citadel Press, 1966), 82; Anne Steinmann and David J. Fox, *The Male Dilemma: How to Survive the Sexual Revolution* (New York: Jason Aronson, 1974), 200; and on the conversion or reversion therapies offered homosexuals, see William H. Masters and Virginia E. Johnson, *Homosexuality in Perspective* (Boston: Little, Brown, 1979).

38. Kaplan, *The New Sex Therapy*, 285; Albert Ellis, *Sex and the Liberated Man* (Secaucus, N.J.: Lyle Stuart, Inc., 1976), 253–54; Gillan, *Sex Therapy Today*, 203–5; Robert Chartham, *The Chartham Letters* (London: New English Library, 1971), 25.

39. Shere Hite, *The Hite Report on Male Sexuality* (New York: Alfred A. Knopf, 1981), 340–53; and see also Inge and Sten Hegeler, *An ABZ of Love*, trans. David Hohnen (London: Neville Spearman, 1969), 186.

40. James Baldwin, *The Fire Next Time* (New York: Dell, 1962), 32, 76, 105; Frantz Fanon, *Black Skin, White Mask*, trans. Charles Lam Markham (New York: Grove Press, 1967), 159, 165, 170; Calvin C. Hernton, *Sex and Racism in America* (New York: Grove Press, 1965), 112; Eldridge Cleaver, *Soul on Ice* (New York: McGraw-Hill, 1968), 170.

41. Steinmann and Fox, *The Male Dilemma* ; Lionel Tiger, *Men in Groups* (New York: Vintage, 1969), 265; George Gilder, *Sexual Suicide* (New York: Quadrangle, 1973), 20, 22–23; Germaine Greer, *The Female Eunuch* (London : MacGibbon & Kee, 1970), 306; and see Sally Robinson, *Marked Men: White Masculinity in Crisis* (New York: Columbia University Press, 2000); Collins, *Modern Love*, 147.

42. David Mace cited in Packard, *The Sexual Wilderness*, 119.

43. Erica Jong, *Fear of Flying* (New York: Holt, Rinehart and Winston, 1973), 96, 97.

44. Kingsley Amis, *Difficulties with Girls* (1981; London: Hutchinson, 1988), 261; Kingsley Amis, *Jake's Thing* (New York: Viking Press, 1978), 31; and see also Zachary Leader, ed., *The Letters of Kingsley Amis* (New York: Harper Collins Publishers, 2000), 806n2; Herb Goldberg, *The Hazards of Being Male: Surviving the Myth of Masculine Privilege* (New York: Nash, 1976), 36.

45. Alberto Moravia, *Two: A Phallic Comedy*, trans. Angus Davidson (New York: Farrar, Straus and Giroux, 1972), 318; and for another Italian novelist's insistence that to be deprived of "screwing" was to be deprived of manhood, see Cesare Pavese, *The Business of Living: Diaries, 1935–1950* (London: Quartet Books, 1980), 32–33, 66.

46. Romain Gary, *Your Ticket Is No Longer Valid*, trans. Sophie Wilkins (New York: Brazillier, 1977) originally published as, *Au-delà de cette limite votre ticket n'est plus valable* (Paris: Gallimard, 1975). A disastrous Canadian film version (dir. George Kaczender) starring Richard Harris appeared in 1979.

47. Philip Roth, *Portnoy's Complaint* (New York: Random House, 1967), 257; Philip Roth, *The Counterlife* (New York: Collins, 1987), 30.

48. Kenneth Tynan, *A View of the English Stage, 1944–1963* (London: Davis-Poynter, 1975), 351; and on war and impotence see Rice, *Sex, Marriage, and Family*, 81, 249–50; E. B. Strauss, "Impotence from the Psychiatric Standpoint," *British Medical Journal* (Mar. 25, 1950): 697–99; Sonya Michel, "Dangers on the Home Front: Motherhood, Sexuality, and Disabled Veterans in American Postwar Films," *Journal of the History of Sexuality* 3 (1992): 109–28; Christina S. Jarvis, *The Male Body at War: American Masculinity During World War II* (Dekalb: Northern Illinois University Press, 2004).

49. Thomas Elsaesser, "Tales of Sound and Fury: Observations on the Family Melodrama," in Gerald Mast, Marshall Cohen, and Keo Braudy, eds., *Film Theory and Criticism: Introductory Readings* (New York: Oxford University Press, 1992), 534.

50. Edward Albee, *Who's Afraid of Virginia Woolf?* (New York: Atheneum, 1978), 28, 188, 189; and see Joan Mellen, *Big Bad Wolves: Masculinity in the American Film* (New York: Pantheon, 1977), 315.

51. Steven Cohen, *Masked Men: Masculinity and the Movies in the Fifties* (Bloomington: Indiana University Press, 1997), 253–54.

52. In *Dr. Strangelove or: How I Learned to Stop Worrying and Love the Bomb* (1964, dir. Stanley Kubrick) a U.S. general is convinced his impotence is due to a Communist conspiracy to contaminate "his precious body fluids."

53. Steven Cohen, "Masquerading as the American Male in the 1950s: *Picnic*, William Holden and the Spectacle of Masculinity in Hollywood Film," in Constance Penley and Sharon Willis, eds., *Male Trouble* (Minneapolis: University of Minnesota Press, 1993), 203–34.

54. Bohumil Hrabal, *Closely Observed Trains*, trans. Edith Pargeter (London: Anacus, 1968), 39, 70; Sandra Wake and Nicola Hayden, eds. *Bonnie and Clyde* (London: Faber and Faber, 1998), 49; Lester D. Friedman, ed., *Arthur Penn's Bonnie and Clyde* (Cambridge: Cambridge University Press, 2000).

55. Tom Kovic *Born on the Fourth of July* (New York: McGraw-Hill, 1975), 98.

56. Mark Elliott, "The Use of 'Impotence' and 'Frigidity': Why Has Impotence Survived?" *Journal of Sex and Marital Therapy* 11 (1985): 51–56; Mace, *Sexual Difficulties in Marriage*, 8.

CHAPTER TEN

1. Bernie Zilbergeld, *The New Male Sexuality* (New York: Bantam, 1999); Meika Loe, *The Rise of Viagra: How the Little Blue Pill Changed Sex in America* (New York: New York University Press, 2004), 133, 169.

2. Meika Loe, "Fixing Broken Masculinity: Viagra as a Technology for the Production of Gender and Sexuality," *Sexuality and Culture* 5 (2001): 98; *Time* (Dec. 5, 1988): 94; Thomas Szasz, *Sex by Prescription* (New York: Anchor/Doubleday, 1980), 86–87.

3. American Medical Systems, *Impotence: Causes and Treatments* (np, nd); Abraham Morgentaler, *The Viagra Myth: The Surprising Impact on Love and Relationships* (San Francisco: Jossey-Bass, 2003), 127; Szasz, *Sex by Prescription*, 83–85; Steven Findlay, "Danger: Implants," *U.S. News & World Report* (Aug. 24, 1992): 62–66.

4. Ronald Virag, "Intracavernous Injection of Papaverine for Erectile Failure," *Lancet* 320 (Oct. 23, 1982): 938; Loe, *The Rise of Viagra*, 36–37.

5. Morgentaler, *The Viagra Myth*, 123–24.

6. David Stipp, and Robert Whitaker, "The Selling of Impotence," *Fortune* (Mar. 16, 1998): 114–16; *New York Times*, July 8, 1995, 7; Aug. 9, 1995, C8; Leonore Tiefer, *Sex Is Not a Natural Act and Other Essays* (Boulder, Colo.: Westview Press, 1995), 144–46; Joseph Weber, "The $665 Million Dollar Market No Body Talks About," *Business Week* (Oct. 30, 1995): 42.

7. David M. Friedman, *A Mind of Its Own: A Cultural History of the Penis* (London: Penguin, 2001), 279; Mels Van Driel, *The Secret Part-A Natural History of the Penis* (Oxford: Mandrake, 2001).

8. Bruce and Eileen MacKenzie, *It's Not All in Your Head: A Couple's Guide to Overcoming Impotence* (New York: E. P. Dutton, 1988); J. Shah, "Erectile Dysfunction through the Ages," *BJU International* 90, no. 4 (Sept. 2002); 433–41.

9. *Time* (Dec. 5, 1988): 94; Helen Singer Kaplan, "My Husband's Vasectomy Ruined Our Sex Life," *Redbook* 173 (Sept., 1989): 22; Margery D. Rosen, "My Husband Can't Make Love," *Ladies' Home Journal* 106 (Sept., 1989): 8; Jan Ziegler, "New Help for Impotence," *McCall's* 117 (Feb., 1990): 88; Kate Nolan, "Is Your Husband Sexually Insecure? (He Won't Tell)," *Redbook* 179 (July, 1992): 82–85.

10. Szasz, *Sex by Prescription*, 9; Friedman, *A Mind of Its Own*, 295; Tiefer, *Sex Is Not a Natural Act*, 160; and see Barbara Marshal, "Hard Science: Gendered Constructions of Sexual Dysfunction in the 'Viagra Age,'" *Sexualities* 5, no. 2 (2002): 131–58; John Bancroft, "Erectile Impotence: Psyche or Soma," *International Journal of Andrology* 5 (1982) 353–55.

11. Leonore Tiefer, "In Pursuit of the Perfect Penis: The Medicalization of Male Sexuality," *American Behavioral Scientist* 29 (1986): 579–99.

12. NIH Consensus Conference, "Impotence," *JAMA* 270 (1993): 83–90.

13. Loe, *The Rise of Viagra*, 43–45.

14. Michael Stroh "The Root of Impotence: Does Nitric Oxide Hold the Key?" *Science News* 42 (July 4, 1992): 10–11; on the scientists involved see "Medicine Nobel Prize Awarded to U.S. Pharmacologists," *Lancet* 352 (Oct. 17, 1998): 1287; and for a fictionalized account see Carl Djerassi, *NO* (Athens: University of Georgia Press, 1998);

15. Friedman, *A Mind of Its Own*, 299; Arthur Wayne Glowka, "Among the New Words," *American Speech* 76, no. 2 (2001): 196–97.

16. Alexandra Alger, "Viagra Falls," *Forbes* 165 (Feb. 7, 2000): 130; Christine Gorman, "A Pill to Treat Impotence?" *Time* (May 20, 1996): 54; John Leland, "A Pill for Impotence?" *Newsweek* (Nov. 17, 1997): 62–66.

17. Edward O. Laumann, John H. Gagnon, Robert T. Michael, and Stuart Michaels, *The Social Organization of Sexuality: Sexual Practices in the United States* (Chicago: University

of Chicago Press, 1994), 375; Lawrence K. Altman, "Study Suggests High Rate of Impotence," *New York Times*, Dec. 22, 1993, C13; Edward O. Laumann, Anthony Paik, Raymond C. Rosen, "Sexual Dysfunction in the United States: Prevalence and Predictors," *JAMA* 281 (1999): 537, 1174.

18. Leonore Tiefer, "Sexology and the Pharmaceutical Industry: The Threat of Co-optation," *Journal of Sex Research* 37 (2000): 273–83; C. Aschka, W. Himmel, E. Ittner, M. M. Kochen, "Sexual Problems of Male Patients in Family Practice, *Journal of Family Practice* 50, no. 9 (2001); 773–78.

19. Stephen Katz and Barbara L. Marshall, "Is the Functional 'Normal'? Aging, Sexuality and the Bio-Marking of Successful Living," *History of the Human Sciences* 17 (2004): 67; Justin Clark, "The Big Turnoff: Stymied by Politics and Viagra, Sex Research Goes Limp," *Psychology Today* 38 (Jan./Feb. 2005): 17–18

20. Bruce Handy, "The Viagra Craze," *Time* (May 4, 1998): 39–45; Robert Langreth, "Hard Sell," *Forbes* 166 (Oct. 16, 2000): 56.

21. Guy Trebay, "Longer Harder Faster," *Village Voice*, Oct. 27–Nov. 2, 1999, 38.

22. Zilbergeld, *The New Male Sexuality*, 319; Irwin Goldstein et al, "Oral Sildenafil in the Treatment of Erectile Dysfunction," *New England Journal of Medicine* 338 (1998): 1397–1404; Jon Cohen, "At the Urologists' Convention, Viagra's Unsung Expert Witnesses," *New Yorker* 74, no. 18. (July 6, 1998): 26; Stuart N. Seidman, Steven P. Roose, and Matthew A. Menza, "Treatment of Erectile Dysfunction in Men with Depressive Symptoms: Results of a Placebo-controlled Trial with Sildenafil Citrate," *American Journal of Psychiatry* 158, no.10 (Oct., 2001): 1623–30.

23. Loe, "Fixing Broken Masculinity," 97–125; J. Tomlinson and D. Wright, "Impact of Erectile Dysfunction and Its Subsequent Treatment with Sildenafil: Qualitative Study," *British Medical Journal* 328 (May 2004): 1037–40.

24. A. Potts, V. Grace, N. Gavey, and T. Vares, "Viagra Stories: Challenging 'Erectile Dysfunction,'" *Social Science and Medicine* 59 (2004): 489–99; Annie Potts, "Deleuze on Viagra or, What Can a 'Viagra-body' Do," *Body and Society* 10 (2004): 18–36; Morgentaler, *The Viagra Myth*, 5, 119.

25. *Toronto Globe and Mail*, March 5, 2005, B4; "Sales of Impotence Drugs Fall, Defying Expectations," *New York Times*, Dec. 4, 2005, A1.

26. Morgentaler, *The Viagra Myth*, 118; Jane Spencer and Scott Hensley, "Falling Down on the Job," *Wall Street Journal*, reprinted in *Toronto Globe and Mail*, May 27, 2005, A13; *Toronto Star*, June 2, 2005, A2.

27. On the critiques of the medical model by "The Working Group on Women's Sexual Problems" led by Leonore Tiefer see Loe, *The Rise of Viagra*, 148; Ray Moynihan, "The Making of a Disease: Female Sexual Dysfunction," *British Medical Journal* 326 (2003): 45–47.

28. Susan Faludi, *Backlash: The Undeclared War against American Women* (New York: Crown, 1991).

29. Leonore Tiefer, "Sexology and the Pharmaceutical Industry: The Threat of Co-optation," *Journal of Sex Research* 37, no. 3 (2000): 273–75.

30. Loe, *The Rise of Viagra*, 23.

31. Douglas Black, "Medicalised Erections on Demand?" *Journal of Medical Ethics* 25 (Feb. 1999): 5–7; Jennifer Baumgardner, "Immaculate Contraception," *Nation* (Jan. 25, 1999): 11–15; Lynne Luciano, *Looking Good: Male Body Image in Modern America* (New

York: Hill and Wang, 2001), 200–201; Paul Rauber, "It's a Man's World," *Sierra*, 83 (Sept.–Oct., 1998): 20–21; Virginia I. Postrel, "Sex Mandates," *Forbes* 163 (May 31, 1999): 121; *New York Times*, April 29, 1998, A1; June 30, 1999, A1.

32. Barbara Marshall and Stephen Katz, "New Sex for Old: Lifestyle, Consumerism and the Politics of Aging Well," *Journal of Aging Studies* 17 (2003): 12; Andrew Bainham, "Sexualities, Sexual Relations and the Law," in Andrew Bainham, Shelley Day Sclater, and Martin Richards, eds., *Body Lore and Laws* (Oxford: Hart Publishing, 2002), 174–75; Susan Bordo, *The Male Body: A New Look at Men in Public and Private* (New York: Farrar, Straus and Giroux, 1999), 42–43; and for the sardonic observation that Viagra was sold as a sort of "denture adhesive" to hold fragile marriages together, see Laura Kipnis, *Against Love* (New York: Random House, 2003), 46.

33. Laumann, Gagnon, Michael, and Michaels, *The Social Organization of Sexuality*, 87, 114, 370, 375; and see also Kaye Wellings, Julia Field, Anne M. Johnson, and Jane Wadsworth, *Sexual Behaviour in Britain: The National Survey of Sexual Attitudes and Lifestyles* (London: Penguin, 1994), 138.

34. Susan Faludi, *Stiffed: The Betrayal of the American Man* (New York: William Morrow, 1999); Sally Robinson, *Marked Men: White Masculinity in Crisis* (New York: Columbia University Press, 2000); Lynn Segal, *Slow Motion: Changing Masculinities, Changing Men* (London: Virago, 1997); Anthony Clare, *On Men: Masculinity in Crisis* (London: Chatto and Windus, 2000); Kenneth Clatterbaugh, *Contemporary Perspectives on Masculinity: Women, Men and Politics in Modern Society* (Boulder, Colo.: Westview Press, 1997); Frank Mort, *Cultures of Consumption: Masculinities and Social Space in Late Twentieth-Century Britain* (London: Routledge, 1996).

35. Jennifer R. Fishman and Laura Mamo, "What's in a Disorder: A Cultural Analysis of Medical and Pharmaceutical Constructions of Male and Female Sexual Dysfunction," *Women and Therapy* 24, nos. 1 and 2 (2001): 184; Laura Mamo and Jennifer R. Fishman. "Potency in All the Right Places: Viagra as a Gendered Technology of the Body," *Body and Society* 7, no. 4 (2001): 13–35.

36. Bordo, *The Male Body*, 59; Morgentaler, *The Viagra Myth*, 135.

37. Annie Potts, *The Science/Fiction of Sex: Feminist Deconstruction and the Vocabularies of Heterosex* (London: Routledge, 2002), 146; Annie Potts, "The Essence of the 'Hard On': Hegemonic Masculinity and the Cultural Construction of 'Erectile Dysfunction,'" *Men and Masculinities* 3 (2000): 85–103.

38. Peter F. Murphy, *Studs, Tools, and the Family Jewels: Metaphors Men Live By* (Madison: University of Wisconsin Press, 2001).

39. Zilbergeld, *The New Male Sexuality*, 63; Potts, "The Essence of the 'Hard On,'" 98–99.

40. Loe, *The Rise of Viagra*, 78.

41. Mason cited in Walter Leavy, "Brothers (and Sisters) and the New Sex Pill," *Ebony* 53 (July 1998): 157; George Edmond Smith, *More than Sex: Reinventing the Black Male Image* (New York: Kensington Books, 2000), 3–4, 124.

42. Susan C. Vaughan, "The Hard Drug," *Harper's Bazaar* (Feb., 1998): 82; Sheryl McCarthy, "The Hard Facts," *Ms.* 8 (May–June 1998): 96; Lynn Snowden, "Viagra Nation: Men Take; Women Reap the Benefits," *Mademoiselle* 103 (Aug., 1998): 55.

43. James R. Petersen, *The Century of Sex: Playboy's History of the Sexual Revolution, 1900–1999* (New York: Grove Press, 1999), 495; Leonore Tiefer, "A New View of Women's Sexual Problems: Why New? Why Now?" *Journal of Sex Research* 38, no. 2 (2001): 89–96.

44. Warren St. John, "In an Over-sexed Age, More Guys Take the Pill," *New York Times*, Dec. 14, 2003, 9:1–2; Loe, *The Rise of Viagra*, 173; Faludi, *Stiffed: The Betrayal of the American Man*, 543; Segal, *Slow Motion: Changing Masculinities*, 213–14.

45. Loe, *The Rise of Viagra*, 113; Bordo, *The Male Body*, 60.

46. Martin cited in John Tierney, "The Aging Body," *Esquire* (May 1982): 55; Gail Sheehy, *Understanding Men's Passages: Discovering the New Map of Men's Lives* (New York: Random House, 1998), 187–91; Judith A. Levy, "Sex and Sexuality in Later Life Stages," in Alice S. Rossi, ed., *Sexuality Across the Life Course* (Chicago: University of Chicago Press, 1994), 287–313.

47. Katz and Marshall, "New Sex for Old," 12; and see also Barbara L. Marshall and Stephen Katz, "Forever Functional: Sexual Fitness and the Aging Male Body," *Body and Society* 8, no. 4 (2002): 43–70; Leslie Laurence and Lani Luciano, "The Aging Face of AIDS," published on World AIDS Day 2000 by the Henry J. Kaiser Family Foundation, http://www.kaisernetwork.org/Daily_reports/rep_index.cfm?DR_ID=1370 (accessed February 1, 2006).

48. A. Vermeulen, "The Male Climacterium," *Annales of Medicine* 25 (1993): 531–34; John Hoberman, *Testosterone Dreams: Rejuvenation, Aphrodisia, Doping* (Berkeley: University of California Press, 2005); Malcolm Carruthers, *Male Menopause: Restoring Vitality and Virility* (London: HarpersCollins, 1996); *Vancouver Sun*, Feb. 2, 2005, 26; Barbara L. Marshall, "Climacteric Redux? (Re)medicalizing the Male Menopause," *Men and Masculinities* (forthcoming 2006).

49. Jennifer R. Fishman and Laura Mamo, "What's in a Disorder: A Cultural Analysis of Medical and Pharmaceutical Constructions of Male and Female Sexual Dysfunction," *Women and Therapy* 24, no. 1 and 2 (2001): 184–85; Bob Adams, "Keeping It Up," *Advocate*, Nov. 11, 2003, 38, 40, 42; *Toronto Globe and Mail*, Jan. 10, 2004, F6.

50. Sean G. Swearingen and Jeffrey D. Klausner, "Sildenafil use, sexual risk behavior, and risk for sexually transmitted diseases, including HIV infection," *American Journal of Medicine* 118, no. 6 (June, 2005): 571–77.

51. Morgentaler, *The Viagra Myth*, 144.

52. One is reminded that in the nineteenth century a "good death" meant enduring suffering as a test for fitness for heaven; by the late twentieth century it meant a quick and painless end. See Peter G. Filene, *In the Arms of Others: A Cultural History of the Right-to-Die in America* (Chicago: Dee, 1998).

53. David B. Morris, *Illness and Culture in the Postmodern Age* (Berkeley: University of California Press, 1998).

54. Gail Hawkes, *Sex and Pleasure in Western Culture* (Cambridge; Polity, 2004); Graham Hart and Kaye Wellings, "Sexual Behaviour and Its Medicalisation: In Sickness and in Health," *British Medical Journal* 324 (2002): 899; Jonathan Michel Metzl, *Prozac on the Couch: Prescribing Gender in the Era of Wonder Drugs* (Durham, N.C.: Duke University Press, 2003).

55. John Taylor, "The Long, Hard Days of Dr. Dick," *Esquire* (September 1995): 120–30; Elizabeth Haiken, "Virtual Virility, or Does Medicine Make the Man?" *Men and Masculinities* 2 (2000): 388–409; Vernon Rosario, "Phallic Performance: Phalloplasty and the Techniques of Sex," in Christopher Forth and Ivan Crozier, eds., *Body Parts: Critical Explorations in Corporeality* (New York; Lexington Books, 2005), 177–90.

56. Bruce Handy, "The Viagra Craze," *Time* (May 4, 1998): 44; Carl Elliott, *Better Than Well: American Medicine Meets the American Dream* (New York: Norton, 2003).

57. Peter Lefcourt, *The Woody* (New York: Simon and Schuster, 1998); *Toronto Globe and Mail*, July 29, 2003, A1.

CONCLUSION

1. See the film *Quartier Mozart* (1992, dir. Jean-Pierre Bekolo); and on the similar Asian belief in "Koro," the disappearance of the male genitals, see Robert E. Bartholomew, *Exotic Deviance: Medicalizing Cultural Idioms from Strangeness to Illness* (Boulder: University Press of Colorado, 2000); Sheung-Tak Cheng, "Epidemic Genital Retraction Syndrome: Environmental and Personal Risk Factors in Southern China," *Journal of Psychology and Human Sexuality* 9 (1997): 57–70; Mai Ghoussoub, "Chewing Gum, Insatiable Women and Foreign Enemies: Male Fears and the Arab Media," in Mai Ghoussoub and Emma Sinclair-Webb, eds., *Imagined Masculinities: Male Identity and Culture in the Modern Middle East* (London: Saqi Books, 2000), 227–35; Judith Farquhar, *Appetites: Food and Sex in Post-Socialist China* (Durham: Duke University Press, 2002), 269–71.
2. David D. Gilmore, *Manhood in the Making* (New Haven: Yale University Press, 1990).
3. J. G. Peristiany, "The Sophron-a Secular Saint? Wisdom and the Wise Man in a Cypriot Community," in J. G. Peristiany and Julian Pitt-Rivers, eds., *Honor and Grace in Anthropology* (Cambridge: Cambridge University Press, 1992), 103–27.
4. Marilyn Yalom, *A History of the Breast* (New York: Alfred A. Knopf, 1997).
5. Shere Hite, *The Hite Report on Male Sexuality* (New York: Alfred A. Knopf, 1981), 459–62.
6. Naomi Pfeffer, "The Hidden Pathology of the Male Reproductive System," in *The Sexual Politics of Reproduction* (London: Gower, 1985), 30–44; Charles E. Rosenberg and Janet Golden, eds., *Framing Disease: Studies in Cultural History* (New Brunswick: Rutgers University Press, 1992).

INDEX